PRACTICAL PAEDIAT

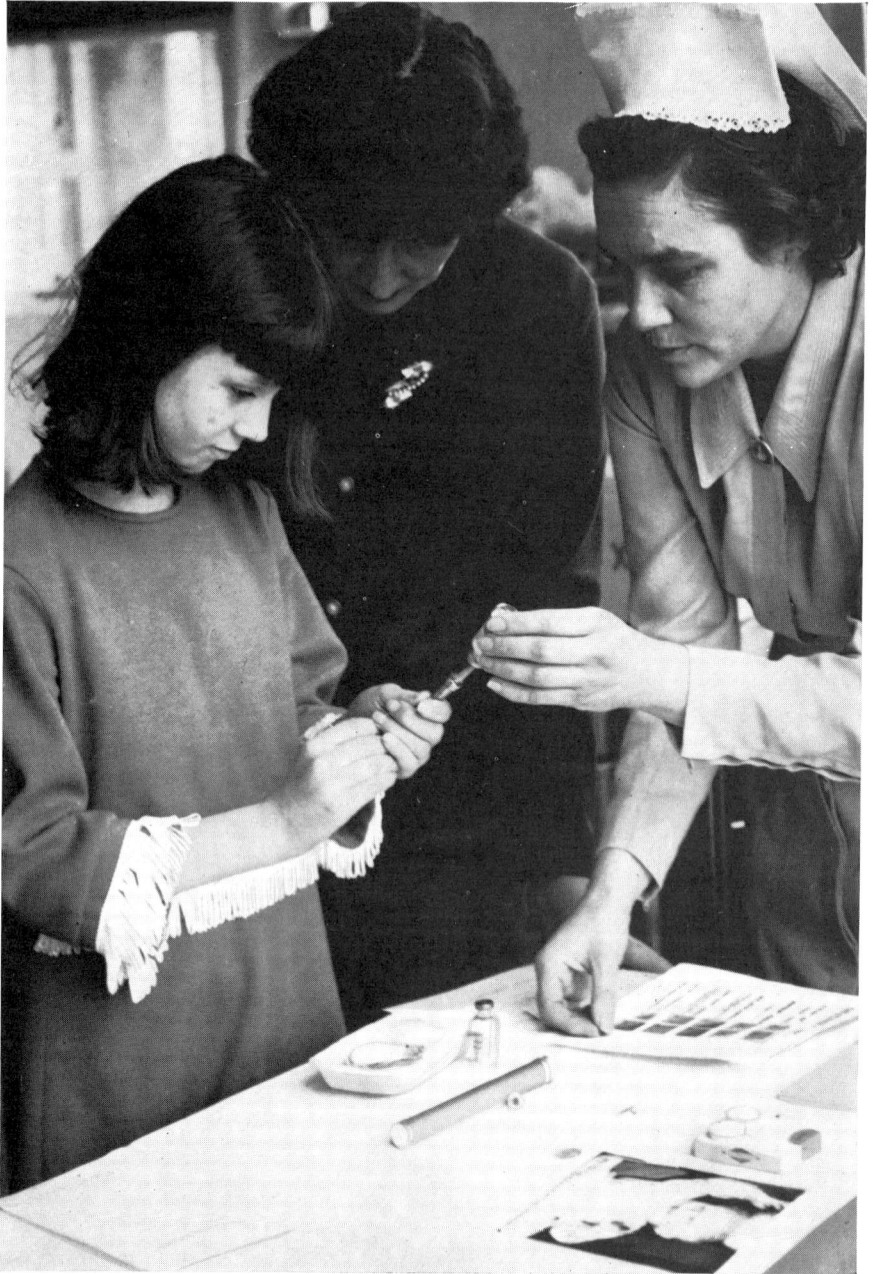

Frontispiece. Education for her new life as a diabetic.
Wendy, aged nine years, was admitted in coma ten days before this picture was taken. With her mother, she is taught how to draw up the correct dose of insulin into a unit syringe.

Practical Paediatric Nursing

SHEILA M. BATES
S.R.N. R.S.C.N. S.C.M.
Sister Tutor's Diploma, (University of London)

*Examiner to the General Nursing Council
for England and Wales*

*Senior Tutor (Paediatrics),
The Queen Elizabeth School of Nursing, Birmingham*

REVISED REPRINT

BLACKWELL SCIENTIFIC PUBLICATIONS
OXFORD LONDON EDINBURGH MELBOURNE

© 1971 by Blackwell Scientific Publications
Osney Mead, Oxford
85 Marylebone High Street, London W1
9 Forrest Road, Edinburgh
P.O. Box 9, North Balwyn, Victoria, Australia

ISBN 0 632 07800 6

First published 1971
Reprinted 1975

Distributed in the U.S.A. by
J. B. Lippincott Company, Philadelphia
and in Canada by
J. B. Lippincott Company of
Canada Ltd, Toronto

Printed and bound in Great Britain by
William Clowes & Sons, Limited,
London, Beccles and Colchester

To all who have the care
of sick children

Contents

Foreword

Looking after children is becoming more specialized, and newer methods of diagnosis and treatment make increasing demands on nursing staff. Paediatricians have always depended on nurses to help children to settle into hospital, to win the confidence of parents and to take the mother's place when she has to be separated from her baby. Nowadays the paediatric nurse is expected to do so much more than provide for the needs and comfort of the sick child, though this is fundamental. She has to be a keen observer, recognising when something is amiss, and she has to keep accurate records; she has to help in the collection of specimens for all kinds of purposes; she must be ready to help when she takes a child to the X-ray department or operating theatre; she may be called upon to deputize for the physiotherapist or to work in an intensive care unit.

Miss Bates has had a distinguished career as nurse, ward sister and tutor. She has worked and examined for the General Nursing Council in a number of paediatric units in Great Britain, and she is well qualified to discuss these matters. Her object has been to describe in detail what a sick children's nurse is expected to do, how it should be done, and why. Within the compass of a relatively small volume she has considered all the procedures that a nurse is likely to have to carry out.

There is room for an up-to-date and authoritative treatise on paediatric nursing. This book should meet that need.

CLIFFORD G. PARSONS
October 1971

Preface

This comprehensive textbook of modern paediatric nursing has been written to provide the learner with a nursing companion to the wide range of paediatric medical and surgical textbooks available to-day. The short first part is concerned with the healthy child and protection of his health. The rest of the book concentrates on those aspects of nursing detail which the paediatric nurse needs to know.

This book has not been written to provide a substitute for careful instruction and demonstration by an experienced paediatric nurse, but to complement such teaching making learning more meaningful. Technical procedures can be mastered only by careful practice supervised by one skilled in the performance and are of greater value to the learner than the content of any book.

Technical efficiency, however, is only part of good nursing care. Children, whether well or sick, are, by reason of their age, entirely dependent on the staff of a paediatric unit for fulfillment of their needs—physical, emotional, social, educational as well as related to their medical or surgical condition. Interpersonal relationships are acquired by imitation and example and cannot be adequately described in words.

Registration by the General Nursing Council for England and Wales as a sick children's nurse is coveted by students from many parts of the world. Qualifying as a Registered Sick Children's Nurse marks a milestone in the long process of learning and much in the content of this book will prove of value to staff nurses, ward sisters and nursing officers who have the care and welfare of sick children at heart.

I am grateful to Miss P. Greening, Miss D. M. Hilditch, Miss H. Jukes, Miss I. Peebles, Miss D. M. Rea and Miss F. M. Wheeler for help with the subjects on which they are experts; to Miss A. Roberts and Mr. J. Dowse for their time and patience in perfecting the original line drawings, and to the Department of Medical Illustration, The United Birmingham Hospitals for many of the photographs and to the Board of Governors for permission to publish them.

I am indebted to many of my friends and colleagues for their help, advice and constructive criticism, especially to Miss B. Bates, Miss E. R. D. Bendall, Miss C. G. L. Clamp, Miss R. M. Maddever, Miss R. Spalton and to Dr. C. G. Parsons who, in spite of his busy life as Senior Consultant Physician at the Birmingham Children's Hospital, has found time to read the text.

To Mrs. Betty Fox, I shall remain indebted for her devotion to the task of typing the drafts and the final manuscript, and to Blackwell Scientific Publications Ltd. for their co-operation and advice.

Last, but by no means least, I thank all who have, knowingly and unknowingly, influenced what I have written—to the tutors and ward sisters who taught me during my very happy student days at the Birmingham Children's Hospital, to my ward sister and staff nurse colleagues and to our student nurses whose need for a new look at paediatric nursing I have endeavoured to fulfill.

SHEILA M. BATES
June 1971

CHAPTER ONE

The Healthy Child

Growth and Development

Growth may be defined as an increase in size and is just one aspect of development. Development refers to increasing maturity—physical, mental or intellectual, social and emotional.

The growth and development of any infant depends both on his innate potential and the influence of his immediate environment which can only improve his performance to his maximum developmental potential.

Unlike the offspring of other species, the human infant takes sixteen to twenty years to achieve adult stature and maturity. This slow continuous process adopts the same sequence of events from conception through foetal life, birth, infancy, childhood and adolescence to full maturity. No two children are alike but all follow the same pattern of development. The milestones or norms are passed in the same order, but the age at which they are achieved differs within certain normal limits.

An essential factor in the learning of new skills is the maturation of the nervous system and no amount of practice will make a child carry out a new skill before that part of the nervous system is ready. This fact is often not appreciated by over-anxious parents whose child may not be up to their great expectations.

AVERAGE STANDARDS

One only has to observe the variation in stature and behaviour of a class of healthy five-year-olds to realise the range of normality. Many detailed studies of healthy children have been made in an endeavour to establish average norms or milestones of physical growth and mental development at any given age. Variations of up to 10–15% above and below these average standards fall within the normal limits, although a child's steady progress compared with his previous achievements is often of far more significance than conformity within a rigid standard.

1

Name .... Date of Birth .... Reg. No. ....

GIRLS

Weight

Single-Time
Standard
(cross-sectional)

97
50
3

Age, years

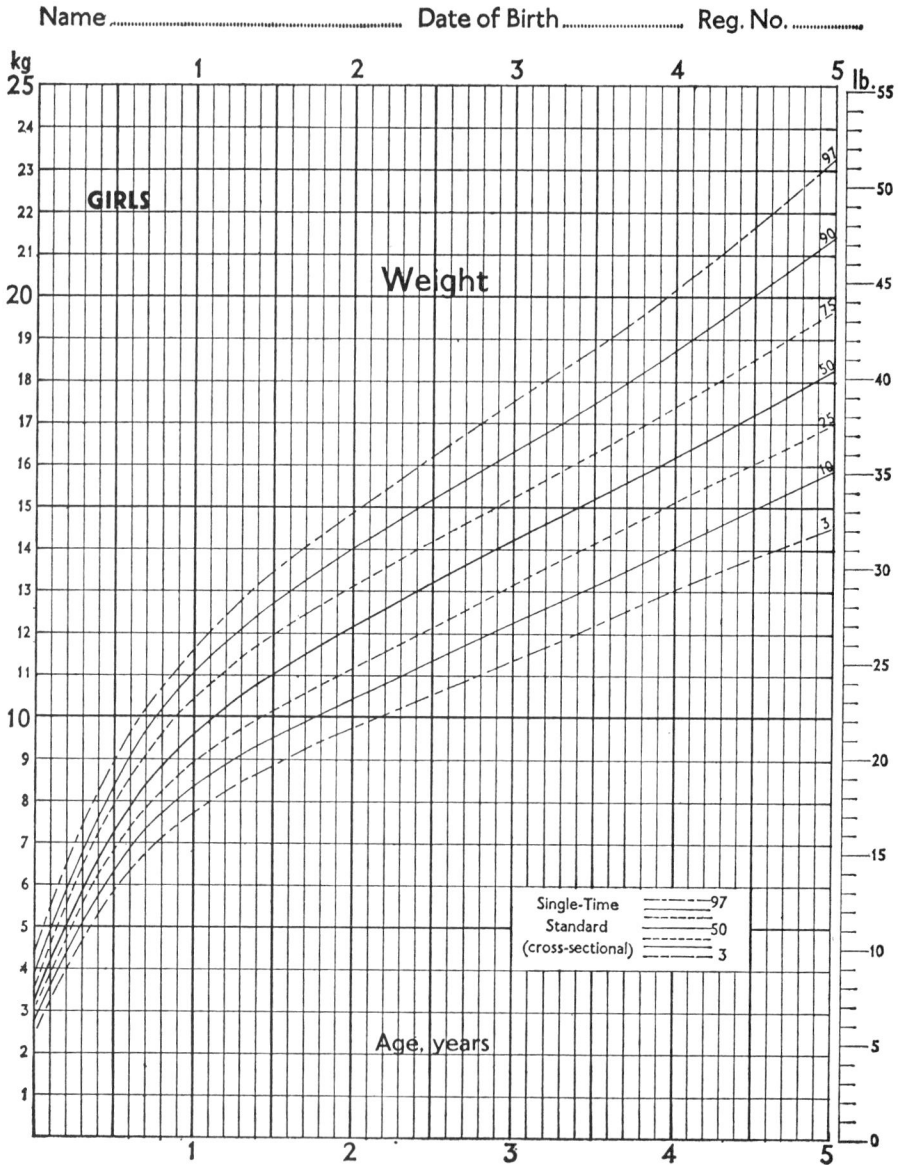

FIG. 1. Weight Standard Chart, Girls 0–5 Years. (Reproduced by kind permission of Professor J. M. Tanner, University of London, Institute of Child Health for the Hospital for Sick Children Great Ormond Street, London and Creaseys of Hertford Ltd., England.)

PHYSICAL GROWTH

Charts are designed with the child's progress recorded as a percentile of the average for his age and sex.

Example: With reference to FIG. 1 (weight chart of a girl 0–5 years) it will be seen that an average eighteen-month-old girl weighs about 11kg, If she weighs 9·5kg, she would not be exceeding the tenth percentile—-a weight not exceeded by 10% of all eighteen-month-old girls. Similarly, if an eighteen-month-old girl weighs 12·6kg, she would be of the ninetieth percentile, because her weight is not exceeded by 90% of all eighteen-month-old girls. Both fall into the wide range of normality as their respective weights are within 10–15% of the average weight for their age and sex.

Values below the third and above the ninety-seventh percentile are considered unhealthy until proved otherwise.

DEVELOPMENTAL QUOTIENT

Many parameters have been used to assess the progress in development of small children. All tests are graded in difficulty and could be achieved by a normal child of a given age. To assess a wide range of attainments during the first two years of life, a table similar to TABLE 1 may be used and the mental age in months estimated by recording each achievement as one and dividing the score by four.

Example: The mental age of a nine-month-old infant who can only achieve the requirements of a six-month-old in locomotor, social and co-ordination, but can say 'mama'—a normal achievement of his age—would be as follows:

Mental age in months

$$= \frac{\text{score}}{4}$$

$$= \frac{6+6+9+6}{4}$$

$$= \frac{27}{4}$$

$$= 6\tfrac{3}{4} \text{ months}$$

INTELLIGENCE QUOTIENT

Once language is acquired, intelligence is assessed on the child's powers of understanding and reasoning and his capacity to deal effectively with a new situation. Many tests have been designed for children of varying age groups and the Intelligence Quotient (I.Q.) is calculated by dividing mental age by the chronological age and multiplying by 100. All tests are graded so that the I.Q. of average children of the same age is about 100.

$$\text{I.Q.} = \frac{\text{Mental age}}{\text{Chronological age}} \times 100$$

TABLE 1.   Normal Development in the First Two Years*

Age in Months	Locomotor	Social	Hearing and Speech	Co-ordination of Eye and Hand
1	Head erect for few seconds	Quietened when picked up	Startled by sounds	Follows light with eyes
2	Head up when prone (chin clear)	Smiles	Listens to bell or rattle	Follows ring up, down and sideways
3	Kicks well	Follows person with eyes	Searches for sound with eyes	Glances from one object to another
4	Lifts head and chest when prone	Returns examiner's smile	Laughs	Clasps and retains cube
5	Holds head erect with no lag	Frolics when played with	Turns head to sound	Pulls paper away from face
6	Rises on to wrists	Turns head to person talking	Babbles or coos to voice or music	Takes cube from table
7	Rolls from front to back	Drinks from a cup	Makes four different sounds	Looks for fallen object
8	Tries to crawl vigorously	Looks at mirror image	Shouts for attention	Passes toy from hand to hand
9	Turns around on floor	Helps to hold cup for drinking	Says 'Mama' or 'Dada'	Manipulates two objects at once
10	Stands when held up	Smiles at mirror image	Listens to watch	Clicks two bricks together
11	Pulls up to stand	Finger feeds	Two words with meaning	Pincer grip
12	Walks or side-steps around pen	Plays pat-a-cake	Three words with meaning	'Holds' pencil meaningfully
13	Stands alone	Holds cup for drinking	Looks at pictures	Preference for one hand
14	Walks alone	Uses spoon	Recognises own name	Makes marks with pencil
15	Climbs up stairs	Shows shoes	Four to five clear words	Places one object upon another
16	Pushes pram, toy horse etc.	Tries to turn door knob	Six to seven clear words	Scribbles freely
17	Climbs on to chair	Manages cup well	Babbled conversation	Pulls (table) cloth to get toy
18	Walks backwards	Takes off shoes and socks	Enjoys pictures in book	Constructive play with toys
19	Climbs stairs up and down	Knows one part of the body	Nine words	Tower of three bricks

* As printed in *A Paediatric Vade-Mecum*, 7th edition (1970), by kind permission of B. S. B. Wood and Lloyd-Luke (Medical Books) Ltd.

TABLE 1—*continued*

Age in Months	Locomotor	Social	Hearing and Speech	Co-ordination of Eye and Hand
20	Jumps	Bowel control	Twelve words	Tower of four bricks
21	Runs	Bladder control by day	Two word sentences	Circular scribble
22	Walks up stairs	Tries to tell experiences	Listens to stories	Tower of five or more bricks
23	Seats himself at table	Knows two parts of body	Twenty words or more	Copies perpendicular stroke
24	Walks up and down stairs	Knows four parts of body	Names four toys	Copies horizontal stroke

Example: A child of 12 years who has a mental age of an 8-year-old would have an I.Q. of:

$$\frac{8}{12} \times 100$$

$$= \frac{2}{3} \times 100$$

$$= 67$$

RANGE OF INTELLIGENCE QUOTIENT AND EQUIVALENT PERCENTILE RATING

I.Q.	Percentile
over 130	98
over 120	90
over 110	75
90–110	50
below 90	25
below 80	10
below 70	2 (educationally subnormal)

The example given above falls below the second percentile as he has an I.Q. below 70, i.e. he is educationally subnormal.

Physical growth

At birth, the head is approximately a quarter of the body length and has a greater circumference than that of the thorax. The trunk is comparatively short as the legs account for more than half the remainder of the infant's length.

Physical growth is not evenly distributed through the childhood years. During

Innate Potential

Congenital abnormalities.
Metabolic ⎫
Chromosomal ⎰ disorders.

Pre-Natal   Post-Natal

Poor nutrition.
Stress.   GROWTH   Lower social classes.
Viral infections.   ──── AND ◄──── Poor economic status.
Certain drugs.   DEVELOPMENT   Limited parental care:
Radiation.   – physical;
                                                                     – emotional.
                                                         Illness.
                                                         Accident.
                                                         Separation from home.

                                 Natal

Premature delivery.
Cerebral damage,
anoxaemia and
haemorrhage.

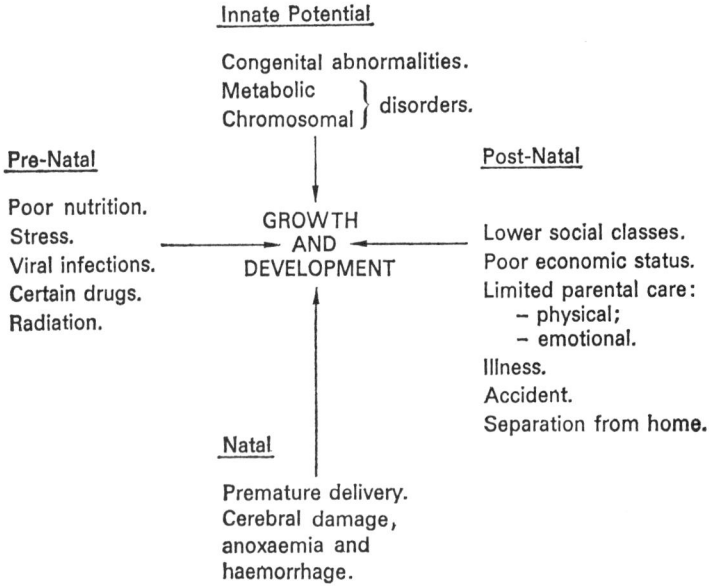

FIG. 2. Adverse factors affecting growth and development. (Biological, social, economical and medical.)

the first two years there is a period of intense growth in length and weight. This is followed by a much slower rate of growth until the onset of puberty when there is a further growth spurt.

Just as physical growth is not at a constant rate throughout childhood, the time and growth rate of the different parts of the body vary considerably. For example, growth of the trunk is rapid in the first two years of life, leaving the limbs well behind. This is followed by a period of rapid growth of the limbs, so that by the age of four years the same size trousers can be worn, but they do little to protect the now lengthy thighs. Similarly, by the age of six years the central nervous system is 90% developed and the skull has grown in size accordingly, but the genital organs remain in their dormant state until stimulated by the sex hormones heralding the onset of puberty.

Boys and girls grow at a similar rate during the pre-pubertal years—boys tending to be slightly larger than girls of the same age. The onset of puberty in girls is earlier—ten-and-a-half to thirteen years—(tending towards an earlier onset of four months in every ten years) than in boys—thirteen to fifteen years—although there is considerable variation in time. This results in girls being temporarily superior in size and strength than boys of the eleven to thirteen years age group. With increased muscular and skeletal growth associated with puberty in the male, boys develop considerable strength and an increase in size which remains 10% or so greater than that of their female contemporaries.

FACTORS INFLUENCING NORMAL GROWTH

1 Birth weight.

2 Sex—boys tend to be slightly larger than girls.

3 Hereditary pattern—parents of small stature tend to breed children of small stature, and vice versa.

4 Racial factors—some races are of small and others of large stature.

5 Endocrine activity—nitrogen retention and physical growth are dependent on growth hormone. The growth spurt at puberty is dependent on sex hormones.

6 Environmental factors, especially nutritional differences and maternal efficiency, affect the growth pattern. Essentially due to better nutrition, the average height is now 7·6cm (3 inches) greater than it was at the turn of the century.

7 Illness, e.g. defective absorption, congenital heart disease, kidney dysfunction and conditions demanding prolonged steroid therapy all retard growth.

WEIGHT

A newborn infant weighs between 2·5kg (5½lb) and 4·5kg (10lb) with an average weight of 3·4kg (7½lb). By definition, an infant weighing 2·5kg or less at birth is regarded as a 'premature infant'.

During the first few days of life there is a weight loss of 10% which is usually regained by the tenth to fourteenth day. From then on, average weight gain is at the rate of 200g (7oz) per week for the first four months; 150g (5oz) for the second four months; and 90g (3oz) per week for the last four months of the first year (TABLE 6, page 53).

EXPECTED WEIGHT GAIN

Birth weight × 2 at 4–6 months
× 3 at 12 months
× 4 at 24 months (2 years)

From the age of 3 years the approximate expected average weight can be calculated as follows:

Weight in kg = (age in years × 2) + 8

Example: at 8 years a child can be expected to weigh approximately:

$$(8 \times 2) + 8 = 24kg$$

Weight in pounds = (age in years + 3) × 5

Example: at 8 years a child can be expected to weigh approximately:

$$(8 + 3) \times 5 = 55lb$$

HEIGHT

A newborn full-term infant measures approximately 50cm (20 inches).

EXPECTED GROWTH RATE IN LENGTH

Height in Centimetres:

> Length at
> birth   = 50cm
> 12 months = 75cm
> 2 years   = 85cm
> 3 years   = 95cm
> 4 years   = 100cm (1m)

From the age of 4 years to puberty, the *approximate* average height can be calculated as follows:

$$\text{Height} = 1m + [(\text{age in years} - 4) \times 6]cm$$

Example: at 8 years a child can be expected to measure approximately:

$$1m + [(8-4) \times 6]cm$$

$$= 1m + 24cm \text{ or } 124cm$$

Height in Inches:

> Length at
> birth   = 20 inches
> 12 months = 30 inches
> 2 years   = 35 inches
> 3 years   = 38 inches

The birth length is doubled during the fourth year. Thereafter, the child grows approximately 2 inches a year until puberty.

HEAD CIRCUMFERENCE

A tape measure passed around the brows anteriorly and the occipital protuberance posteriorly records the following average head circumference at different ages:

> Birth   33–35·5cm or 13–14 inches
> 3 months 41cm or 16 inches
> 6 months 43cm or 17 inches
> 12 months 46cm or 18 inches
> 2 years   48cm or 19 inches ⎫ anterior
> 3 years   50cm or 20 inches ⎬ fontanelle
>   ⎭ closed

DENTITION

There is much variation in the time of onset and rate of eruption of the twenty teeth in the first or deciduous dentition, and the thirty-two in the second or permanent dentition.

The usual pattern of eruption and loss is as follows:

DECIDUOUS DENTITION

Upper jaw	Time of Eruption in Months		Time of Loss in Years
Central Incisor	8–11	a a	6–8th
Lateral Incisor	10–13	b b	10th
Canine	16–20	c c	12th
First Molar	13–17	d d	11th
Second Molar	23–26	e e	11th

Lower jaw			
Second Molar	23–26	e e	11th
First Molar	13–17	d d	10th
Canine	16–20	c c	12th
Lateral Incisor	10–14	b b	7–8th
Central Incisor	6–10	a a	6–8th

PERMANENT DENTITION

Upper jaw	Time of Eruption in Years	
Central Incisor	6– 8	1 1
Lateral Incisor	7– 9	2 2
Canine	11–12	1 1
First Premolar	9–11	1 1
Second Premolar	10–12	2 2
First Molar	6– 7	1 1
Second Molar	11–14	2 2
Third Molar	16–21	3 3

Lower jaw		
Third Molar	16–21	3 3
Second Molar	11–13	2 2
First Molar	6– 7	1 1
Second Premolar	11–12	2 2
First Premolar	10–12	1 1
Canine	9–10	1 1
Lateral Incisor	7– 8	2 2
Central Incisor	6– 7	1 1

Development

In the Formative Years (First Five)

To be born into a family is the birthright of every child, both mother and father taking a share in the child's physical care and mental development.

The newborn infant is a completely helpless creature with a reflex behaviour pattern peculiar to this age group. Reflexes essential for survival are present in a mature infant. Like most small mammals, when the cheek is touched the head is reflexly turned towards the stimulus—the so-called rooting or searching reflex. The sucking and swallowing reflexes are present from about the thirty-second week of gestation. Other neonatal reflexes include the Moro reflex—when startled by a sudden noise, bright light or a fear of falling, the arms are extended with the fingers separated (FIG. 3); the grasp reflex—a finger or other object

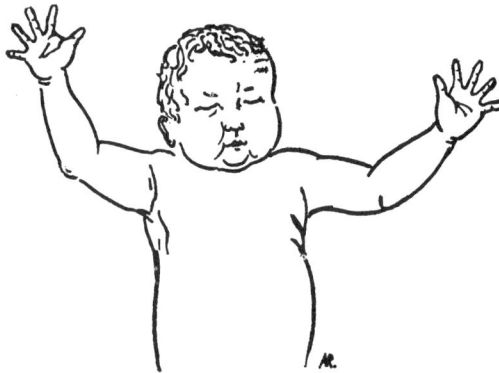

FIG. 3. Moro reflex.

placed across the palm is grasped, and the stepping reflex in which the infant makes stepping movements when supported in an upright position with his feet on a firm surface.

For the first few weeks of life, the child's immediate environment continues to be his mother. In fulfilling her infant's physical needs and desires at guaranteed regular intervals, the mother is fulfilling her own, thus creating an effective bond of love and security so necessary for satisfactory emotional development. Her child's future stability and security within the family unit rests on this early establishment of a satisfactory mother-child relationship.

For emotional security, the small child needs:

i   sustained understanding parental affection, initially from his mother, but with father taking an increasingly prominent part in his physical care and mental development;

ii to belong to a small intimate family unit who have a genuine interest in the care and welfare of each other;

iii scope for self-expression—physical, emotional, social and intellectual;

iv guidance and direction into acceptable channels of sociable behaviour.

A child is essentially a product of his home environment—adverse or otherwise. During his formative years it is the way of family life—the so-called emotional climate—that has the greatest influence in moulding him into the accepted standards and expectations of the family and national culture. Failure to provide for his emotional needs, or an imbalance in the way they are provided, leads to insecurity. Manifestations of such insecurity are seen in the characteristic emotional reactions of small children considered to be normal behaviour for the age group concerned, but unacceptable as normal at a later age.

Sibling rivalry is not uncommon. A small child needs very careful handling to prevent jealousy—sometimes of a malicious nature—towards an addition to the family. He may resent this intruder demanding so much of his mother's love and care. Extra attention and reassuring love by understanding parents are necessary to help him accept this new situation. Regression to infantile behaviour, a manifestation of insecurity, is common and is a means of getting extra parental attention. Deliberate naughtiness and food fads are other attention-seeking devices. Activities, such as head-banging and masturbation in the two to three-year-olds, and nose-picking and nail-biting in the older child, are exhibited by an insecure child and are a means of overcoming inner aggression. Once the underlying cause is overcome, the behaviour pattern is dropped, but if allowed to persist, nail-biting can become a habit difficult to cure.

During the late second and third years of life, the less dependent child develops and exhibits a strong will of his own, seen as frequent outbursts of temper or obstinacy. These temper tantrums are often related to toilet training and occur at meal-times or in response to frustrating restricted activity. Breath-holding attacks may give rise to parental alarm, especially when accompanied by cyanosis and convulsive movements.

Fears are the normal response to danger and are very common and real to the three-year-old. These fears, usually transitory, must be respected and appreciated by sympathetic parents. Fear of the dark is very common and a reassuring nightlight may help a child to overcome this dread.

Correction, if necessary, should be severe enough to hurt and given immediately so that the child realises the reason for his mother's rebuke or withdrawal of a privilege. The matter is then best forgotten.

HABIT TRAINING

The very young (and old) are secure in a regular pattern of activity. The establishment of good habits which form part of this secure routine are essential for the formation of character and personality. The mere mention of habit training immediately brings to most minds the toilet training of the young, but entails much wider training than this.

Sleep. The pattern of the small infant's day is essentially sleep, disturbed only for feeding and changing with their associated love and care.

Growth is rapid during the first months of life, so long hours of sleep are necessary. By the age of one year, the twenty-one hours of sleep necessary for the newborn infant are reduced to sixteen to eighteen hours, taken as a twelve to fourteen hour night and one or two naps during the day. By the age of four to five years, the daytime sleep is dropped and the child is tucked up with his favourite toy for a twelve to fourteen hour night. A warm bath, a quiet game or listening to a suitable story, all help the active small child to unwind before going to bed. Bad habits of sleep can be learned by the child demanding a parent to sit with him until he falls asleep or to fetch him downstairs for more attention. Most children outgrow this phase very quickly. Many children like a comforter in the form of a piece of cloth, old rag doll, thumb, fingers or dummy.

Meals. Meal-times give opportunity for teaching acceptable standards of table manners. The child, by encouragement and example, learns to hold his cup, feed himself with a spoon and later a knife and fork, sit at the table and learn to wait until others have finished eating. Regular eating habits are established in the young. Snacks between meals are invariably of high carbohydrate content and are of detriment to both teeth and weight.

Cleanliness. Children are not naturally fond of water for washing purposes, especially as they become older, but water to play in fascinates children from a very early age. Good personal hygiene is established in the home, and a small child can be taught from a very early age to wash his hands after visiting the toilet and before meals, and to brush his teeth night and morning.

Toilet Training. Micturition and defaecation are spontaneous reflex actions which a child must learn to inhibit to become socially acceptable. During the first year of life, an infant may be sat on a pot following a feed or meal, and frequently soiled napkins are avoided. At this stage he is unable to appreciate the meaning of his 'sit', but is quick to detect his mother's reactions to an empty pot and subsequent soiled napkin.

By the age of fourteen to eighteen months, reflex inhibition is achieved and micturition and defaecation become under the control of the will. If potty-training is fraught with maternal emotions, or if the toddler is insecure in his home environment, reversion to wet and soiled napkins results. Usually by the age of eighteen months to two years a child can tell his mother he is wet or that he wants his pot, and if his needs are met, he can be expected to be clean and almost dry during the day. Most children have bladder control for the full twenty-four hours by the age of three years, although there is wide variation in the age of this attainment.

TABLE 2. Summary of Average Rate of Growth and Physiological Performance.

	Birth	3 months	6 months	1 year	2 years	3 years
Height to nearest						
cm	50	60	66	75	85	95
inches	20	24	26	30	35	38
Weight in						
Boys kg	3·4	5·7	7·8	10·3	12·7	14·7
lb	7½	12¾	17¼	22¾	28	32½
Girls kg	3·4	5·2	7·3	9·6	12·0	14·1
lb	7½	11½	17	21¼	26½	31¼
Head circumference						
cm	33–35·5	40·6	43·2	45·7	48·3	50·8
inches	13–14	15	17	18	19	20
Haemoglobin grams %	18–22·0	10·5–12·5	11·8	12·3–13·8	12·3–13·8	12·3–13·8
Pulse rate per minute	150–130	130–110	120	115	110–100	100–90
Respiratory rate	60–30 irregular	50–30	45–30	30–25	30–25	25
Urine output ml/24 hours	90–120	250–450	450–500	450–600	500–700 Bladder control (day)	500–700 Bladder control (day and night)
Bowel actions number per day	4–5	3–4	3–4	2	1–2	1
First dentition	—	—	2	10	20 complete	

PLAY

Through play, a small child discovers himself and comes to terms with the nature of his surroundings.

At first, an infant is satisfied to play by himself, gradually gaining strength and neuromuscular co-ordination in constant mouthing and manipulation of his fingers, toes and safe toys of different bright colours, textures, shapes and noises. With increasing awareness of his surrounding environment, he responds to and enjoys adult attention at regular intervals during his play.

For the first three years or so, play is absolutely self-centred (egocentric). Gradually, the toddler discovers the advantages of shared play and group activities with increased social contacts. He should learn to give and take, to seek the approval of his playmates, and generally learn to get on with his friends. Through play, a child is able to release his emotions in realistic and imaginative circumstances. To the small child, imaginary situations are as real as life itself.

Toys are the essential tools of play but are not a substitute for love and security of which the child needs constant reassurance. All must be safe and suitable for the age, interest and ability of the child. Frequently, the simple cheaper play materials are appreciated more than elaborate expensive ones. Light washable toys are ideal for a beginner. Very small toys, or parts of toys, should be avoided as they may be swallowed or inhaled or pushed into a nostril or an ear. Paint should be lead-free and sharp objects avoided. Play materials giving scope for constructive, destructive, imaginative and creative play are necessary as the trial and error learning of the young is gradually replaced by more meaningful learning with understanding.

The School Years

During the pre-school years, the small child has learned about himself, what he can do, to understand and reason with people, to control his emotions and become reasonably independent as far as toilet and dressing needs are concerned.

His first day at school, usually talked about for weeks before, is a memorable occasion for the family, but often not remembered by the child concerned. For possibly the first time in his life he is faced with unfamiliar surroundings in the absence of his mother. His freedom may be restricted by a comparative stranger whom he has to share with a large number of other children of different sizes abilities and backgrounds.

The infant school years form a bridge between the affectionate security of a small family unit and true learning. Most children quickly adapt to the widening horizon of school and benefit from increased social contact which the learning process of school life affords. Fleeting friendships are made with class-mates; lasting friendships, on the whole, are made much later. Learning is essentially by doing, with frequent changes of activity. The excessive energy of this age group calls for opportunity during school sessions to release their boisterous nature.

By the age of seven years, the average child is well settled into the competitive life of a school routine. Powers of sustained concentration are improved and he is quick and keen to learn. Both school and out-of-school activities encourage group and team activities, fostering interest in nature and the value of our heritage. Greater independence is encouraged and the child is taught to save up for his pleasures from his weekly pocket money. With the assurance of a secure, loving home in the background, most children find this is a happy, carefree period of life; the standards set by the family and society have been accepted, but as yet they are too young to be accepted as responsible members of society.

Senior school life is essentially an extension of this continuing learning process.

Further interests and activities are fostered as greater independence is sought. Our educational system may well create a teenager who is intellectually superior to his less privileged parents and this may lead to parental resentment. All have need to contribute, and many do, to less fortunate members of society if guided into the right channels. Advice regarding a desirable career is important at an early stage so that senior school work can be in accordance with individual aspirations.

Adolescence

This complex stage of development, when physical, mental and emotional changes are rapidly taking place, forms the bridge between the dependency of childhood and the independency of adulthood.

With the earlier onset of puberty in both girls and boys, physical development is in advance of emotional development, which may leave the adolescent in social and moral danger unless adequately instructed in such responsibility. A natural interest in the body starts during the very early years of life; at puberty, the child becomes self-conscious of the body's changing form and possible physical awkwardness. The attitude and interest shown by the parents to their child's previous infantile masturbatory activity may well affect the adolescent's reactions to sex. If no satisfactory instruction is given at home he will seek information elsewhere.

The adolescent begins to challenge the attitudes of both parents and teachers assimilated during his childhood years and this is often revealed as rebellious or moody behaviour. Conformity to the fashions and interests of the moment is vital for acceptance in a group. Teachers, dignitaries and pop stars are 'hero-worshipped' by this age group seeking a true meaning for life.

For Further Reading

ILLINGWORTH R. S. (1970). *The Development of the Infant and Young Child: Normal and Abnormal*, 4th edition. E. & S. Livingstone, Edinburgh.
ILLINGWORTH R. S. (1968). *The Normal Child*, 4th edition. J. & A. Churchill, London.
ANON (1966). *The Seven Ages of Man—A survey of the development of man through life—his body, his personality and his abilities*. New Society—New Science Publications Ltd., London.

CHAPTER TWO

Safeguarding the Child's Health

Since the turn of this century, Great Britain has seen a vast improvement in the health of the nation in general and its children in particular. The infant mortality rate, an index of living standards, has fallen from 153 in 1900 to 18 per 1,000 live births in 1969. The expectation of life is now sixteen to eighteen years longer than it was for a person born in 1900. Diphtheria, typhoid, tuberculosis and other virulent infectious diseases are now rare, and account for but a few deaths, while accidental death and malignancy take an increasing toll.

There are many factors which have assisted in increasing the standard of living, thus reducing infant mortality and improving the health of the individual:

1 Environmental—pure water supply, clean air, better sanitation, better housing—less overcrowding, control of milk supplies and food inspection.
2 Economic security—less unemployment and better pay and social security benefits—unemployment pay, pensions, family allowance, etc.
3 Compulsory education from five to fifteen years.
4 Marked decrease in size of family—active birth control.
5 Awareness of the need for preventive medicine provided by the social services.
6 Immunization controlling many diseases which carry high mortality and morbidity rates, i.e. whooping cough, measles, diphtheria, typhoid, poliomyelitis, tetanus, smallpox and tuberculosis.
7 A reduction in the virulence of some micro-organisms, as for example, the streptococcus.
8 Knowledge of disease, its causation, detection, prevention, treatment and follow-up.

Maternity and Child Welfare

There are many services designed to promote positive health and prevent disease. These services extend to before the birth of an infant and sometimes before conception. No child asks to come into the world, but all too often children are

16

born unwanted and unloved. If put into practice, the contraceptive advice offered by a family planning clinic or prescribed by the family doctor frequently prevents conception of an unwanted child.

Genetic counselling, available in a few centres, advises parents regarding the desirability of a future pregnancy following the birth of one or more abnormal infants, or if there is a history of a familial hereditary disorder.

Antenatal Care

Antenatal care aims at prevention and early detection of the complications of pregnancy which are of detriment to maternal health and the developing infant, and to advise and educate the mother for her new role of motherhood.

Once pregnancy is confirmed and the expected date of delivery estimated, the woman is advised regarding hospital or home delivery. Hospital confinement is becoming more commonplace, but as yet this facility is not available to all. Those given priority include mothers expecting their first, fifth and subsequent infant, those over the age of thirty-five years, those with a history of previous abnormality of pregnancy or labour, the unmarried, and others living in undesirable social circumstances. Individual antenatal care is then the responsibility of either the family doctor and district midwife, or the antenatal clinic run by the maternity unit in which she is to be delivered.

On her first visit, a family and personal medical history and previous and the present obstetric history are recorded, and a general medical examination is undertaken to exclude previous undetected illness. An early chest X-ray is requested to exclude tuberculosis. Blood is withdrawn to determine the haemoglobin content and blood group and to exclude hidden infection of syphilis (Wassermann test). The blood pressure is recorded, the woman weighed and a clean specimen of urine tested for the presence of protein and sugar. Advice regarding further visits, mothercraft sessions, minor ailments, financial benefits and the necessity for dental care, rest and a well-balanced diet concludes her first visit to the clinic.

On subsequent visits to the antenatal clinic the woman is questioned about her health and welfare, and the appropriate advice is offered. She is weighed, her blood pressure recorded, urine tested for the presence of protein, and her legs examined for signs of oedema. A marked increase in weight, rise in blood pressure, proteinuria and oedema are signs of pre-eclampsia. Examination of the abdomen determines the size of the uterus and later the size, position and heart rate of the developing foetus. Towards the end of pregnancy, cephalo-pelvic disproportion is excluded. If the maternal blood group is Rhesus negative and the father Rhesus positive group, maternal blood will be taken at intervals to determine any rise in the antibody titre indicating maternal-foetal Rhesus incompatibility.

Attendance at mothercraft classes prepares the mother for labour, and advice is given about the care, feeding, clothing and other requirements necessary for her new infant.

Care at Birth

Unforeseen obstetric complications occur in the most unsuspected circumstances and the possibility should always be anticipated. With a few accidental exceptions, women are delivered by a doctor or practising midwife with the services of a skilled obstetrician available in complicated cases. Cerebral anoxaemia and haemorrhage occurring during delivery account for more deaths than any other single cause during the neonatal period and for many children and adults with cerebral palsy living today. The need for skilled personnel speaks for itself. Premature delivery accounts for many neonatal deaths, some morbidity and many hours of skilled nursing care and observation. The cause is often unexplained, but good antenatal care and advice regarding diet and early detection of pre-eclampsia can help to reduce the incidence. It is preferable for premature delivery of an infant to take place where good facilities are available for his controlled birth, resuscitation and subsequent special care.

The hospital or domiciliary midwife has the care of both mother and infant up to the tenth day following delivery. The medical officer of health for the area must be notified of the infant's birth and this information is passed on to the local health visitor who is to supervise the welfare of the child during his pre-school years.

Care of the Pre-School Child

It is the health visitor's function to promote physical and mental health of the whole family, and it is usually the arrival of a new infant that brings her into close contact with all members of a household. Once a good relationship has been established, the health visitor is a welcome adviser to mothers on all health matters and has an excellent opportunity for health education both in the home and at the well-babies clinic held regularly in all areas. Her work includes visiting homes where there are children under five-years-of-age and encouraging attendance at the clinic. Screening tests for phenylketonuria, congenital dislocation of the hip and hearing defects are made, and advice regarding feeding, weaning and immunization is given. Her frequent contact with the child ensures that he is receiving adequate care and that normal physical growth and mental development are being attained. Any suspected deviation from the normal is referred to the clinic or family doctor, and the child's name is included in the 'At Risk' register, if necessary.

Well-babies clinics give opportunity for regular contact with the health visitor and doctor as necessary, and for the sale of dried milk preparations, cereals and vitamins. Some immunizations are given and health education is continued in the form of demonstrations, informal discussions and the use of film strips.

The individual records maintained by the health visitor are passed on to the school medical service once full-time education is commenced.

Benefits

A *Maternity Grant* is available on a husband's or the mother's (if unmarried) insurance if national insurance contributions are satisfactory. This lump sum of money (£25 in 1971) can be claimed after the thirty-first week of pregnancy to help meet the extra expense of having an infant.

A *Maternity Allowance* is paid only on the wife's national insurance contributions for an eighteen week period starting eleven weeks prior to the expected date of delivery. This allowance relieves a working mother of financial difficulties at a time when work would affect not only her health, but that of her unborn child. (£5 a week for eighteen weeks in 1971.)

Family Allowance—a weekly sum of money available to benefit the family as a whole can be claimed by a mother with the right number of children of the right ages, i.e. more than one child under the age of fifteen years—or older if still dependent.

As soon as pregnancy is confirmed, and until her child is five-years-of-age, a needy mother can claim a free bottle of *milk* daily. This helps initially to ensure that the maternal calcium intake is adequate for her growing infant's needs, thus protecting her teeth from decalcification and decay, and that the subsequent growth of her child is not affected.

Dental treatment is free during pregnancy and for the year following delivery.

No charge is made for *drugs* prescribed by the doctor for expectant mothers. Iron in the form of ferrous sulphate pills is usually prescribed for the expectant mother. This maintains a satisfactory maternal haemoglobin level to meet the demands of the developing infant.

Vitamin supplements are available at a reduced cost at maternity and child welfare clinics both for the expectant mother and for her pre-school child.

The Unsupported Mother and her Child

An average of 8·3%* of live births in England and Wales are illegitimate, causing psychological and social trauma to the mother, and if the child is not adopted, a greater hazard to his normal development, unless the necessary social services are available:

i Daily child-minders are required to register with the local health authority who exact a certain standard of requirements with regard to health, housing and food hygiene;

* Registrar General's Report 1969.

ii   Day nurseries may be provided by the local health authority, and the cost of maintaining priority places for unsupported children may be subsidized.

Knowledge of the pregnancy may be concealed, particularly when the mother is under sixteen-years-of-age, and antenatal care may be neglected. Social attitudes are undergoing change and rejection of the unmarried mother by her family is now less common. Local authorities are providing more accommodation for these girls in flats with day nurseries attached to them, instead of unmarried mother and baby homes as used to be the pattern. More frequent use of contraceptive advice and the Abortion Act has also lessened the problem.

When the unmarried mother applies for help, she needs advice regarding antenatal care and future rehabilitation. Mothers who decide, often most reluctantly, that adoption would give their child better opportunities are referred to the diocesan social worker or the Department of Social Services. The mother may be required to care for her infant for the first six weeks, unless an initial fostering arrangement is made and supervised by the Department of Social Services. A mother who decides to keep her child may require help from the local authority or her family to care for the child during her absence at work. She may remain at home with her infant and claim social security benefits, but there is a danger that she may become isolated from the community and subject to emotional stress which may adversely affect the child's development.

Care of the Child Deprived of a Normal Home Life

The Children's Act, 1948, put into effect the recommendations laid down in the Curtis Report (H.M.S.O. 1946). Under this act, local authorities are empowered to take into their care any child under the age of seventeen years who is deprived of a normal home life, i.e. one who has no parents or guardian, or who has been abandoned, or whose parents are unwilling or unable to provide for him temporarily or permanently. Every effort is made to keep a child in his home environment, or to return him to it when the crisis is over. Children removed from their parents following ill-treatment or neglect are retained in the care of the Department of Social Services until a satisfactory standard of parental care is assured.

The aim of the local authority is to give the children in their care as near normal a home life as possible. Suitable children are boarded out with foster parents, who receive a maintenance allowance for their care. If a foster home is not available, or the child not suitable for boarding out, he is cared for in a children's home maintained by the local authority or by one of the several voluntary organizations. Here, a group of twelve or so children of various ages are cared for by a house-mother, or house-parents with the husband following his own occupation. The children attend the local school and are encouraged to participate in the activities of the local community. Both foster care and accommodation in a children's home afford opportunity for individual care from a mother-substitute, so necessary for the development of personality and individual interests.

In addition to direct placement, and care and supervision of deprived children, the Department of Social Services supervise provision for residential care made by voluntary organizations and day care provided by daily child-minders. Adoption of eligible children is arranged by and through the department or adoption society and, until legally adopted, a child remains the department's responsibility. Reports of suspected cruelty or neglect reported by the National Society for the Prevention of Cruelty to Children, or individuals, are investigated by the staff. Delinquent children and young persons under the age of eighteen years needing care and protection are committed to their care by juvenile courts. Under the Childrens and Young Persons Act, 1963, the staff of the department have had their work extended to include taking measures to prevent, as well as rectify, the breakdown of family life in 'problem families'.

Resistance to Infection (Immunity)

Congenital (Innate) Immunity

An infant is born with a high degree of resistance to a wide range of micro-organisms. This innate immunity is non-specific, i.e. it will protect the child from all micro-organisms, and not just one, as in specific acquired immunity.

The means by which the body is able to defend itself against invasion by micro-organisms include:
i   an intact skin and mucous membrane;
ii   secretions of the body containing lysozyme;
iii   bacteriolysins, e.g. complement and properdin;
iv   phagocytic action of structures forming the reticulo-endothelial system and the polymorphonuclear leucocytes;
v   cilia lining the respiratory tract;
vi   normal bacterial flora of the large intestine.

Acquired Immunity

Active Immunity
Most children experience some infectious diseases during their early years of life. The dangers of some, such as German measles, mumps and chickenpox, lie in their complications and are best avoided until over the age of two years when the child is better equipped to tolerate the consequences. As a result of contracting the disease, the child produces his own lasting supply of antibodies to protect him from a further attack (active immunity, naturally acquired).

Diphtheria, whooping cough, smallpox, poliomyelitis and measles can all be prevented, or the symptoms attenuated, by the introduction of small quantities of sufficiently potent antigen to stimulate the formation of antibodies, but modified so that active disease will not result (active immunity artificially acquired). In addition, protection against tetanus (tetanus toxoid) is given early in life to avoid the necessity of injecting anti-tetanus serum, with its associated risks, should the need arise. Protection against tuberculosis (B.C.G.—Bacille Calmette-Guérin) is given to infants where there is particular risk of exposure, and to older school children who are tuberculin negative.

This artificial production of immunity is of greatest value in protecting a child against a number of diseases which previously carried high mortality and morbidity rates. During this century, there has been a marked decrease in the incidence of some diseases, due largely to the protection of the population by immunization and vaccination and not due to the disappearance of the disease. Because a disease is now uncommon, many parents consider immunization unnecessary. As the number of inadequately protected children increases, so the risk of a serious epidemic with its associated parental panic increases.

Summary

Active Immunity.
(Production of
own antibodies
in response to
antigen.)

	Naturally acquired.			Artificially acquired.	
Manifesta-tion of the disease.	Subclinical infection.	Repeated contact with infec-tion.	Living anti-gen, e.g. Smallpox vaccine.	Dead antigen, e.g. Whoop-ing cough vaccine.	Toxoid, e.g. Tetanus.

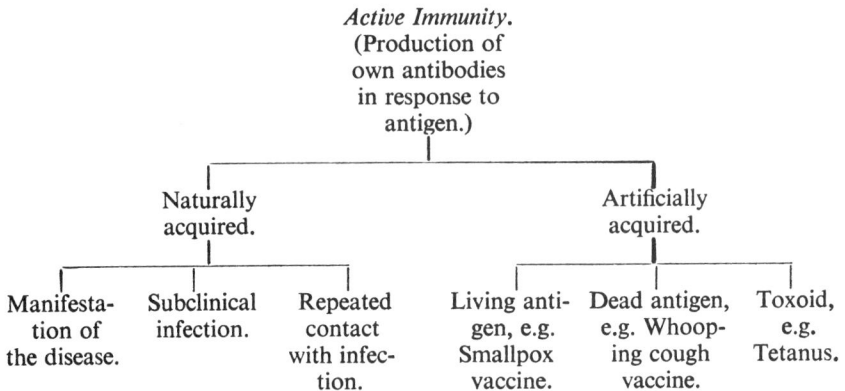

PASSIVE IMMUNITY

A newborn infant is endowed with specific antibodies against infectious diseases experienced by his mother (passive immunity, naturally acquired). Protection is temporary, lasting six to nine months. This emphasizes the necessity for the child to start producing his own antibodies at an early age in response to a controlled immunization programme.

Antibodies produced by other human beings (pooled human gamma globulin) or another species—usually equine (anti-tetanus and anti-diphtheria sera)—give temporary (three weeks) immunity (passive immunity—artificially acquired).

Summary.

Passive Immunity.
(Antibodies
produced
elsewhere).

Naturally
acquired

Artificially
acquired

Via the placental
barrier

In breast milk.

Pooled human
gamma globulin
(non-specific).

Antitoxins (speci-
fic), e.g. Diphtheria
and tetanus.

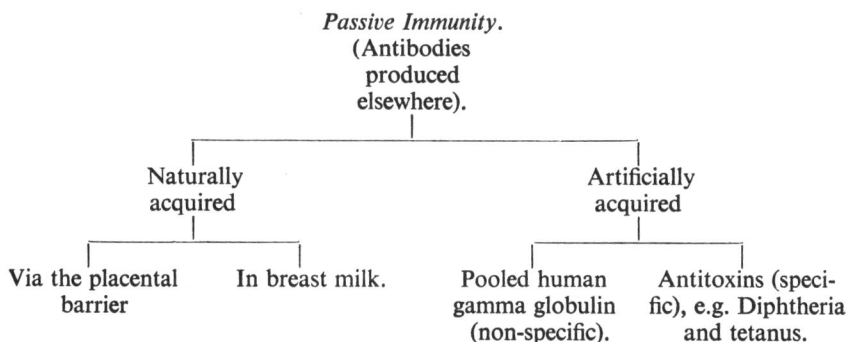

Immunization

Artificial immunization is recommended to all parents of young children, but is not compulsory in this country. The complications of immunization are few, and are far out-weighed by the advantage of having a protected child population.

PRINCIPLES OF IMMUNIZATION

Doses of antigen are given at intervals over a period of months so that the child produces a high antibody level. Subsequent reinforcing (booster) doses of antigen ensure that the antibody level is maintained.

An immunization schedule is adopted by each local authority and is carried out at well-babies clinics.

To avoid the need for multiple injections, three antigens—tetanus, diphtheria and whooping cough—are combined in one injection (Triple Antigen).

Diphtheria, Tetanus and Whooping Cough. It is important that a small infant is protected against an attack of whooping cough. Three injections of Triple Antigen are given at intervals between the ages of six to fourteen months of life. Diphtheria and tetanus reinforcing doses are given on entry to school. A booster dose of tetanus toxoid may then be given at any time when the child has suffered accidental injury. Whooping cough immunization is omitted after the second year of life.

Poliomyelitis antigen. This may be given orally on a sugar lump in three doses at intervals after the age of six months. Reinforcing doses are given during the second year and on entry to school.

Smallpox. Unless earlier protection is required by travel and contact, smallpox vaccine is given sometime during the second year of life, but not less than four weeks before or after any other immunization. It may be repeated once during the school years and as travel and contact demand.

Tuberculosis. B.C.G. vaccine to tuberculin negative children is given during the latter years at school, or earlier where the risk to exposure is great. Contact with a sufferer of open tuberculosis for the following six weeks should be avoided.

Measles. An attack of measles is particularly dangerous in the first two to three years of life. The vaccine is usually given after the age of ten months and not less than one month after other forms of immunization.

German Measles. Although German measles is a comparatively mild infection, maternal infection during the first trimester of pregnancy results in a high incidence of foetal abnormality. Vaccine is now available to all girls of eleven to thirteen-years-of-age to ensure that they are protected before reaching the normal child-bearing age.

TABLE 3. Suggested Immunisation Programme

Age	Vaccine	
6 months	Diphtheria/Pertussis/Tetanus Poliomyelitis Oral	First dose
8 months	Diphtheria/Pertussis/Tetanus Poliomyelitis Oral	Second dose (2 months later)
14 months	Diphtheria/Pertussis/Tetanus Poliomyelitis Oral	Third dose (6 months later)
14 months	Attenuated Measles	
1–2 years	Smallpox	
4–5 years	Diphtheria/Tetanus Poliomyelitis Oral	Booster dose 4 years after
11–13 years	German Measles	(Girls only)
13 years	B.C.G. (if Heaf or Mantoux negative)	

CONTRA-INDICATIONS TO ARTIFICIAL IMMUNIZATION

Contra-indications to any form of artificial immunity include:

i   untoward reactions to previous immunization;
ii   active infection at the time;
iii eczematous conditions contra-indicate vaccination;
iv   convulsions in early life.

Education

The Education Act, 1944, laid down that 'it shall be the duty of the local education authority for every area so far as their powers extend, to contribute towards the spiritual, moral, mental and physical development of the community by securing that efficient education throughout the school years shall be available to meet the needs of the population of their area.' Every parent is required to submit his child to full-time education suitable to his age, ability and aptitude between the ages of five to fifteen years. This may be taken in publicly maintained or assisted schools, independent schools, day and residential special schools, at home or in hospital. Transport to and from state schools is provided free to children living outside a certain radius.

Nursery Schools

Children between the ages of two and five years can attend nursery schools, or a nursery class in an infants school, provided by the local education authority. These schools give opportunity for constructive play and group activities organized by teachers with the help of nursery assistants. Improved facilities for compulsory education have been expanded at the expense of nursery education. The all too few vacancies available are reserved for children with a special need. Priority cases include children from crowded living conditions, the handicapped, or those with a behaviour disorder, and others recommended by the family doctor, health visitor or other authoritative person. Attendance is free.

To compensate for the lack of nursery schools, private nurseries and pre-school play groups have been started by local groups of mothers or other women, with the knowledge and approval of the local health authority.

Special Schools

Facilities for the education of physically and educable mentally handicapped children may be available within the area controlled by the local authority or financed in another area, or provided by a specific voluntary organization. Depending on the nature and degree of severity of the handicap, the child may be educated:

i   in an ordinary day school;
ii in a special class in an ordinary day school;
iii in a day special school;
iv in a residential special school;
v   in a hospital school;
vi at home.

A handicap of sufficient severity to inhibit a normal school life must be diagnosed as early as possible, and the parents given all the help and guidance necessary to bring their child to his full developmental and intellectual potential. Early residential education may be advised which the parents may find difficult to accept.

The Blind. Total blindness is usually detected early and these children are educated by non-visual methods. The Royal National Institute for the Blind have Sunshine Homes where children from two to five years can start their special training. Separation from home is unfortunately inevitable in most instances as day schools for blind children are only available in a few densely populated cities.

Partially Sighted. With some eyesight, and the use of special equipment, partially sighted children may be taught in small numbers, using visual methods, either in a special school or small class attached to a day school.

The Deaf. Children with no auditory activity are naturally dumb but, with modern teaching methods, they can be taught to speak. Most deaf children are educated in residential schools and their education is started before the age of five years.

Partially Deaf. With some hearing and the use of hearing aids, these children are taught in small classes in day or residential special schools.

The Delicate. This group consists of children with a multiplicity of conditions which would interfere with normal education. Many are unable to tolerate the pace of the school and play life of their healthy counterparts, while others, because of their disability, experience many interruptions in the continuity of education. Children with chest conditions, e.g. asthma, cystic fibrosis, bronchiectasis or with heart lesions (both congenital and rheumatic), bleeding disorders, e.g. haemophilia and Christmas disease, may need educating in a residential or day special school, or in some instances at home under the guidance of a home teacher.

The Educationally Subnormal. Children of low mental ability (I.Q. 55–70) are unable to take advantage of the normal educational facilities. Suitable education is provided in special (E.S.N.) schools or in a special class in an ordinary day school where the pace of work is much slower.

The Maladjusted. These children are the so-called 'problem children'—usually emotionally unstable, often the product of an unstable home environment, and possibly suffering from a psychiatric disorder. They are referred for special treatment from child guidance clinics or centres and their subsequent future in relation to education and psychiatric treatment is planned. Separation from a normal school life is avoided as far as possible.

The Physically Handicapped. Many children with mild physical handicaps can be very satisfactorily educated in an ordinary day school, with the possible addition of special transport to and from home. Residential and day special schools cater for the very severely handicapped child. Children suffering from non-progressive illnesses are encouraged to as near independence as is practical and receive an education to allow them to take their place (even though possibly sheltered) in the outside world. This group includes the increasing number of children surviving with spina bifida, the cerebral palsied and other brain damaged children.

The Epileptic Child. Unless an epileptic child has frequent convulsions or is emotionally unstable, education in an ordinary day school is advisable. Residential schools and colonies are available for the education of children who have frequent convulsions or who are emotionally unstable.

Speech Defect. About 1% of all children have a speech defect, usually a stammer, which may quickly develop into a nervous phenomenon if not corrected by a speech therapist. Education is in an ordinary school but under the close supervision of a speech therapist.

The Ineducable Mentally Subnormal Child. Under the age of sixteen years the ineducable mentally subnormal child is provided for in either a junior training centre or in a hospital for the mentally subnormal where training in sociability and independence encourages self-respect and greater acceptance in the community.

The School Medical Service

The local education authority is essentially concerned with compulsory education but, in addition, continues the promotion of positive health provided by the local health authority for the pre-school child.

The school medical service is essentially a diagnostic service. Routine medical inspections are carried out at intervals during the child's school career, i.e. on entering school and again at the ages of eight, eleven and fourteen, or so. Children with a disability are examined at yearly intervals between. Close liaison between the school doctor, family doctor, parents and teacher ensure that adequate treatment and follow-up is given. Reinforcing doses of vaccines are given and the B.C.G. vaccine is offered to tuberculin negative school leavers. Regular inspections by the school nurse ensure that personal cleanliness is maintained at a high level. The hair is inspected for head lice (3% of the child population harbour head lice), the skin for scabies and the feet for verrucae. Appropriate deinfestation of the whole family is arranged for the first two mentioned, and children with verrucae are treated at the school clinic or by their family doctor. Dental, ophthalmic, orthopaedic, foot and child guidance clinics are supplied by most local education authorities.

Positive health education should play an integral part in the school curriculum. Subject-matter includes such topics as personal cleanliness, dental hygiene, eating habits, use of leisure hours, and self-discipline related to relaxation, sleep, sex, smoking, alcohol and drugs.

School meals are provided at a reduced cost to all, and at no cost to particularly needy children, or the members of a large family. One third of a pint of milk is provided free in all state schools to the age of seven years. When the family income is insufficient to meet the demands for adequate clothing and shoes, their cost may be met at the discretion of the local education committee.

Moral and Physical Protection

Many laws have been made to safeguard the health and welfare of children and young people from the physical dangers, exploitation and vices of modern society. To mention just a few—it is, for example, unlawful to employ a child under the age of thirteen years; to serve alcohol to an unaccompanied child under the age of eighteen years; to sell cigarettes to anyone under the age of sixteen years; to allow a girl under the age of sixteen years into a brothel or to be subjected to sexual intercourse, or for a drunken person to be in charge of a child.

In recent years, there has been increasing awareness of the problem of young children who are deliberately injured by their parents. If no preventive action is taken when these cases come to light, the child may be at risk of further physical injury and other children in the family may be similarly maltreated. If suspicions of the battered baby syndrome are aroused, the Department of Social Services should be informed and the consultant paediatrician may feel it necessary to inform the police.

Accidents—Environmental and in the Home

In spite of preventive measures, death by accident carries an increasing toll. In 1969, 764 under fifteen-years-of-age died in road accidents and many more were seriously injured. Accidents—road-traffic, drowning and in the home— account for more deaths than any single cause in the five to fourteen years age group.

These statistics speak for themselves. Road safety should be taught early and at every possible opportunity by parents. School visits by the local police and organization of cycle proficiency tests encourage road safety as well as improve the child's relationship with the law. Swimming instruction given in schools ensures that most children can swim from an early age.

Accidents in the home are common and usually preventable. Many children are seriously injured, physically and psychologically scarred, and sometimes incapacitated for life as the result of parental carelessness or ignorance. In 1969, 159 children died from burns and scalds, and hundreds more suffered permanent disfigurement. Accidental poisoning accounted for 43 deaths and 780 children died of asphyxia due to drowning, inhalation, and suffocation. Because of their natural desire for adventure, small children are particularly vulnerable.

Accident prevention should be taught at every opportunity by all personnel concerned in positive health and preventive medicine. Health visitors who regularly visit homes have an excellent opportunity to educate the family. Advice includes the dangers of polythene bags and plastic sheeting; small, sharp and lead-painted toys; saucepan handles; hanging table cloths; hot-water bottles; matches; unguarded fires; windows and stairs; berries; use of pillows for the infant; and the safe storage of disinfectants, cleansing agents, fertilizers, cosmetics and medications.

Legislation has attempted to reduce the number of tragic deaths due to burning. For example, a child should have reached the age of thirteen years before being sold fireworks, and gas, electric and paraffin fires for sale must conform to safety regulations. It is now illegal for shopkeepers to sell nightdresses, or material for children's nightdresses, which are not flameproof. Failure to guard an open fire or heating appliance will cause the parents a fine *but only* if a child under the age of twelve years is killed or severely injured as the result of burns.

Minor Ailments of Childhood

The presence of animal parasites in the hair, clothing or intestine is referred to as infestation. Infection is due to the presence of pathogenic micro-organisms— bacteria, viruses, protozoa or fungi.

Infestations

THREADWORMS
Nocturnal irritability may suggest that a young child is harbouring intestinal threadworms. During the hours of sleep these white parasites (0·4–1·2cm in length) lay their eggs in the perianal area from where they are scattered into personal and bed linen and find their way to the child's mouth by way of the exploring finger nails. The swallowed eggs allow adult worms to develop in the intestine and so auto-infestation continues. If not treated, the infestation usually dies out within three months.

Specific treatment includes administration of piperazine, usually given in combination with Senokot as Pripsen. One dose is usually sufficient.

A high standard of personal hygiene helps to discourage auto- and cross-infestation:
1 Use of individual towels for each member of the family.
2 Meticulous care with handwashing before meals and after visiting the toilet.
3 Finger nails kept short and clean, and direct anal scratching discouraged by the use of tight-fitting pants and cotton gloves.
4 The infested child should have his own bed.
5 Underwear, nightwear and bedclothes require frequent, careful laundering to avoid scattering the threadworm eggs into the environment.

PEDICULOSIS
Infestation with the head, body and pubic lice occurs in overcrowded, poor living conditions, and in situations where there is little opportunity for personal cleanliness and change of clothing, although a child from the best of homes may acquire the parasite.

The head louse (Pediculus capitis) is a small, greyish-white wingless insect, 1–2mm in length, readily visible with the observant naked eye. It lays its eggs (nits) near to the hair roots of the nape of the neck and behind the ears. Disinfestation and treatment are given on page 123.

SCABIES

Caused by the minute (0·4mm) Sarcoptes scabiei—the 'itch mite', scabies is an infestation manifesting as crops of vesicles in loose areas of skin—between the toes and fingers, in the axillae and on the wrists and elbows—although other parts of the body may be affected.

Each vesicle represents the site where a scabies mite has laid twenty-four or so eggs as she burrowed into the skin. Irritation is intense, scratching inevitable, and secondary infection quickly ensues. Infestation is by direct contact and is essentially indicative of a low standard of personal cleanliness, and affects whole families living in poor living conditions. Eradication, therefore, entails treatment of the whole family:

1   Personal and bed linen removed and laundered.
2   A hot bath is given and the hair is washed.
3   The whole body (excluding the face and scalp) is painted with Lorexane 1% (I.C.I.) or benzyl benzoate 25%, and allowed to dry.
4   Clean personal clothing is worn.
5   The treatment is repeated twenty-four hours later.

Infections

RINGWORM (TINEA)

This highly contagious fungal infection may affect the scalp, body or feet.

Tinea infection of the scalp is characterized by the typical circular patches of lustreless, grey, broken hairs overlying grey-white crusts. The infection is usually of human origin, but the family dog or cat may infect a small child. If left untreated, the infection resolves at puberty.

Tinea infection of the body presents as sporadic irritating red circular discs on the arms and legs.

Prolonged systemic Griseofulvin therapy usually controls both types of infection.

Tinea pedis (athlete's foot) is more common in older children who have greater opportunity to frequent swimming and communal baths. Vesicular lesions between the toes becomes white, macerated, and peel to reveal raw, red areas. To prevent, control and cure the infection, the following foot care is advised:

1   The feet are washed, dried and powdered at night.
2   Socks changed daily.
3   Leather footwear worn.

4 The child is discouraged from walking barefoot in communal wet places, i.e. school shower, swimming and communal baths.
5 Mercurial ointment or powder may be prescribed for local application.

VERRUCAE (PLANTAR WARTS)
Amongst school children, verrucae are common. Due to a viral infection of the dermis, this painful wart is acquired in communal baths and gymnasia where shoes are not worn. The wart is shelled out following prolonged treatment with 3% formalin, or application of carbon dioxide snow. The child is discouraged from walking barefoot.

IMPETIGO
Impetigo is a highly contagious staphylococcal infection of the superficial layers of the skin. An isolated lesion is quickly spread to other parts of the face and scalp by the exploring finger nails. Impetigo is characterized by vesicular and pustular swellings which discharge to form dried crusts on the skin surface. Treatment may be local in the form of antibiotic cream, but systemic antibiotic therapy may have to be prescribed when there is widespread infection. The child must be isolated and restrained from scratching.

Infectious Diseases of Childhood

PRINCIPLES OF MANAGEMENT INCLUDE:
1 Case isolation (Chapter 8).
   i Rest;
  ii Fluids and a light nourishing diet;
 iii Specific care, e.g. local applications to alleviate pruritus. Local heat in relief of pain.
     Antipyretics / Sedatives / Antibiotics } as ordered by the doctor.
2 Protection of vulnerable contacts by gamma globulins or by oral antibiotics as in gastro-intestinal infections.
3 Examination of all contacts for evidence of the carrier state.

For Further Reading

MEREDITH DAVIES, J. B. (1965). *Preventive Medicine for Nurses and Social Workers.* English Universities Press Ltd, London.

TABLE 4. Infectious

Disease	i Causative Agent ii Mode of Spread	i Incubation and ii Segregation Period	Clinical Manifestations
CHICKEN POX† (VARICELLA).	i Virus. ii Airborne. Contact (of high infectivity).	i 14–21 days. ii Until lesions healed.	Rash first sign. Slight pyrexia.
RUBELLA (GERMAN MEASLES).	i Virus. ii Airborne.	i 14–21 days. ii Until rash has faded.	Mild pyrexia, malaise. Enlarged suboccipital glands.
MUMPS (EPIDEMIC PAROTITIS).	i Virus. ii Airborne.	i 14–28 days. ii 7 days after swelling subsides.	Unilateral or bilateral parotid swelling → trismus. Slight fever and lassitude.
MEASLES* (MORBILLI).	i Virus. ii Airborne (of high infectivity).	i 7–14 days. ii Not less than 5 days after rash faded.	4 days of coryza, photophobia, conjunctivitis, dry irritating cough, misery + + ↑ temperature. 2nd day Koplik spots on buccal mucous membrane— diagnostic of infection.
WHOOPING* COUGH (PERTUSSIS).	i Bordetella Haemophilus pertussis. ii Airborne (of high infectivity).	i 6–18 days. ii 6 weeks.	Coryza → chest infection → productive cough becoming paroxysmal associated with vomiting and classical whoop. Lymphocytosis and reduced erythrocyte sedimentation rate (E.S.R.).
SCARLET* FEVER (SCARLATINA).	i Haemolytic Streptococcus, Lancefield Group A. ii Airborne. Contaminated milk. Inanimate objects. From case or carrier.	i 1–7 days. ii Until throat swab is clear—usually 6–10 days.	Pyrexia, headache, tonsilitis, malaise.
DIPHTHERIA*	i Corynebacterium Diphtheriae (Klebs-Loeffler bacillus). ii Direct. Airborne. Inanimate objects. Contaminated milk—from case or carrier.	i 1–6 days. ii At least 4 weeks and until 2 consecutive negative throat cultures.	Toxaemia + + Lassitude. Grey membranous patches on tonsils. Low grade pyrexia. Tachycardia.
ANTERIOR* POLIOMYELITIS	i Virus types. 1, 11, 111. ii Airborne Ingestion.	i 7–14 days. ii At least 3 weeks.	Symptoms of 'summer 'flu'. Pyrexia, headache, sore throat → neck and back stiffness → flaccid weakness or paralysis of muscles.

* Notifiable to the Medical Officer of Health.   † Notifiable during a smallpox outbreak.

Diseases of Childhood.

Rash Type and Distribution	Complications	Treatment	Prevention
Centripetal distribution of irritating superficial uniocular pink macules → papules → vesicles → pustules → scabs by 5th day. (Multiocular of centrifugal distribution in smallpox (Variola).)	Rare. Scarring. Encephalitis. Could be fatal to child receiving steroid therapy.	Symptomatic to prevent scarring.	Segregation of susceptible. Case isolation.
Generalised small discrete pink macules becoming confluent—fading in 2 days.	Foetal developmental abnormalities if infected in first trimester of pregnancy.	Symptomatic.	Active immunization for girls. Attenuated rubella vaccine. Gamma globulin to susceptible pregnant women.
None.	Rare. Encephalitis. Orchitis. Pancreatitis.	Symptomatic in relief of discomfort.	Case isolation.
4th day. Minute red spots → dusky red blotchy macular rash behind ears and on forehead spreading over body → desquamation.	Not uncommon. Otitis media. Broncho-pneumonia. Encephalitis. Strabismus. Gastro-enteritis and Croup in infancy.	Symptomatic. Sedation for misery. Antibiotics for secondary infection.	Attenuated measles vaccine in 2nd year of life. Human gamma globulin to vulnerable contacts 0·25 ml./kg.
None.	Not common: Spontaneous pneumothorax. Broncho-pneumonia. Subconjunctival haemorrhages. Hernia. Anoxaemic convulsions.	Symptomatic. Sedatives. Chloramphenicol.	Killed haemophilus vaccine in Triple Antigen.
2nd day generalised punctate erythema → scarlet rash → desquamation. Strawberry tongue.	Toxic: Acute glomerular nephritis. Rheumatic fever. Bacterial: Otitis media. Sinusitis.	Symptomatic. Sulphonamides. Penicillin.	Prophylactic sulphonamides.
None.	Paralyses. Myocarditis. Asphyxia. Often fatal.	Diphtheria antitoxin. Penicillin or Erythromycin. Rest → myocarditis. Tracheostomy → respiratory obstruction.	Diphtheria toxoid in Triple Antigen.
None.	Paralysis. Respiratory insufficiency.	Symptomatic. Physio-therapy. Aids to respiration.	Oral live attenuated vaccine (Sabin) or killed vaccine (Salk).

The Quarantine Period when enforced is the longest incubation time + 3 days.

CHAPTER THREE

Caring for Small Infants

Every newborn infant is examined carefully to ascertain normality and to exclude obvious and suggestive evidence of abnormality. Some serious congenital abnormalities are not obvious at birth, and it is only with careful observation of the infant that their presence can be suspected.

Examination of the Newborn

Characteristics of the full-term newborn infant are to be found on page 67.

1 An antenatal history of German measles in the first trimester, hydramnios or administration of certain drugs call for particular scrutiny of the newborn infant. For example, the possibility of oesophageal atresia in an infant born to a mother with hydramnios is excluded by the passage of a fairly rigid, sterile radio-opaque catheter (Plate 15).

2 Obvious congenital abnormalities such as cleft lip and palate, spina bifida, varus deformity of the feet, imperforate anus, extra digits, syndactyly and hypospadias are excluded, the femoral pulses palpated, and the hips examined for evidence of dislocation.

3 Manifestations such as ears set at a low level, the presence of a single umbilical artery, extra digits and syndactyly are suggestive, but not by any means conclusive, of hidden congenital abnormality—often of the urinary tract.

4 Congenital deformity or damage to the central nervous system, due to haemorrhage or anoxaemia, is assessed by observing the infant's posture and movements and eliciting the primitive reflexes.

5 Some physical defects, e.g. congenital heart disease, intestinal atresia, diaphragmatic hernia, choanal atresia, urethral valves, and some chromosomal and metabolic disorders may not be apparent at birth, but many may be suspected soon after birth, while others may not be revealed until months or even years later.

Care of the Umbilical Cord

The umbilical cord consists of two umbilical arteries (1 in 150 have only 1) and an umbilical vein supported in a greyish-white connective tissue called Wharton's jelly. Following delivery, the cord is clamped and the blood vessels occluded, using a disposable umbilical clamp, latex band or two linen thread ligatures—tied in reef knots—according to the practice of the authority. The cord is then shortened to within 3–5cm, or 1–2 inches, of the infant's abdomen.

Frequent cord inspection during the first forty-eight hours of life is necessary to detect slackening of a ligature as the Wharton's jelly shrinks, and a further ligature may be required. Haemorrhage must be prevented at all costs—remembering that the blood volume of the newborn infant is only in the region of 80ml/kg. To facilitate the process of necrosis and to prevent the entry of micro-organisms, the cord is kept clean and dry and treated with an antiseptic spirit

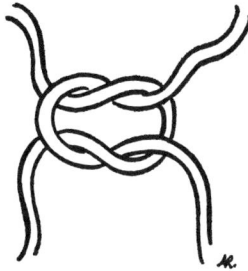

FIG. 4. Reef knot.

solution, such as triple dye or tincture of chlorhexidine 0·5%, at birth and again at intervals until spontaneous separation of the cord occurs five to ten days later. This natural process should not be expedited as haemorrhage may occur or infection may be introduced. After the cord has separated, a residual granuloma may be treated with silver nitrate.

Fullfilling the Infant's Needs

The newborn infant is a helpless individual, completely dependent on his mother, or mother substitute, for the fulfilment of his basic needs:
1 Establishment and maintenance of a clear airway.
2 Warmth.
3 Rest and sleep.
4 Nourishment (Chapter 4).
5 Exercise.

6 Love and affection—security.
7 Protection.
8 Cleanliness.
9 Excretion.

Establishment and Maintenance of a Clear Airway

Establishment and maintenance of a clear airway is of prime importance in the immediate care of the newborn. When resuscitation is slow, the clinical condition of the infant may be evaluated using the Apgar score one minute and five minutes after birth (TABLE 5). This evaluation gives the paediatrician an indication of the infant's ultimate prognosis. Each individual observation is scored as 0, 1 or 2. A total score of 10 indicates that the infant is in the best possible condition. With a score of less than 7, the infant will require close observation and follow-up.

TABLE 5. Apgar Scoring System
(Evaluation of the Newborn Infant One Minute and Five Minutes after Birth)

Score	Colour	Heart Rate	Reflex Irritability*	Muscle Tone	Respiratory Effort
2	Pink	100–140	Normal cough/sneeze	Good	Normal cry
1	Body pink, extremities blue	Below 100	Moderately depressed (Grimace)	Fair	Irregular and shallow
0	Cyanotic	No beat obtained	Absent	Flaccid	Apnoea for more than 60 seconds

* Response to catheter in nostril after clearance of oro-pharynx.

Many newborn infants are admitted to a paediatric unit when the airway still requires special care. To facilitate drainage of mucus from the mouth and to prevent inhalation of vomitus, the infant is nursed on one side with the foot of the cot or incubator tray slightly elevated unless contra-indicated by brain damage. Careful use of a mucus aspirator or suction apparatus turned to minimal negative pressure may be necessary to prevent inhalation of excessive secretion. Damage to the delicate lining of the nose and mouth must be prevented by careful aspiration. Oxygen should not be given until a clear airway is ensured.

Cyanotic attacks due to periods of apnoea are more common in the infant of low birth weight, and if central cyanosis is seen in the full-term infant, this is frequently due to inhalation of foreign matter and demands prompt removal. Peripheral cyanosis is common in the first hour or so of life (page 148).

Warmth

The heat-regulating centre of the newborn infant is immature, and variation in body temperature may be sudden and considerable. Chilling of the newborn infant must be avoided. For the first forty weeks of life, the infant has been in the warm, wet environment of the uterus where a stable body temperature has been maintained. After such comfort and the shock of being born, the infant is thrust out into a cooler environment, and his immature heat-regulating centre takes over the maintenance of a stable temperature, regardless of the temperature of the environment. A certain amount of exposure at birth is inevitable and this time increases if active resuscitation is necessary. Chilling is avoided by maintaining the delivery room temperature at 18–21°C or 65–70°F, and wrapping the infant in a warm towel or tinfoil before placing him in a warmed cot.

Every effort should be made to maintain a constant warm environment for a newborn infant. Nursed in a warm room, the personal clothing and cot linen can be light. Neonatal hypothermia (page 72) occurs when a small infant is nursed in a room where the temperature fluctuates according to the time of the day. A cot temperature of around 21°–23°C or 70°–75°F can be maintained by the discriminate use of adequately protected hot-water bottles. Securing an infant tightly in a wrapper anchored by tight bedclothes is not the best way to keep him warm. Activity of his small body encourages the production of heat which is conserved in the air spaces between layers of light clothing. Light, loose clothing and wrapping with little restraint is, therefore, preferable.

Unless a basin type cot is used, care should be taken to see that the infant is not in a draught between the window, door or fireplace. A screen around a drop-side cot excludes draughts.

Overheating is not uncommon and can be avoided by adjusting the personal and bed clothing according to the temperature of the environment.

Rest and Sleep

The newborn infant spends twenty-one or so hours in twenty-four asleep, waking only for food. Quiet wakefulness in the newborn period is often a sign of intracranial damage, demanding medical attention. An infant of low birth weight and one suffering from physiological jaundice may be very drowsy, not bothering to wake for nourishment.

Exercise

A certain amount of freedom of expression is important at all ages, and no less so in the first few weeks of life. Crying is the only means by which an infant can make his feelings known, and this is often accompanied by much activity of the limbs when he is truly cross.

Provided the room is warm, the small infant benefits from increasing periods of time when, free from restrictive clothing, he can kick his legs and begin to discover his body.

There is usually some good reason for an infant to exercise his lungs, and his crying should never pass ignored. Most infants are pacified by fulfilment of their need for food, warmth or a love and a cuddle without the risk of forming bad habits.

Love and Affection

In normal circumstances, a close mother–child relationship is established within the first few days of birth. When the infant has had his mother's instinctive care substituted for the skilled nursing care of the staff of a special care baby unit or neonatal surgical unit, this relationship may be difficult to establish. Regular physical maternal contact with her infant should, therefore, be encouraged as soon as possible after birth.

Protection

1 INFECTION
All newborn infants are susceptible to infection as their only defence consists of immunological gamma globulins inherited from the mother. Minor skin, nail-bed, mouth and eye infections are not uncommon, but should be confined to the affected infant by practising a good barrier nursing routine to prevent cross-infection.

2 SUFFOCATION
A young infant is unable to change his position should he roll over on to his face. A pillow in the cot or pram is not necessary and is potentially dangerous.

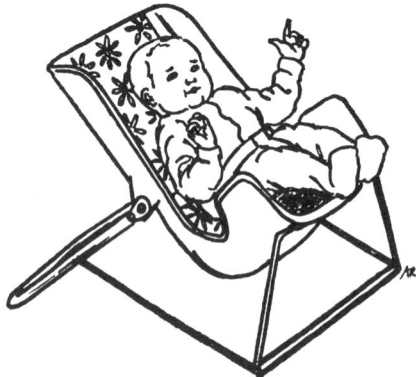

FIG. 5. Safe Sitter (Mothercare).

Under the age of one year, the head and upper part of the body can be elevated by raising the head of the cot on blocks or placing a firm pillow under the mattress, rather than altering the position of the infant.

When a small infant is suffering from dyspnoea due to respiratory difficulty, or cardiac failure, or persistent vomiting due to hiatus hernia, he may be strapped securely in the upright position in a Safe Sitter chair (Mothercare) (FIG. 5).

Inhalation of vomitus is avoided by nursing the small infant on alternate sides, and ensuring that he breaks wind before being returned to his cot after feeding. Under no circumstances should an infant be allowed to feed himself from a bottle propped up in his cot. This is a potentially lethal practice in the early weeks of life, and deprives the infant of physical contact with his mother.

3 BURNS

Hot-water bottles must be used with great caution. They should preferably be removed from the cot before the infant is tucked in. Where their constant use is recommended, a canvas lining to the cot allows hot-water bottles to be placed in the pockets.

After two-thirds filling with hot water, the screw should be firmly secured and the bottle protected in a thick cover. It is then placed in the pocket with the open end away from the infant. If a cot lining is not available, at least two thick layers of blanket are necessary to prevent the hot water bottle from burning the infant.

4 OTHER TRAUMA

Prolonged indiscriminate use of knitted mittens is not recommended. A fine strand of fibre has been known to cause constriction of the terminal phalanx, resulting in oedema, gangrene and even traumatic amputation.

Cleanliness

Most authorities are now of the opinion that bathing of newborn infants is not necessary. 'Top and tail' procedure is adequate until the umbilical cord has separated, the infant's condition is satisfactory, and the environmental temperature is of a sufficiently high level to allow exposure. To prevent cross-infection where small infants are crowded together, communal baths and changing tables are not used. The infant is attended to in his cot, preferably by his own mother or on the knees of a gowned nurse.

Bathing an Infant

To avoid prolonged exposure of the infant, all requirements are put within easy reach of the nurse. The windows are closed and the area screened if there is a tendency to draughts. The room temperature should be at least 21°C or 70°F, otherwise the infant is best just 'top and tailed'.

REQUIREMENTS
Low nursing chair.
Bath or large bowl.
Bath thermometer.
Flannel, bath towel, bath blanket.
Cotton wool, receptacle of boiled or tap water.
Clinical rectal thermometer. Wool balls. Soft yellow paraffin.
Soap, talcum powder, cream, hair brush.
Napkin, gown (vest), jacket.
Receptacle for soiled swabs.
Receptacle for napkin.
Receptacle for infant's personal clothes.

METHOD
The bath water is prepared to a temperature of 40°C (104°F) and the bath thermometer removed.

Before touching the infant or his bedclothes, the nurse washes and dries her hands and puts on the barrier gown. The infant's pulse and respiration rates are counted before he is disturbed. Waterproof protection for the nurse's uniform is necessary. Cotton barrier gowns are not waterproof, and contamination of the nurse's dress could lead to cross-infection. If the infant is nursed on a waterproof square, this is placed under the buttocks on the nurse's knees. The infant's clothing is removed, with the exception of the napkin, and he is securely wrapped in the bath blanket.

Several cotton wool balls are moistened in the receptacle of water and the face and ears are washed and dried, and the swabs discarded. Individual swabs may be used for the eye-lids of small infants or for those with a little discharge—each one being used once only to cleanse the lids from within, outwards. If the nostrils contain dried secretions, the infant may be encouraged to sneeze by stimulating the anterior nares with a wisp of cotton wool. If this method fails to clear the nostrils, small moistened cotton wool pledgets can be used with care.

Supporting the infant's head over the bath, the hair is wetted, washed with a small amount of soap and thoroughly rinsed before drying. The pulsating fontanelle of a small infant often causes unnecessary anxiety to the young mother, who may avoid touching the area. Gentle application of warm olive oil the night before will soften resistant scurf, allowing removal the following day.

The napkin is removed and the buttocks cleansed with the clean corners of the napkin. The rectal temperature is recorded at this stage, if necessary. With well-soaped hands, the infant is washed, commencing at the neck and progressing to both axillae, arms and hands. After soaping the trunk and groins, the nurse slips her hands beneath the infant's trunk and rolls him towards herself into the prone position. The back, legs and buttocks are then soaped. The soap is removed from the bath water and the nurse rinses her hands. The now slippery infant is gently lowered into the bath water, his left arm held in the nurse's left hand. The infant's head and shoulders are thus supported by the nurse's left forearm. The under aspect of the infant's left thigh is grasped by the nurse's right hand (FIG. 6). Once safely in the water, the nurse can free her right hand for rinsing the soap from all areas. If the atmosphere is warm and the infant enjoys his bath, he should be given opportunity to exercise his legs in the water.

Grasping the distal arm and leg as before, the infant is lifted out of the bath on to the bath towel and dabbed dry, working from the neck downwards, avoiding unnecessary exposure. Particular attention is paid to skin creases, i.e. under the chin, axillae, groins, natal cleft and between fingers and toes. When thoroughly dry, talcum powder is applied to the trunk and barrier cream is applied to the napkin area. The napkin is secured in position and the infant dressed. The hair is brushed, the nails inspected and trimmed with small scissors, and the infant returned to his warm cot.

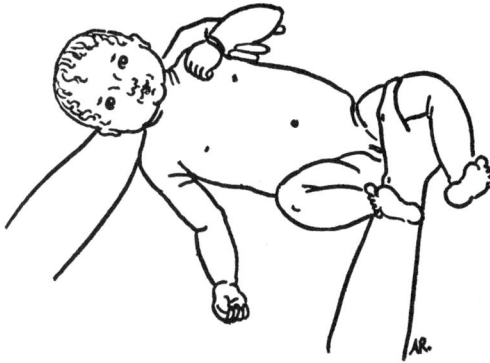

FIG. 6. Lowering an infant into the bath.

The equipment is returned to the infant's locker, and the bath or bowl is cleaned. The nurse washes and dries her hands, removes her gown and leaves the cubicle to record any necessary observations. The soiled napkins, swabs and linen are removed from the area in the accepted routine.

'Top and Tail' Procedure

This can be carried out with the infant remaining in his cot or incubator, or on the nurse's knees. The procedure is carried out twice a day unless substituted for a daily bath.

Requirements for the procedure are as for bathing an infant, with a small bowl substituted for the infant's bath.

METHOD

The infant's clothing is removed, with the exception of the napkin and vest, and the infant is protected in the bath blanket.

Using cotton wool moistened in warm tap water, the face and ears are washed and dried with dry wool. Care is taken to see that the skin folds under the chin are washed and thoroughly dried. The axillae are inspected. The napkin is removed, the bath towel placed under the infant's buttocks, and the area thoroughly cleansed with soap and water, rinsed well and dried. A fine sprinkling of talcum powder or barrier cream may be applied to the area and a clean napkin is applied and the infant dressed. Unless adequately washed, rinsed and dried, the skin creases may become red and infected. This is particularly so when the infant has been allowed to become overheated in the humid atmosphere of an incubator. Clothing of an infant nursed in a cot should be light, but adequate, to prevent this sweat rash developing. Vernix may be removed from the body creases by gentle massage with soaped finger tips.

Bootees, mittens and elbow restraint if worn, should be removed at this time and the toes and fingers inspected and exercised. An enclosed extremity requires washing and drying at least once daily.

Excretion

The newborn infant must be carefully observed for evidence of satisfactory excretory functioning.

Urine is frequently passed at the time of delivery, and if not, the napkin must be checked at four hourly intervals. Small quantities of urine are passed at frequent intervals, with dry periods between. Red 'cayenne pepper' deposits, due to the presence of uric acid crystals, may be seen in the wet napkin during the first few days of life. Once distinguished from blood, there is no cause for alarm.

The thick, green, tenacious first stool of the newborn (meconium) should be passed within the first twenty-four hours or so of life. The examining finger, or rectal thermometer, will usually provoke a bowel action. A thin smear of Vaseline previously spread over the buttocks, and prompt attention, will facilitate easy cleansing following passage of meconium. A disposable lining to the napkin will reduce laundering effort. (For description of stools during infancy, see page 151).

FOLDING AND APPLICATION OF NAPKINS

Where disposable napkins are in use, their application is easy, allowing for little variation.

Soft Harrington squares are ideal for the small infant, whose skin is delicate and may reject the more harsh Turkish towelling napkin. If lined with a soft disposable nappy-liner, or silicone-impregnated (therefore, water-repellent) napkin, direct contact of the towelling napkin with the infant's skin is prevented. *The Triangular Method.* This method is suitable for small infants. The napkin, folded cornerwise, is placed under the infant's buttocks and a single fold (1) is brought well up between the infant's legs (FIG. 7). Corners (2) and (3) are then brought, one at a time, between the infant's legs and tucked under the opposite buttock. Corner (4) is then brought between the legs and the napkin secured with one safety-pin inserted horizontally. In this way, the napkin is used to best advantage. When soiled, corners (2), (3) and (4) can be used to remove excessive faecal matter, thus avoiding extravagant use of cotton wool.

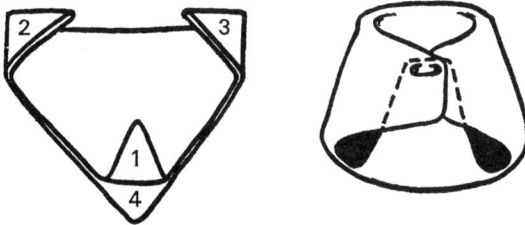

FIG. 7. Triangular method of folding napkins.

The Pilch Method. The square napkin is folded as in FIG. 8 and the broad end placed under the infant's buttocks. (A) and (B) are brought over the infant's abdomen and the narrow portion (C) is brought between the infant's legs. Two safety-pins are used to secure the napkin in position. This method is suitable for infants of all ages, but particularly for the more active, larger infant.

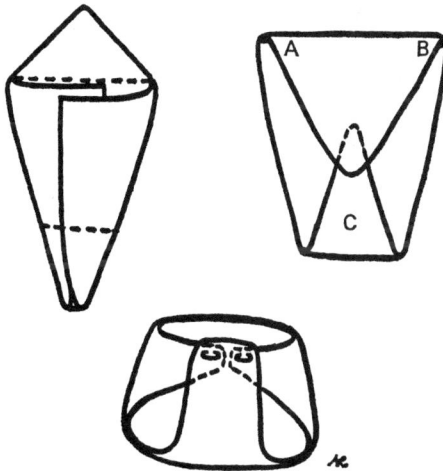

FIG. 8. Pilch method of folding napkins.

Changing Soiled Napkins. On removing a wet or soiled napkin, it should be immediately placed in a suitable covered receptacle to be subsequently washed, or dispatched to the laundry, or to be incinerated if disposable. The hands should be thoroughly washed and dried before attempting another procedure.

Some Minor Deviations from the Normal

In Relation to the Head

Over-riding of the skull bones in the moulding process necessary for passage of the head through the birth canal gives the newborn infant's head a characteristic shape. There is considerable variation in the size of the anterior fontanelle which can be seen and felt to pulsate. Depression is suggestive of dehydration, while an increased intracranial pressure increases the tension of the fontanelle. Superficial oedema of the presenting part—a caput succedaneum—is caused by temporary local congestion of the venous return and disappears as the head adopts a normal shape within the first few days of life. Another less common swelling (or swellings) due to subperiosteal haemorrhage—a cephalhaematoma— may occur soon after birth and may take up to one year for the blood to be reabsorbed. This swelling is confined by the sutures of the skull.

In Relation to the Skin

The infant's skin is delicate and readily becomes excoriated by urine, faeces, vomit and mucus. A smear of Vaseline on the dependent cheek and immediate removal of a damp sheet will prevent mucus excoriation of the face in the first hours of life. Peeling (exfoliation) of the extremities is common in the first week of life, while postmature and other infants starved in utero tend towards more extensive peeling.

Innumerable whitish-yellow pinhead-sized spots on and surrounding the nose disappear within the first two weeks of life. These milia, as they are called, are due to obstructed sebaceous glands. 'Stork marks' seen as faint mauve staining on the forehead above the nose and suboccipital region usually fade within the first few months of life, but the suboccipital staining, conveniently covered by hair, may persist throughout life.

Skin rashes are common. Wool often produces irritating, blotchy, red (erythematous) patches, particularly if the infant is overheated. Calamine lotion applied locally and use of a cotton vest will help the infant to become less irritable. A sweat rash, seen as pin-point cream spots in the reddened skin folds of an overheated small infant, is liable to monilial infection. Meticulous care with cleanliness in washing, drying and powdering, and clothing the infant according to the environmental temperature will prevent as well as treat this minor disorder.

Sore Buttocks

With careful consideration of the following points, sore buttocks can often be prevented:

1 Napkin changed when wet or soiled,
2 Area washed and dried at every changing.
3 Cream protection of sensitive skin.
4 Use of soft, laundered napkins—soap powders (not detergents) used and napkins thoroughly rinsed and dried slowly.
5 Plastic pants used only for special occasions.

The cause of sore buttocks is often suggested by the typical distribution of erythema.

AMMONIACAL DERMATITIS

This is not common in the first few weeks of life, but presents later as painful erythema leading to excoriation and ulceration over the napkin area, due to liberation of ammonia from the bacterial decomposition of urea. The skin creases are not affected.

The condition is prevented by maintaining a high standard of napkin care (see above) and treated in addition as follows:
1 Napkins boiled, or disposable variety used.
2 Extra fluids given to avoid concentration of urine.
3 Zinc and castor oil with benzoin cream applied to area.
4 Exposing the buttocks to a warm atmosphere.

PERIANAL EXCORIATION

Frequent loose, frothy, acid stools cause the anal area to become excoriated. Frequent changing is necessary and the cause treated. Often this is due to a misunderstanding regarding feeding—too much sugar or too high a concentration of feed being given.

Exposure of the buttocks and protection of the perianal region with white of egg or silicone cream will allow the area to heal more rapidly.

EXPOSURE OF THE BUTTOCKS

Air and heat allow the skin of the buttocks to heal more readily. Exposing the buttocks to the air is quite safe in the home environment, but in a paediatric unit the safety of the other infants must be considered. Cross air-currents could cause the spread of a gastro-intestinal infection unless suitable precautions are taken.

Ideally, the infant free from gastro-intestinal infection should be in a warm, single cubicle, ventilated to the exterior. He is secured in the lateral position by clove hitch restraint to his legs, if necessary, and kept warm by use of bootees and adequate protection of the rest of the body. A small bed-cradle may be placed over a small infant to prevent chilling while allowing free circulation of air around the buttocks.

Sunlight may be used, but it is usually more practical to expose the buttocks for fifteen to twenty minutes at four hourly intervals to the warmth radiated from a 40 Watt electric light bulb placed along-side the buttocks at a distance of at least 30cm (12 inches). This treatment requires care and discretion in use and the infant should not be left unattended. The anglepoise lamp is not placed directly above the infant in case the hot bulb should fall on the infant's skin. Similarly, the warm air discharged from a hair-drier, held at a suitable distance to avoid discomfort or burning, can be used effectively for five to ten minutes every four hours.

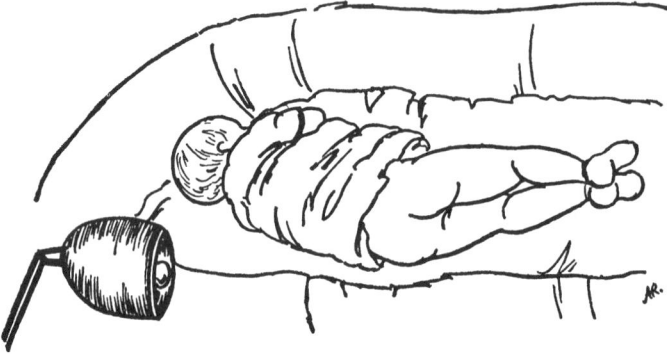

FIG. 9. Exposure of sore buttocks. Note, the anglepoise lamp is placed at least 30 cm along-side and not directly above the infant's buttocks.

Dehydration Fever

If the fluid intake is inadequate, or loss excessive, larger infants may become pyrexial on the third and fourth days of life. This is prevented and remedied by offering an increased fluid intake and avoiding overheating.

Physiological Jaundice

Almost half of all full term infants develop jaundice on the second or third days of life. This physiological jaundice is due to the breakdown of excess red blood cells no longer required by the infant and to inadequacy of the glucuronyl transferase enzyme system of the liver to conjugate the bilirubin for excretion (page 395). The infant becomes drowsy and reluctant to feed. Extra fluids are necessary to avoid haemoconcentration, an increase in the serum bilirubin level (hyperbilirubinaemia) and bile-staining of the basal ganglia (kernicterus). The jaundice usually fades by the end of the first week with no further treatment. Jaundice persisting beyond this time requires further investigation.

Pseudomenstruation

The mucus discharged per vaginum during the first three to four days of life may be blood-stained and is sometimes referred to as pseudomenstruation. This is normally due to withdrawal of circulating maternal oestrogens from the infant's circulation.

Engorgement of the Breasts

For the same reason as above, engorgement of the breasts of either sex may occur within the first week of life. To prevent mastitis, expression of 'witch's milk' is discouraged.

Infant Baptism

When admitting an infant to hospital, it is usual to obtain the parents' wish regarding baptism, and to fulfil the request should their child's life be in danger. When the need is urgent in the absence of the hospital chaplain, holy baptism must be administered reverently and in all sincerity by a Christian member of the nursing staff.

METHOD

A container of warm water and a small towel are placed on a clean white cloth covering a small clear surface.

If the infant is too sick he must remain in his cot, otherwise he is cradled in the nurse's left arm. The head is sprinkled with water three times as the nurse says the words ' . . . (Name) I baptise you in the Name of the Father, and of the Son, and of the Holy Spirit. Amen.' Afterwards, she should make the sign of the cross on the infant's forehead and then say the short prayer: 'The Lord bless you and keep you, the Lord make His face to shine upon you and give you peace, today, and for evermore. Amen'.

The infant's name should then be entered in the register of baptisms and a certificate of baptism given to his parents. The appropriate chaplain should be informed.

For Further Reading

CRAIG W. S. (1970). *Care of the Newly Born Infant*, 4th edition. E. & S. Livingstone, Edinburgh.

ILLINGWORTH R. S. (1968). *Babies and Young Children: feeding, management and care*, 8th edition. J. & A. Churchill, London.

CHAPTER FOUR

Principles of Infant Feeding

Breast Feeding

The composition of breast milk is ideal to meet the needs of the average healthy infant. There are still many advantages of breast feeding but, as the hazards of artificial feeding have been minimized, more women prefer to bottle feed their infants with one of the many modified cow's milk preparations available today.

No mother should be made to feel that she is depriving her infant of his birthright if she does not wish to, or succeed in breast feeding. It is essential that a mother is given every help and encouragement to fulfil this natural function if she so desires and to be given advice and guidance about artificial feeding when and if the need arises.

Advantages of Breast Feeding

The constant composition of breast milk is suited to the infant's needs and digestion. It is cheap to produce, delivered at the correct temperature and free from micro-organisms. The infant receives warmth, comfort and love at the breast which enhance the mother–infant relationship. Breast-fed infants have a greater resistance to infection during the first year of life—gastro-enteritis is rarely seen in breast-fed infants.

The mother, too, benefits from breast feeding. She experiences a gratifying sense of achievement that she has fulfilled her role as a mother. A feed during the night is simple, with little disturbance to the rest of the household. Contraction and involution of the uterus are encouraged by reflex action which results when her infant is feeding at the breast.

Any breast milk produced in excess of her own infant's needs may be collected, pasteurized, stored and distributed for the benefit of sick and small infants whose mothers have not been able to establish lactation in their absence. Breast milk banks are centred in a few large maternity hospitals and limited supplies of breast milk can be bought for feeding 'priority' infants. This is an expensive service but of great value to special care baby units and neonatal medical and surgical units.

Contra-Indications to Breast Feeding

If the infant is too immature, weak or ill to make the necessary effort to obtain milk from the breast, milk may be expressed and given to him by an easier method. Severe deformity of the lip, palate or lower jaw will make breast feeding impossible.

As far as the mother is concerned, she may suffer from general poor health due to chronic kidney or heart disease or diabetes mellitus. Nature does not often give her the opportunity to breast feed as lactation is rarely established in such cases. The infant is in danger if the mother suffers from tuberculosis, epilepsy or psychosis. The infant of the tuberculous mother must be separated from his mother for six weeks following B.C.G. vaccination. An epileptic mother may have a fit while breast feeding, and the life and health of the infant may be in danger if the mother is psychotic.

Local conditions of the breast, such as deformed nipples and breast infections, contra-indicate breast feeding. Failure of lactation in an otherwise healthy mother is rare, but when it does occur, artificial feeding is instituted.

Lactation may not be encouraged for social reasons. If the mother has the care of a very large family, her lactation may well fail on resuming her home duties. If the infant is born to an unmarried or working mother, or is to be adopted, then breast feeding is not usually encouraged.

Preparation for Breast Feeding

Preparation for this natural function starts in the antenatal period. The breasts enlarge in pregnancy, this being one of the very early signs of pregnancy. The breasts, and particularly the nipples, are examined early to ensure that everything possible is done to encourage successful breast feeding. The nipple must be erect for the infant to be able to withdraw milk, and Waller's shells may be worn inside an adequate supporting brassière during pregnancy to withdraw inverted or retracted nipples. Towards the end of pregnancy, the mother may be instructed how to express the colostrum, the first sweet viscid secretion produced by the breasts.

For the first two to three days following delivery, only colostrum is available in very small quantities. From the third day onwards, milk is produced, often in large amounts, causing painful engorgement of the breasts. Sympathetic care is required at this time to prevent unnecessary physical or psychological trauma which may completely discourage the mother from breast feeding.

Breast feeding may have to be established in a paediatric unit following a period of separation of a newborn infant from his mother. Depending on the cause for the separation, the mother may have been encouraged to establish lactation in the absence of her infant or she may have had her lactation suppressed. Naturally, establishment of lactation is discouraged when the survival of an ill infant is in grave doubt. Breast milk is cheap to produce but expensive to buy. It is an advantage if the mother is able to produce and express breast milk for her infant in the hope that lactation can be sustained until the infant is strong and well enough to feed at the breast. The suckling infant is the best stimulus for the production of milk and in his absence milk production may fail.

Management of Breast Feeding

Time and patience are essential for creating a satisfactory harmony between mother and infant. The hands and breasts are washed and dried well before starting the feed. The mother is encouraged to position herself comfortably on a low nursing chair and to cuddle her infant in the crook of one arm. For the first feed, it is advisable to wrap the infant so that arms and legs are secure until he is safely fixed at the breast. Free movement of arms and legs can then be encouraged.

Both breasts are offered at each feed, using each first at alternate feeds. To prevent the nipples becoming sore, the length of time at each breast is short in the early days, the time increasing to a maximum of ten minutes at each breast.

The infant draws the nipple to the back of his tongue so that the nipple and the areolar (the pigmented area around the nipple) are in his wide open mouth (Fig. 10). A vacuum is created, and the infant's gums compress the ampulla,

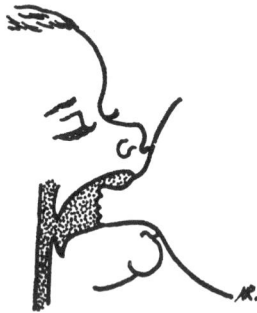

Fig. 10. Infant suckling at the breast.

pushing the milk forward. The tongue pushes the nipple against the hard palate, expelling the milk into his mouth. The infant should not be allowed to chew the nipple as this will cause the nipple to become sore. Expressing a small quantity of milk from the nipple may encourage the infant to fix securely at the breast.

It is necessary for the mother to retract the breast tissue from the infant's nostrils so that respiration is not impeded.

The majority of a feed is taken in the first few minutes at the breast. The infant should not be left too long at the breast or he will use it as a pacifier and swallow large quantities of air. After feeding at each breast, the infant is encouraged to break wind. To release the infant from the breast, gentle pressure is applied to the lower jaw, thus releasing the suction.

On completion of the breast feed, the mother should empty the breasts by manual expression or with the assistance of a hand or electric breast pump. Expressing the residual milk will help to encourage lactation. Manual expression is done by gently but rapidly squeezing behind the nipple between the thumb and the forefinger to compress the ampulla and expel the milk.

The mother must have plenty of rest and a good diet containing adequate protein, iron, calcium and vitamins. Additional fresh fruit and vegetables increase the vitamin C content of the breast milk. Her fluid intake should be increased according to her need. Smoking suppresses lactation and is therefore discouraged. Most drugs, including alcohol, find their way into breast milk and may affect the infant.

BREAKING WIND

All the air in an infant's stomach has been swallowed and is not the result of digestion. When feeding an infant, air swallowing should be minimal, and for the infant's comfort and the parent's rest, eructation should be encouraged. The infant is supported either over the protected shoulder or held with the back straight on the mother's knees. This allows the air bubble to rise to the cardia of the stomach for ready exit. Gentle massage of the infant's back in an upward direction may encourage eructation, but patting is unnecessary and to be avoided (FIG. 11).

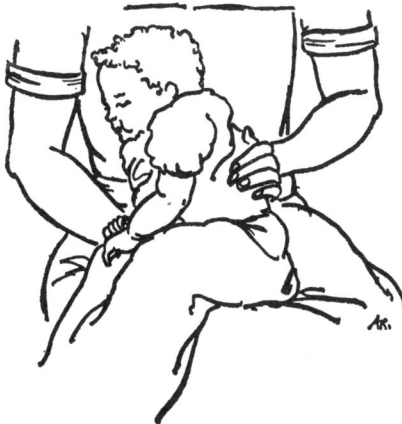

FIG. 11. Breaking wind.

This procedure is necessary half-way through the feed, or the stomach may become distended with wind and the infant reluctant to take the rest of his feed, and at the end of the feed before the infant is laid flat, to prevent the air passing into the intestine, causing colic.

UNDERFEEDING

Underfeeding is fairly common in breast-fed infants. If lactation is inadequate or the infant unable to obtain the milk from the breast, this may be shown by the infant's behaviour. To prevent underfeeding, the breast-fed infant should be weighed at weekly intervals. If underfeeding is suspected, the infant may be test-fed over a twenty-four hour period.

Signs of underfeeding:

1   The infant tends to be restless and to cry a lot. Not all underfed infants behave in this way, however. Some of the smaller infants may be well satisfied with the small amount of milk available to them and behave in a fairly normal manner.
2   The infant appears ravenous but fails to gain weight.
3   The stools are dark, sometimes green, infrequent and small (starvation stools).
4   The urine output is scanty.

TEST FEEDING

When the milk supply is good, the breast-fed infant takes varying quantities at each feed. To obtain an accurate estimate of his intake, the infant must be weighed before and after each feed during a twenty-four hour period. The fully-clothed infant is weighed before being fed at the breast and again, wearing the same clothes, at the end of the feed, i.e. without changing the napkin if it becomes wet or soiled. The difference between the two weights indicates the amount of milk obtained from the breast.

COMPLEMENTARY FEEDING

If underfeeding is suspected, the infant may be offered a small quantity of milk mixture immediately after his deficient breast feed. The amount of feed offered varies with the age of the infant, but should be sufficient to fulfil his need. When complementary feeds are offered to young infants, the milk mixture should not be too sweet and the hole in the teat not too large or the infant may prefer the bottle to a breast feed. Some authorities may prefer to offer complementary feeds using a cup and spoon. Complementary feeding is used as a temporary measure when lactation is inadequate. If the supply of breast milk does not improve, bottle feeding is usually introduced.

SUPPLEMENTARY FEEDING

If the mother of a breast-fed infant has to be separated from her infant at a feeding time, a feed of milk mixture may be offered to the infant. This is referred to as a supplementary feed.

OVERFEEDING

Overfeeding is characterized by crying and vomiting with loss of weight in an infant who has previously made a satisfactory weight gain. Overfeeding a healthy infant is rare, however, as most infants will discontinue sucking when sufficient feed has been taken to satisfy their need, or regurgitate any feed taken in excess.

Number of Feeds in Twenty-Four Hours

The healthy infant is offered his full fluid and energy requirement for the twenty-four hours in divided amounts during an eighteen hour, or so, period. As most parents know only too well, this does not guarantee an undisturbed night's sleep, particularly in the early days of life. Gradually, the infant fits into a more acceptable routine, sleeping for a longer period. Allowing an infant to cry during the night is of no benefit to the child or his parents. He should be offered an additional feed, as water will rarely pacify a hungry infant. This is not habit-forming in any way, and sooner or later the infant will sleep through the night.

Four hourly feeding is suitable for infants of 3·4kg (7½lb) or over; the twenty hour feed requirement being divided between five feeds.

Six feeds at three hourly intervals are preferable for smaller and ill infants.

At home, a mother is able to feed her infant as demanded by his need and not by the clock. This demand feeding may not fit into the household routine at first, but gradually an acceptable pattern is adopted. There is no place for demand feeding of ill or small infants.

Expected Weight Gain

An infant loses up to 10% of his birth weight during the first twenty-four hours or so of life which is regained ten to fourteen days later. His average expected weight gain from this time is shown in the following table:

TABLE 6. Expected Weight Gain

Age in months	Weight gain per week in grammes	Weight gain per week in ounces
2 weeks–4	200	7
4–8	150	5
8–12	90	3

TO CALCULATE THE EXPECTED WEIGHT OF AN INFANT

INFORMATION REQUIRED:

1 The age of the infant.

2 His birth weight.

3 Knowledge of expected weight gain.

4 Remember that the infant does not regain his birth weight until the age of ten to fourteen days.

5 A knowledge of imperial and metric equivalents may be necessary until such time as the metric system is used exclusively (Appendix 1).

Example 1. (Using kilogrammes and grammes)

Infant's age	8 weeks
Infant's birth weight	3400g (3·4kg)
200g gain per week for (8 − 2) weeks	
= 200g × 6 = 1200g	1200g
Therefore, expected weight of infant =	4600g (4·6kg)

Example 2. (Using pounds and ounces)

Infant's age	8 weeks
Infant's birth weight	7lb 4oz
7 oz gain per week for (8 − 2) weeks	
= 7oz × 6 = 42oz	2lb 10oz
Therefore, expected weight of infant =	9lb 14oz

Fluid and Energy Requirements

To maintain a satisfactory weight gain, the average healthy full-term infant requires approximately:

150ml
110kcal* } per kilogram of expected body weight per day.

2½oz
50kcal* } per pound of expected body weight per day.

It is reasonable to estimate the feed requirement of a healthy infant by calculating his fluid and energy requirement according to his actual weight, but it is imperative that sick and underweight infants are fed according to their expected body weight.

On the first day of life, the infant requires 1/7 of this requirement; on the second day 2/7, and so on, until by the end of the first week the infant's full requirement is met.

Breast milk, cow's milk and most reconstituted modified cow's milk preparations used in infant feeding produce approximately:

* A kilocalorie (kcal) is the amount of heat necessary to raise the temperature of 1kg of water through 1°C.

65–70kcal/100ml

20kcal/oz

The infant's energy requirement is, therefore, fulfilled if the feed is calculated in terms of fluid requirement.

Feed Requirements (Using Examples 1 and 2 above)

Example 1.

Infant's age	8 weeks
Birth weight	3400g (3·4kg)
Expected weight	4600g (4·6kg)
Feed requirement =	150ml/kg/day
	110kcal/kg/day

Therefore, $150 \times 4·6 =$ ml fluid required in 24 hours

$= 690$ml fluid required in 24 hours.

Infant would be offered 5 feeds, each of 140ml, i.e. 140ml, 4 hourly for 5 feeds. *For quick calculation:* If the infant is to receive 5 feeds a day, the number of millilitres to be given at each feed is the weight in kilogrammes multiplied by 30, i.e. our infant weighing 4·6kg. requires $4·6 \times 30 = 138$ml per feed.

Example 2.

Infant's age	8 weeks
Birth weight	7lb 4oz
Expected weight	9lb 14oz
Feed requirement =	$2\frac{1}{2}$oz/lb/day
	50kcal/lb/day

Therefore, $2\frac{1}{2} \times 10 =$ oz fluid required in 24 hours

$= \frac{5}{2} \times 10 = 25$oz fluid required in 24 hours

Infant would be offered 5 feeds each of 5 oz, i.e. 5 oz, 4 hourly for 5 feeds. *For quick calculation:* If the infant is to receive 5 feeds a day, the number of ounces to be given at each feed is half the infant's weight in pounds, i.e. our infant weighing 10lb therefore requires $10 \div 2$oz $= 5$oz per feed.

Artificial Feeding

Milk can be a dangerous medium where micro-organisms will thrive and multiply. Although modified cow's milk preparations used for artificial feeding have improved in content and bacteriological safety, more intelligence on the part of the mother is required to bottle feed an infant. Scrupulous cleanliness in preparation and in feeding is essential to ensure that the milk or the utensils do not become contaminated.

There is no perfect substitute for breast milk but many efforts have been made to simulate its content. Most of the proprietary feeds available have been derived from cow's milk and are suitable for healthy infants. Special milk substitutes are available for those infants who are unable to tolerate cow's milk, e.g. Velactin, Minafen, Allergilac, Galactomin, etc.

Most infants will thrive on all the common brands of modified cow's milk preparations available as long as the fluid and energy requirements of the infant are met. The choice of feed for a healthy infant is a matter of personal preference, availability and advice. Most maternity hospitals and paediatric units have a standard feed which is given to all artificially-fed infants, unless contra-indicated. A more expensive feed is not necessarily superior, as is often believed by mothers who naturally want to give their infants only the best.

Differences in the Content of Human and Cow's Milk

1 *Protein.* Lactalbumen is the main protein found in breast milk and is readily digestible. There is six times more caseinogen in cow's milk than in human milk. It is not readily digested by the human stomach where it forms large, indigestible curds. Allergy to caseinogen may be seen in artificially-fed infants.

2 *Fat.* Although the fat content of the two milks is similar in quantity, the quality is quite different. The fat in breast milk is split into small globules forming an easily digested emulsion. The fat in cow's milk is in the form of large fat globules which are indigestible to young infants. Half cream feeds are often recommended for small and sick infants for this reason.

3 *Sugar.* The sugar (lactose) content of cow's milk is deficient.

4 *Mineral salts.* The phosphorus content of cow's milk is several times greater than in breast milk and may account for the increasing number of young artificially-fed infants suffering from neonatal tetany. The iron content of both milks is low, but is slightly higher in breast milk.

5 *Vitamins.* The vitamin D content of breast milk is higher than in cow's milk.

TABLE 7. Percentage Composition of Human Milk Compared with Cow's
Milk (i.e. per 100ml)

(Figures in brackets indicate approximations)

Human Milk		Cow's milk
1·5 (2)	Protein	3·5 (4)
3·5 (4)	Fat	4·4 (4)
7·0 (6)	Carbohydrate	4·5 (4)
0·2	Mineral Salts	0·75
0·1	Iron	0·04
0·4–10·0 I.U.	Vitamin D	0·3–4·4 I.U.
85·0	Water	85·0
65/100ml	Kilocalories	65/100ml
(20/oz)		(20/oz)

Choice of Milk for Artificial Feeding

1   Reconstituted dried milk—full cream, half cream.
2   Evaporated milk—full cream, half cream.
3   Suitably diluted fresh cow's milk.
4   Special feeds to meet specific needs (see Chapter 10).

DRIED MILK PREPARATIONS
Modified dried milk powders are available as full and half cream preparations. They are processed in such a way that the protein is made more digestible and the powder is rendered free from micro-organisms, unless subsequently contaminated. Most dried milk preparations are dried to 12·5% (1/8) of their volume and fortified with vitamins and iron. 100ml of fresh milk, therefore, becomes 12·5g and 1oz, 1 drachm.
For reconstitution:
    12·5g of milk powder + 100ml boiled water = 100ml milk
    1 drachm (scoop) milk powder + 1oz boiled water = 1oz milk.
When reconstituted 1:8, i.e. 12·5g to 100ml or 1 scoop to 1oz:
    100ml of Full Cream Milk Mixture produces approximately 63kcal
    and 1oz of Full Cream Milk Mixture produces approximately 18·9kcal
    100ml of Half Cream Milk Mixture produces approximately 56kcal
    and 1oz of Half Cream Milk Mixture produces approximately 16·8kcal.
To increase the energy value of some milk mixtures to 70kcal/100ml (20kcal/oz) it is necessary to add sugar. The sugar content of an unfamiliar feed should always be checked before adding more. Too much sugar in the feed will cause abdominal colic and passage of frothy, acid, loose stools. Cane sugar is used unless the infant has a tendency to be constipated when demerara sugar may be substituted.

When the carbohydrate content of the feed is low, sugar is usually added in the following proportions:

    Full Cream—1 part sugar to 6 parts dried milk, i.e. 4g (1 teaspoon) per
        180ml (6oz) of feed.
    Half Cream—1 part sugar to 4 parts dried milk, i.e. 4g (1 teaspoon) per
        120ml (4oz) of feed.

Example: To make up a 180ml feed using Full Cream National Dried Milk:
As full cream milk mixtures are rich, and may not be tolerated as 12·5% or 1:8 mixtures, it is usual to prepare a 10% solution, or omit one scoop from each feed. The infant's energy need will be met in cereals.

Milk powder	18g	95kcal	5 scoops
Sugar	4g	16kcal	1 teaspoon
Boiled water	180ml	—	6oz
	180ml	111kcal	6oz

Example: To make up a 120ml (4oz) feed using Half Cream National Dried Milk

Milk powder	15g	72kcal	4 scoops
Sugar	4g	16kcal	1 teaspoon
Boiled water	120ml	—	4oz
	120ml	88kcal	4oz

EVAPORATED MILK

If a mother wishes to use evaporated milk, a refrigerator is an essential piece of equipment. Evaporated milk has had approximately 60% of its water removed and is reconstituted by adding water in a 1:3 or 1:2 ratio. Sugar is added in the same proportions as for full and half cream dried milk preparations respectively. For reconstitution, it is advisable to refer to the dilution formula given on the tin

Example: To make up 180ml (6oz) of Full Cream Evaporated Milk

Evaporated Milk	60ml	100kcal	2oz
Sugar	4g	16kcal	1 teaspoon
Boiled water	120ml	—	4oz
	180ml	116kcal	6oz

COW'S MILK

Liquid cow's milk is not a popular choice of milk for artificial feeding of a small infant in this country. After the age of four to six months, milk may be given whole after boiling, but dilution is necessary in the first months of life. Dried milk preparations have many advantages over the use of liquid cow's milk.

To use liquid cow's milk for feeding to young infants:

1   The fresh milk is diluted 2:1 or 3:1 with water to dilute the protein and mineral salts.
2   4g (1 teaspoon) of sugar producing 16 kcal is added to each 120ml (4oz) of feed to increase the carbohydrate content and energy value of the feed.
3   The mixture is brought to the boil to make it bacteriologically safe and to denature the protein. Browning of the feed can be avoided by adding the sugar after boiling.

Example: To make up 120ml (4oz) feed:

Cow's milk	90ml	60kcal	3oz
Sugar	4g	16kcal	1 teaspoon
Water (boiled)	30ml	—	1oz
	120ml	76kcal	4oz

SPECIAL MILK MIXTURES

When an infant is unable to tolerate milk feeds, special feeds are prescribed by the doctor, most of which are available on prescription—E.C.10. Most are reconstituted as a 12·5% or 1:8 solution as for other dried milk preparations, but confirmation of the dilution will be found on the packing.

THICKENING FEEDS

Thickened feeds may be used to discourage vomiting when the possibility of an underlying cause has been excluded, and as a means of increasing the energy value of the feed. Nestagel and arrowroot are suitable for thickening milk feeds. Nestagel has no energy value; arrowroot produces 3·5kcal/g (100kcal/oz).

CLEAR FLUID FEEDS

To maintain hydration when milk feeds are not tolerated, a clear fluid of 5% sugar in N/5 saline, or just 5% sugar may be prescribed (page 177).
Example: To prepare 100ml of 5% sugar in N/5 saline:

Sugar	5g	20kcal	1 teaspoonful (slightly more than level)
Salt	0·18g	—	A pinch
Boiled water	100ml	—	100ml
	100ml	20kcal	100ml

Vitamin Supplements

An infant's requirement of vitamins A, D and C is not fully met by milk feeding. The healthy infant requires:

Vitamin A 2500 I.U.
Vitamin D 400–800 I.U. }daily
Vitamin C 30–50mg

Vitamin supplements are commenced four to six weeks after birth, and are given as concentrated multivitamin preparations. Hypervitaminosis must be avoided and the vitamin D content of fortified dried milk preparations taken into account when deciding on the amount of vitamin supplement to be given. Vitamin C may be given as diluted orange juice, rose hip syrup or blackcurrant juice.

All infants receiving synthetic milks such as Minafen, Velactin, Edosol, Galactomin, etc. need additional vitamin supplements. These are supplied by giving Ketovite syrup 5ml together with three Ketovite tablets daily.

Introduction to Mixed Feeding

A healthy infant is usually satisfied with milk feeding for the first three months or so of life, by which time he weighs about 5kg (11lb). The breast-fed infant is often satisfied for longer, and weaning may be delayed until he is four to five months old.

Introduction to mixed feeding is usually started with one of the available pre-cooked fortified cereals given at the morning and evening feeds. One teaspoonful mixed with a small quantity of the feed is offered to the infant on a small spoon. Gradually, the amount of cereal is increased to three teaspoonfuls at any one time and different varieties are introduced over a period of time. Cereal is essentially of carbohydrate content (1 teaspoonful producing 16kcal). Too much cereal will cause the infant to become overweight. Overweight infants should be offered the minimum amount of cereal and introduced to less fattening strained broth and vegetables at an early age.

When the infant has become accustomed to less liquid nourishment, small quantities of puréed meats and vegetables should be introduced at lunch-time. These may be prepared at home by reducing the family diet to a purée, or they may be purchased from the wide range of strained foods available to the busy mother. As the iron store of the infant reaches a very low level by the age of three months, the introduction of foods containing iron, such as meat, vegetables and egg yolk, should be made early.

The additions to his diet are gradually increased in amount and variety, with a corresponding decrease in milk requirement. As long as the infant receives one pint of milk daily, his additional fluid requirement may be given as orange juice. Feeding from a cup should be encouraged, but it may take many months before the infant is willing to part with his bottle at bed-time.

Once the infant starts teething, he will enjoy a hard rusk to chew. Gradually, mashed and minced foods replace the puréed foods so that he is encouraged to use his newly-erupted primary teeth. His vitamin supplements are continued to the age of two years.

By the age of nine months, the infant should be having three good meals a day with one pint of milk and his vitamin supplements. He is gradually encouraged to feed himself with a spoon and to drink from a cup, but will still appreciate a love and cuddle while he drinks from a bottle at bed-time.

Preparation of Feeds

When a home is without a refrigerator, each individual feed should be made up immediately prior to feeding time. This will reduce the risk of contamination and multiplication of micro-organisms.

In hospital, the feeds for each infant are usually prepared every twenty-four hours and stored in clearly labelled bottles in a refrigerator. With the introduction and increasing use of pre-packed feeds in disposable bottles and envelopes, mass preparation of infants' feeds by the hospital staff may well prove outmoded in the not too distant future.

Central Milk Kitchen

In units where large numbers of feeds are prepared daily, there is usually a specially designed central milk kitchen with its own staff trained for their responsible task. The milk kitchen should consist of two separate areas, a 'clean area' where the feeds are prepared and a 'dirty area' where the equipment used for the preparation of feeds, and the bottles returned from the wards, are washed and sterilized.

The used feeding bottles are rinsed on the wards and in some instances may be immersed in Milton 1:80 for $1\frac{1}{2}$ hours before being returned to the central area for thorough washing and sterilization. Unless a rigid routine is adopted, the central milk kitchen could be a source from which infection could be disseminated throughout the hospital, with catastrophic results.

The alternative to this method is for each ward to be responsible for the preparation of its own feeds. This is uneconomic in time and resources, and means that the nurse who is preparing the feeds may also be working with infants suffering from gastro-intestinal infections. However, if scrupulous attention is paid to personal hygiene and sterilization of equipment, this appears to be a satisfactory alternative.

Preparation of Equipment

All equipment used in the preparation and administration of feeds must be sterilized before use. Whichever method of sterilization is chosen—Milton 1:80 for $1\frac{1}{2}$ hours, or boiling for 5 minutes—the equipment must be washed and rinsed thoroughly before being completely immersed. Where large numbers of feeds are prepared, the equipment may be sterilized by autoclaving. In some maternity and paediatric units, the feeds are prepared and terminally sterilized in their bottles prior to refrigeration.

REQUIREMENTS
Bowl or basin.
Graduated jug (preferably Pyrex).
Whisk or fork.
Teaspoon.
Knife.
Granulated sugar.
Liquid or dried milk preparation.
Hot, boiled water.
Feeding bottle(s).
Funnel.
Weighing scales (if feeds for 24 hours are to be made).

METHOD

Scrupulous cleanliness must be observed in the preparation of the infant's feeds. The area used, whether it be the kitchen of a home, a ward kitchen or a specially designed central milk kitchen, should be well ventilated, free from dirt and dust, and contain a well illuminated, clean, smooth working surface. The people concerned in the preparation of feeds should wear masks, gowns and caps, and wash and dry their hands thoroughly before starting the preparation.

METHOD OF PREPARING FEEDS FOR TWENTY-FOUR HOURS

The feed formula is read carefully, and the dried milk powder and sugar carefully weighed and emptied into the bowl. Hot, boiled water is poured into the graduated jug to the required level. This is poured slowly over the milk powder while whisking to prevent the formation of lumps. The feed is strained if necessary and poured from the graduated jug into the feeding bottles with the help of a funnel. The bottles are then sealed with a valve or tin-foil cap, labelled with the infant's name or number, and placed into the refrigerator to promote rapid cooling. The feeds remain in the refrigerator until just before administration.

If terminal sterilization is used, the bottle is sealed with a tin-foil cap, with or without the teat, prior to the autoclaving process and refrigeration.

METHOD OF PREPARING ONE FEED

To prepare one feed, the appropriate number of level scoops of dried milk powder are measured, using the standard scoop and a knife. Sugar is added as required, and the hot, boiled water is added as above. The feed is poured into the bottle to the appropriate level and the teat put on to the bottle and covered with a sterile cover, e.g. a medicine measure, until required.

Feeding an Infant

REQUIREMENTS

Jug of hot water or electric feed-warmer containing feeding bottle.
Tray.
Teat (in Milton 1:80, or boiled).
Infant's bib, napkin and blanket.

METHOD

Whenever possible, an infant is taken out of his cot for feeding. If he is very uncomfortable with a wet or soiled napkin, this should be changed before the feed is taken to his cot side. If the infant has a tendency to vomit, then it is preferable to change his napkin before feeding to prevent undue disturbance when his stomach is full. The feed is placed on the infant's locker, the protective seal removed from the bottle, and the cover removed from the teat container.

The nurse then washes and dries her hands and before touching anything else, takes the teat from the container and attaches it to the feeding bottle. If the infant is barrier nursed, the nurse then puts on her gown before wrapping the infant in a light blanket. The nurse makes herself comfortable on a low nursing chair and cuddles the infant in the crook of one arm. The mouth is checked for evidence of thrush. If the mouth is sore, the infant will find sucking painful. The temperature of the feed is checked by inverting the feeding bottle over the visible veins of the wrist. The hole in the teat should be large enough to allow one drop of feed per second to fall. Too large a hole will cause the infant to choke and the teat should be discarded. Too small a hole results in overtiring the infant and large quantities of air being swallowed, causing subsequent abdominal discomfort. A small hole can be enlarged with a red hot needle. Any medicines are given from a 5ml spoon before the feed is commenced.

When the feed feels comfortably warm to the nurse's wrist, the teat is introduced into the infant's mouth, ensuring that it is on top of, and not underneath, the tongue. Small or lethargic infants have a tendency for the tongue to be 'sealed' to the roof of the mouth; the tongue is released by gentle pressure on the chin. It is unhygienic to place a finger in the infant's mouth, although the hands have been thoroughly washed. The bottle is held at an angle steep enough to prevent the infant sucking air (FIG. 12). The bottle may be held so that the

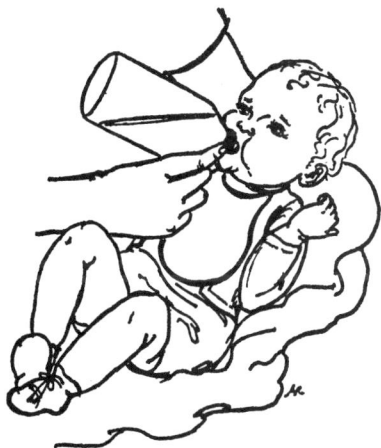

FIG. 12. 'Milk—not air'.

index finger, placed under the chin of a drowsy or small infant, can give any necessary reminder (FIG. 13). To prevent a vacuum replacing the milk, the bottle is gently twisted from time to time to allow air to enter the teat. An older infant will release the teat at frequent intervals for the same purpose.

At least once during the feed the remaining feed is kept warm while the infant is encouraged to break wind. At the end of the feed, the infant should give two good burps before being placed on his side in his cot. The whole feed should take no longer than fifteen to twenty minutes.

The bottle is rinsed with cold water and the teat throughly cleansed of milk, both inside and outside, before being boiled or returned to the container of Milton. The feed equipment is left aside while the infant's napkin is changed. After washing her hands, the nurse removes her barrier gown and washes and dries her hands again. She then records the amount and nature of the feed taken, and bladder and bowel functioning, in the appropriate columns on the infant's fluid balance chart.

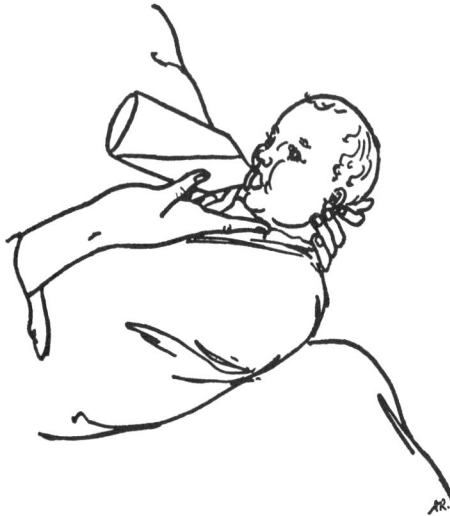

FIG. 13. An index finger, placed under the chin of a drowsy or small infant, can give any necessary reminder.

Some Feeding Difficulties

REFUSAL TO FEED

There are several reasons why an infant may be unwilling to take the feed he is being offered:

1   He may be too hot, too cold, uncomfortable with a wet or soiled napkin, wind or constipation, or just feel insecure in the arms of an inexperienced person. Air entry may be inadequate due to blocked nostrils. His mouth may be sore, making sucking a painful operation.

2   The feed may be too hot or too cold.

3   The teat may be too large for his small mouth, or the hole too large or too small.

4   Failure to feed may be the first indication that the infant is unwell.

VOMITING

Vomiting may range from excessive possetting at the end of a feed, to effortless or projectile expulsion of all or most of the feed. Vomiting in the first twenty-four hours of life is not uncommon. If the vomitus contains mucus or altered blood, then a gentle gastric washout is often effective treatment.

Swallowing an excessive amount of air results in vomiting on eructation at the end of a feed and abdominal colic. Underfeeding often results in a fretful infant who is unable to obtain his feed quickly enough and has a tendency to gulp large volumes of air while sucking his fingers or fist. An excessive amount of air is swallowed if the hole in the teat is too small or if the nostrils are blocked. Ephedrine $\frac{1}{2}\%$ in normal saline nasal drops prior to feeding may be prescribed by the doctor to relieve the latter situation. Excessive handling after feeding is sometimes the only cause for vomiting.

Pathological causes of vomiting are also seen in the early days of life and require the appropriate treatment once a diagnosis has been confirmed, e.g. intestinal obstruction, hiatus hernia, milk intolerance, infection, congenital hypertrophic pyloric stenosis and cerebral trauma.

COLIC

Intestinal colic is usually associated with excessive air swallowing or a faulty feeding formula or technique and is manifested as frequent intermittent flexion of the thighs over a distended abdomen soon after the feed has been given. Release of flatulence relieves the situation. Colic is prevented by treating the cause.

'Three months' colic' is a fairly common transient phenomenon, often occurring between the 18.00 and 20.00 hours feeds until the age of about three months. Its cause is as yet unknown, but not for the need for suggestions, and there is no treatment.

POSSETTING

Possetting is not vomiting, but regurgitation of a mouthful or so of feed. It is a common occurrence in the early weeks of life when encouraging an infant to break wind. It is a safety valve when the infant has taken too much feed, but may occur as the result of excessive handling immediately following a feed.

RUMINATION

Rumination is voluntary regurgitation and may become a habit in an overactive infant. The cumulative loss of feed will result in failure to progress, and the situation demands early recognition. The possibility of an organic lesion such as hiatus hernia or achalasia of the cardia is excluded, and the child is nursed in an upright position and treated with sedatives, alkalies and thickened feeds.

CHAPTER FIVE

The Low Birth Weight Infant

By international agreement, an infant weighing 2,500g (5½lb) or less at birth is called a premature infant regardless of the estimated period of gestation. 6–7% of all live births result in a low birth weight infant requiring special care and observation to detect early deviation from the normal and to ensure that preventable complications do not occur.

Low birth weight infants fall into two categories:

1 Those born before the fortieth week of gestation, therefore, truly premature by dates. This group includes the large but immature infants of diabetic mothers.

2 Those who are of abnormally low birth weight for the estimated gestational age—the 'small-for-dates' or dysmature infants.

Causes of Low Birth Weight

This may be due to premature labour or to malnutrition of the foetus, or a combination of both. Many factors are associated with both prematurity and dysmaturity, but in about 50% of cases, the cause is yet unknown. Predisposing causes include:

1 Socio-economic conditions, such as lower social class, poor housing, malnutrition, neglect of antenatal care, prolonged employment during pregnancy, smoking and illegitimacy.

2 Biological factors, such as race, small size of the mother, maternal age over forty years and birth order.

3 Chronic ill-health in the mother, such as heart or kidney disease, diabetes mellitus or hypertension.

4 Maternal complications of pregnancy, such as pre-eclampsia, antepartum haemorrhage, postmaturity resulting in placental insufficiency.

5 Maternal and foetal complications of pregnancy demanding termination of pregnancy before the fortieth week of gestation, e.g. severe pre-eclampsia, antepartum haemorrhage, Rhesus incompatibility.

6 Multiple pregnancy.

7 Congenital abnormalities.

TABLE 8.

Maturity	Length		Average birth Weight		Head Circumference	
	cm	in	g	lb	cm	in
28 weeks	35	14	1,020	2lb 4oz	25	10
32 weeks	40	16	1,590	3lb 8oz	29	11½
36 weeks	45	18	2,350	5lb 3oz	32	12¾
40 weeks	50	20	3,400	7lb 8oz	33–35·5	13–14

TABLE 9. Comparison between Mature, Premature and 'Small for Dates' (Dysmature) Infants

	Mature	Premature	Dysmature
Length			
cm	50	45 or less	Longer than weight
inches	20	18 or less	alone would suggest.
Weight			
kg	3·4 average	2·5 or less	2·5 or less
lb	(7½ average)	5½ or less	5½ or less
Head Circum-ference			
cm	33–35·5	33 or less	33–35·5
inches	13–14	13 or less	13–14
Skin	Pink and smooth. Some vernix. Subcutaneous fat present. Lanugo minimal. Nails hard and long.	Red and wrinkled. Vernix scanty. Minimal fat. Lanugo plentiful. Nails soft and short.	Pink. Evidence of weight loss. Exfoliation of skin creases.
Vitality	Strong and active. Wakes for feeds. Feeds well. Lusty cry. Normal temperature.	Drowsy and feeble. Readily tires. Mewing cry. Subnormal temperature.	Fairly alert. Often ravenous. Feeds hungrily. Feeble cry.
Genitalia			
female	Labia majora cover labia minora.	Labia minora exposed.	Labia minora usually covered.
male	Testicles in the scrotum.	Scrotum usually empty.	Testicles in the scrotum.

Estimation of Maturity

Many physical and neurological parameters are used for determining the maturity of low birth weight infants whose survival does not depend on the birth weight so much as the degree of maturity. The measurement of the length from vertex to heels rather than the weight of the infant is a more reliable means of estimating maturity. After the twenty-eighth week of gestation, when the infant is legally viable, he measures approximately $1\frac{1}{4} \times$ week of maturity in centimetres ($\frac{1}{2} \times$ week of maturity in inches) i.e. an infant of 32 weeks measures $1\frac{1}{4} \times 32 = 40$cm or $\frac{1}{2} \times 32 = 16$ inches.

Causes of Infant Mortality and Morbidity

The more immature the infant is, the greater is the risk of complications. An infant born before the thirty-second week of gestation has a fifty-fifty chance of surviving the hazards of birth and the first week of life.

80% of deaths associated with low birth weight infants occur in the first week of life—50% in the first twenty-four hours. The prime causes of death are, in order of frequency:

1   Atelectasis—primary and secondary—due to idiopathic respiratory distress syndrome, with or without hyaline membrane, account for more than half the deaths of low birth weight infants.
2   Congenital abnormalities.
3   Birth injury—traumatic or anoxaemic.
4   Infection.

Care and Observation of Low Birth Weight Infants

When social circumstances are good and the services of premature baby district nurses are available, the larger low birth weight infant free from complications may be very satisfactorily cared for at home. Home nursing has its advantages. A good mother–child relationship is established from the beginning, and the risk of infection with pathogenic micro-organisms is less. Economically, home nursing is cheaper.

The infant and his mother must be isolated in a room with a temperature maintained at a constant level of 21°C or 70°F, day and night. The mother must be educated in a high standard of personal hygiene and in the aseptic preparation of the infant's feeds. Coping with the infant's care will give her great satisfaction, but prove tiring in the early days.

Breathing difficulties, failure to establish feeding, jaundice and cyanotic attacks are indications that the infant requires the constant observation and care given by the skilled staff of a special care baby unit. The special care of low birth weight infants demands devotion to duty of skilled staff, practising good powers of constant observation and meticulous attention to nursing detail.

General Care

Infants weighing less than 1·8kg (4lb) are best nursed in an incubator. Following delivery, larger infants may be nursed in an incubator but transferred to a cot as soon as their condition is satisfactory. The activity of an infant in an incubator can be reduced by placing a piece of Gamgee over the infant's legs. Procedures are carried out gently, with minimal handling, to prevent physical exhaustion and loss of body heat. The infant is not bathed until he weighs about 2kg or 5lb. Twice daily 'top and tail' with boiled water is adequate. Hexachlorophane baby cream may be used to oil the infant's skin.

The infant is nursed on alternate sides. This position is maintained by placing a rolled napkin parallel with the infant's back. Change of position not only prevents the occurrence of pressure sores and allows expansion of both lungs, but facilitates symmetrical shaping of the soft skull bones. A small infant with respiratory distress may be nursed supine with his head turned to one side. The prone knee-chest position may also give some relief (FIG. 18).

As the infant progresses, he is gradually introduced to a cot in an environment of lower temperature in preparation for his discharge home. Nurseries of differing temperatures allow for this 'cooling off' process.

The staff of a special care baby unit are confronted with four main problems presented by their patients:
1 Their increased susceptibility to infection.
2 Their inability to control body temperature.
3 Respiratory difficulties requiring prevention, early detection and treatment.
4 Feeding difficulties.

Protection from Infection

The low birth weight infant is particularly prone to infection. Each infant should have his own requirements confined to the area around his cot or incubator, and only clean equipment free from pathogenic micro-organisms is taken into the cubicle. Unless infected, two to four low birth weight infants can be nursed in one cubicle. Contact with the adult population should be reduced to a minimum, but not at the exclusion of his mother and father. All personnel attending the infant must observe the rules of isolation nursing given in Chapter 8. Hand washing, the correct use of masks and gowns and absolute integrity with regard to personal hygiene are essentials.

To reduce the risk of infection, infants suffering from an infection or admitted to the unit from home or another hospital are isolated. The staff of the unit must be healthy and free from respiratory, skin and gastro-intestinal disorders. The nursing care of the infant is carried out in his cot or incubator or on the knees of a gowned nurse and not on a communal changing table or bath.

Maintenance of Body Temperature

The low birth weight infant with an immature temperature-regulating centre is unable to produce and conserve body heat, and so adopts a body temperature similar to that of his surrounding environment. This frequently results in chilling, which lessens his chances of survival. Similarly, overheating occurs when over-enthusiastic measures of warming are used.

COT NURSING

A low birth weight infant may be nursed in an open basin type cot in a warm, humid atmosphere. A constant room temperature of 21°–27°C or 70°–80°F is necessary for the smaller infant, with a cot temperature maintained at 29°–32°C or 85°–90°F. Humidity can be achieved by boiling a kettle or drying clean, wet linen in the warm room. Light, loose, warm clothing will ensure that respiratory movements are not impeded. Adequately protected hot-water bottles, preferably placed in the pockets of a canvas lining to the cot, require hourly attention in order to maintain a satisfactory cot temperature. Overheating is a real problem, and a wall thermometer placed between layers of light bedclothes should be read at hourly intervals.

USE OF AN INCUBATOR

Use of an incubator is a much more convenient means of observing a naked infant in a stable, warm, humid atmosphere, isolated from air-borne micro-organisms. The modern 'closed' incubator maintains a pre-set thermostatically controlled temperature with thermal convection, or fan-assisted circulation of moist, filtered air, thus ensuring a constant exchange of air with uniform distribution of heat. Fluctuations in temperature, humidity and oxygen content are reduced to a minimum by attending to the infant's needs through the sleeves or portholes.

Preparation for use. The foam mattress of the incubator tray is covered with a sheet and napkin and tucked under at the sides. Any linen hanging over the sides of the tray will prevent correct circulation of the air. The portholes or sleeves of the clean incubator are closed.

Before switching on at the mains, the humidity tank is filled to the appropriate level with sterile distilled water to prevent incubation of pathogenic micro-organisms and furring of the humidity tank, respectively. Humidification of the atmosphere assists in conservation of body heat and in keeping the respiratory passages moist. A relative humidity of 75–80% adequately fulfils the needs of most low birth weight infants. When a greater water saturation is required, a nebulizer attached to the more recent incubators gives super-saturation.

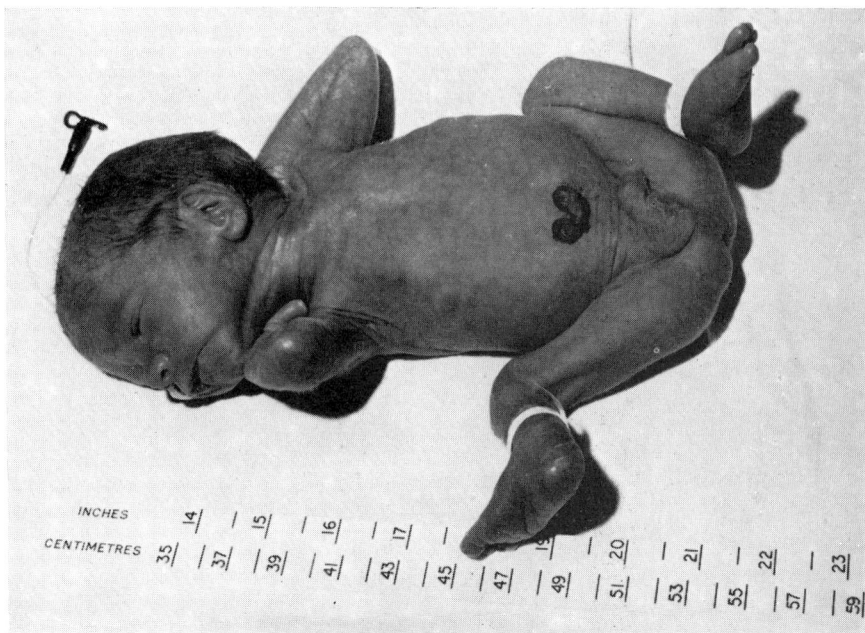

INCHES 14 15 16 17 19 20 21 22 23
CENTIMETRES 35 37 39 41 43 45 47 49 51 53 55 57 59

PLATE 1. Newly born infant of low birth weight.

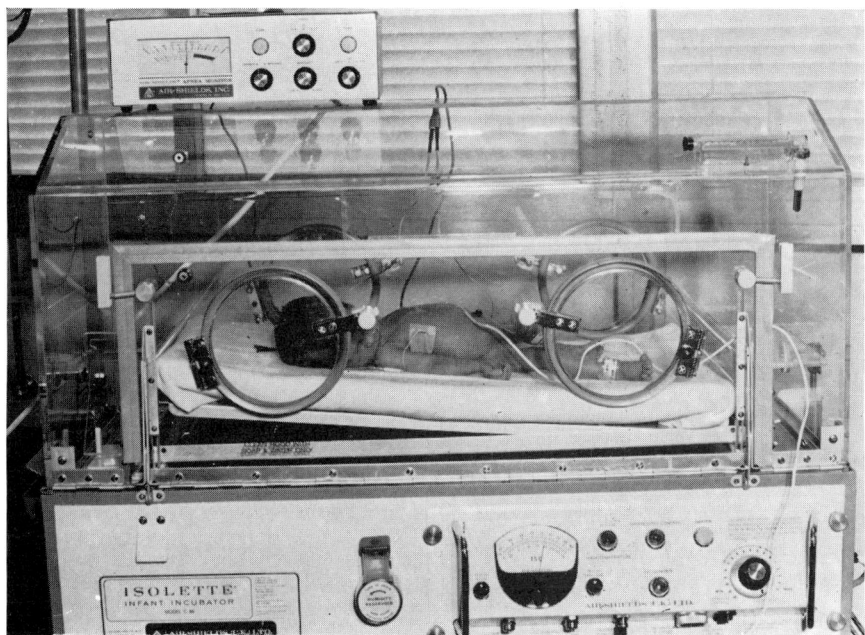

PLATE 2. Isolette Incubator in use (Air-Shields (U.K.) Ltd.)
A Servo temperature control panel is in use. The white lead connects the temperature sensitive thermister attached to the skin of the abdomen to the control panel. Leads from small skin electrodes firmly adhered to the chest wall are connected to an Air-Shields Apnoea Monitor.

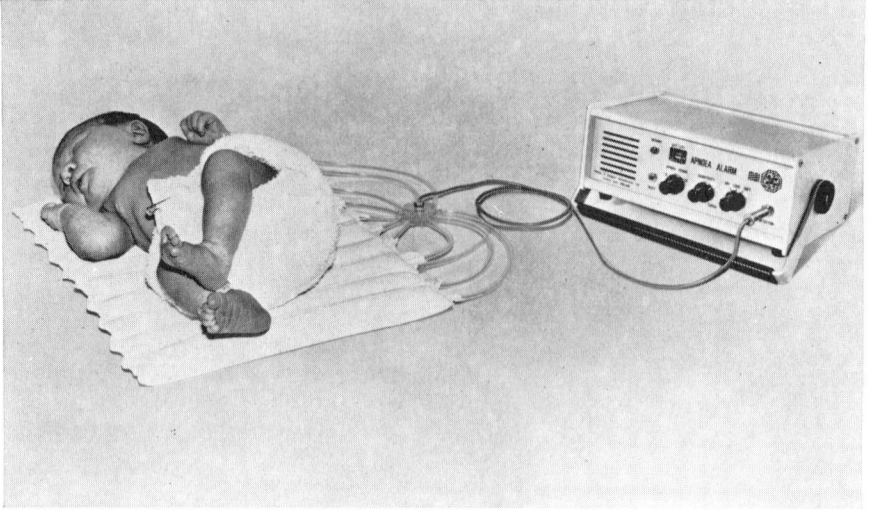

PLATE 3. The M.B.I. Apnoea Alarm Mark II
(Reproduced by kind permission of Medical and Biological Instrumentation Ltd.)

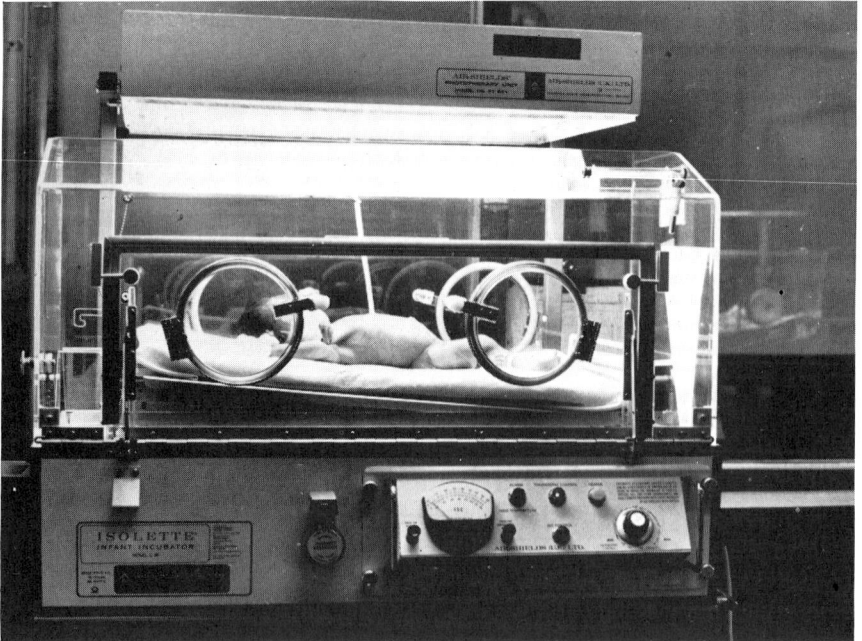

PLATE 4. Phototherapy used to control hyperbilirubinaemia.
Both eyes are completely occluded with gauze covered black paper or special goggles. The infant is wearing Tubegauz mittens.

The temperature of the incubator is pre-set at 32°C or 90°F for the reception of a low birth weight infant. The temperature of the incubator may have to be raised to 35°C or 95°F to maintain the infant's temperature between 35°C–36·6°C or 95°–98°F.

If oxygen is necessary, pressure tubing is attached to the oxygen supply and oxygen inlet nozzle. Unless the air filter is obstructed by the use of a red disc in the more modern incubators, the oxygen concentration will never exceed 35%. Additional oxygen may be administered for short periods by face mask or into an oxygen concentrator if ordered by the doctor in the treatment of cyanosis.

To avoid condensation inside an incubator, the temperature of the cubicle must be maintained above 21°C or 70°F. If the incubator is placed in direct sunlight or near to a hot radiator, overheating will occur, causing the warning bell to ring.

The welfare of an infant is safeguarded by a warning bell which operates for the reasons listed below. This does not, however, do away with the necessity for frequent supervision, as only extreme situations cause the bell to ring.

1   Failure of electricity supply due to:
    i   a power cut;
    ii   a blown fuse in the plug or incubator;
    iii   the wall plug pulled out at the socket;
    iv   the electricity turned off at the socket.
2   Overheating, i.e. temperature above 37°C or 99°F.
3   Failure of correct operation of the fan.
4   Each time the modern Oxygenaire incubator is switched on, the alarm bell rings. This can be rectified by re-setting the button.

Daily care of incubator. The humidity tank should be replenished and the inside and outside of an incubator cleaned with a damp disposable cloth daily. When the infant requires prolonged use of an incubator, this is changed for a clean one every seven days.

Terminal care of the incubator. When the incubator is no longer required, the electricity supply is switched off at the unit and at the mains and the humidity tank is drained. Detachable parts are removed and washed in hot, soapy water, rinsed, dried and placed on a clean surface. The floor of the incubator is thoroughly washed in the same manner and the unit reassembled. Exposure to fresh air and sunshine will facilitate adequate cleansing. The air filter is changed according to the manufacturer's instructions. If the infant has had an infection or occupied the incubator for a long time, the incubator is disinfected to minimize the risk of cross-infection. Swabs are taken for culture and sensitivity before and after disinfection. The manufacturer's instructions should be consulted when disinfection is desirable, as a method suitable for one type of unit could prove disastrous if used for another.

Servo temperature control. Use of a Servo temperature control panel attachment in the more modern incubators allows the very small or very ill infant to control the incubator thermostat, increasing or decreasing the heat so that his skin temperature corresponds to the pre-set temperature (PLATE 2). A temperature-sensitive thermister, or patient probe, is attached to the skin of the infant's abdomen with a length of adhesive tape. The lead is plugged into the control panel, the temperature control switched to Servo, and the dial set to the temperature required—usually 36·8°C or 98·4°F. The temperature recorded by the incubator thermometer is thus ignored.

COLD INJURY

Because of their relatively large surface area for heat loss and immaturity of the temperature-regulating system, newborn infants are liable to become chilled if exposed to low temperatures. The low birth weight infant and others with cerebral birth injury or sepsis are particularly vulnerable.

The affected infant becomes lethargic, reluctant to wake and to feed. His healthy appearance is very deceiving; his skin remains remarkably pink, yet cold and hard to the touch (sclerema). Pitting oedema often develops in the extremities. The rectal temperature may be as low as 26°C or 80°F. Initially, the pulse is rapid, but bradycardia occurs when the rectal temperature falls below 34°C or 90°F.

The hypothermic infant should be warmed up very slowly to enable the body to adjust to the rising temperature. The infant is best nursed in an incubator at a controlled temperature of 1·5°C or 2°F above his body temperature. The temperature is slowly increased over the next thirty-six hours. Rapid overheating increases the mortality rate and the nursing staff have a responsible task to ensure that this does not occur. With the use of Servo temperature control of the incubator this risk is minimized. Glucose fluids may be administered via an indwelling naso-gastric tube, but to avoid the risk of inhalation of regurgitated feed, glucose may be given intravenously. A broad spectrum antibiotic is usually prescribed to protect the infant against secondary bacterial infection.

Observation

Early recognition of complications to which low birth weight infants are prone demands frequent recordings of clinical observations (FIG. 14).

TEMPERATURE

To ensure that the infant's temperature remains within the normal range, 35·5°–36·6°C or 96°–98°F, the rectal temperature is recorded four hourly, using a low-reading thermometer. When Servo control is in use, the skin temperature of the infant is recorded hourly.

PULSE

The heart rate is best recorded by placing a warmed hand, or stethoscope, over the left side of the infant's chest and counting the apex beat for a full minute every hour.

RESPIRATION

Respiratory effort is essentially abdominal, varying in rate, depth and rhythm. Respiratory distress experienced by a high proportion of the smaller infants accounts for much of the mortality and morbidity of low birth weight infants. The irregular respiratory rate is counted for a full minute. A rate exceeding 65/minute is considered a sign that the infant is experiencing respiratory difficulty. The degree of respiratory distress can be evaluated by the use of the Silverman score (TABLE 10). The higher the score, the more severe degree of respiratory distress is present. As an incubator is comparatively soundproof, respiratory effort can only be heard through an open sleeve or porthole.

TABLE 10. Silverman Score.
(Evaluation and Rating of Respiratory Distress)

Score	Movement of Chest and Abdomen (A)	Intercostal Recession (B)	Xiphoid Retraction (C)	Movement of Chin (D)	Expiratory Grunt (E)
0	Rise together.	Absent.	Absent.	No descent of chin.	Absent.
1	Minimal lag.	Slight.	Slight.	Descent lips closed.	Occasionally heard.
2	Maximum lag.	Marked.	Marked.	Descent lips open.	Present with every expiration.

Periods of temporary apnoea are not uncommon in full-term newborn infants and may be prolonged in low birth weight infants, with the risk of cerebral anoxaemia. Monitoring devices are an asset in the detection of respiratory arrest.

MONITORING RESPIRATORY ACTIVITY

Apnoea Monitor (Air-Shields Ltd). This simple, reliable instrument provides both aural and visual alarms in the absence of respiration, and also records the respiratory rate. Two small skin electrodes are attached to the chest wall, one on either side just below each axilla. Care must be taken to see that they are firmly adhered to the skin, or false alarms will be recorded (PLATE 2).

Apnoea Alarm (M.B.I. Ltd). Like the apnoea monitor, this very simple piece of equipment provides aural alarm in the absence of respiration and also interprets respiratory movement by a series of clicks. The infant simply lies on a mattress which is rather like a miniature air-bed attached by a series of tubes to a single, highly sensitive electronic device. Care must be taken to see that the mattress is inflated to the manufacturer's recommended pressure, that the infant lies the length of the inflated mattress, and that the lead is connected, or false alarms will be recorded (PLATE 3).

On both devices, whenever a pre-set period of time has elapsed, i.e. 15, 20 or 30 seconds in which the infant does not breathe, the alarms are activated, summoning the attention of the ward staff. Continuous stimulation or back raising is usually sufficient to stimulate inspiration. Both pieces of equipment are expensive and delicate, and all staff should appreciate their value in the care of low birth weight and sick infants.

BEHAVIOUR

Normally, the low birth weight infant is quiet, responding to external stimulation by weak, purposeless, jerky movements, and an infrequent feeble cry. Excessive involuntary activity of the infant should be reported. A jittery, irritable infant could well be suffering from cerebral irritation, a low blood sugar level (hypoglycaemia) or a low blood calcium level (hypocalcaemia).

If there is history of a difficult delivery, cerebral irritation will be controlled with sedatives.

A Dextrostix estimation of blood sugar level is necessary in the presence of these signs (page 417). 'Small-for-dates' infants, and infants of diabetic mothers are particularly prone. These infants need regular four hourly estimations of the blood sugar level until their energy intake is adequate. The normal blood sugar level of a full-term infant in the first week of life is 50–70mg/100ml. Signs of hypoglycaemia are seen when the level is below 30mg/100ml. The normal range of blood sugar for low birth weight infants is 40–50mg/100ml, with signs of hypoglycaemia observed when the level falls below 20mg/100ml. The risk of preventable permanent brain damage is great, thus emphasizing the importance of early detection and prevention of hypoglycaemia.

Neonatal tetany due to hypocalcaemia is confirmed by estimation of the blood calcium level.

APPEARANCE

Colour. i Physiological jaundice usually develops after the first forty-eight hours of life, reaches its peak towards the end of the first week, then rapidly diminishes in intensity. Compared with the full-term infant, physiological jaundice is more pronounced and prolonged. The depth of jaundice can be roughly estimated by pressing a perspex icterometer against the infant's nose and comparing the colour of the skin with one of the yellow strips of different shades numbered 1–5. When the reading is more than 3, an accurate laboratory estimation of the serum bilirubin is essential. Serum bilirubin levels are estimated at daily or more frequent intervals until the level begins to subside.

ii Cyanosis is an ominous sign. If the airway is clear, it is usually a sign that gaseous exchange at lung level is inadequate to clear the blood of excess carbon dioxide, and oxygen is not getting to the vital structures. Administration of oxygen is dependent on the degree of cyanosis present. A more accurate means of confirming the infant's need for oxygen is for the arterial oxygen pressure (Po_2) to be estimated from a specimen of blood withdrawn from the cannulated umbilical artery.

iii Pallor may indicate blood loss. Vitamin Kl (Konakion) 0·5mg is routinely administered to low birth weight infants to prevent haemorrhage, due to a low prothrombin level (hypoprothrombinaemia). The cord, skin, and excreta should be observed for signs of bleeding.

Oedema, commonly seen at birth, usually resolves in the first forty-eight hours of life. General or localized oedema may occur later, due to a low serum protein (hypoproteinaemia) and/or salt retention.

Abdominal distension is common, especially following a feed, and may super-impose the already present respiratory difficulty. Abdominal distension accompanied by constipation requires immediate medical attention.

FLUID BALANCE

An accurate fluid balance record should be maintained. Small quantities of dilute urine are passed at frequent intervals. Passage of meconium is usually delayed, sometimes long enough to suggest an abnormality of the gastrointestinal tract.

INCUBATOR

The temperature (and humidity) and oxygen concentration of the incubator are recorded at hourly intervals. In the absence of cyanosis, oxygen is potentially dangerous. Blindness due to retrolental fibroplasia will not occur when oxygen is administered for the relief of cyanosis. The oxygen concentration is estimated by using a pyrogallic acid oxygen analyzer or a more modern electro-magnetic device. A 5ml specimen of gas drawn 7–10cm or 3–4 inches from the infant's face is injected into the pyrogallic acid. Alternatively, the aspirator bulb of an electro-magnetic oxygen analyzer is squeezed 4–5 times while the end of the sampling tube is held 7–10cm from the infant's face. The percentage oxygen concentration is seen by reading the position of a light beam on a graduated scale.

Feeding

Opinion differs on the safest time for introducing the low birth weight infant to oral feeding. Although carrying a risk of inhalation of vomitus, most now agree that early feeding, when carried out by an experienced nurse, outweighs the morbid effects of metabolic disturbance arising when feeding is delayed. The need for kilocalories is great, especially if the infant is experiencing respiratory difficulty.

Each infant is an individual, requiring individual consideration. The following

INCUBATOR CHART A
(HOURLY)

Reg. Number: 503694 — Surname: SMITH — Birth Weight: 1.68 kg. — Date of Birth: 1/8/70 — Consultant: DR. WILLIAMS — Time of Birth: 11.15. — Age (in days): 1 — DATE: 1/8/70.

	INCUBATOR					INFANT				SILVERMAN SCORE							
TIME	Normal Temp C°	Setting	Servo Set temp	O2 % conc.	O2 Litres/m	Heart rate	Resp. rate	SKIN temp °C	Rectal temp °C	A	B	C	D	E	Total	COMMENTS	HRS
1																	1
2																	2
3																	3
4																	4
5																	5
6																	6
7																	7
8																	8
9																	9
10																	10
11	On	ADMISSION.	36		2	152	56	34^8	34^2	2	0	2	0	0	4.	Good colour.	11
12			36		2	156.	52.	34^8	—	2	0	2	0	0	4.	Good colour.—mucousy.	12
13			36		2	160.	60.	35^2	—	2	1	2	0	0	5.	Still good colour.—Respirations laboured.	13
14			36		3	152.	64.	35^6	—	2	1	2	0	1	6.	" " Intermittent grunting.	14
15			36		3 +feeds	148.	64.	35^8	—	2	1	2	0	1	6.	Pale. Intermittent grunting.	15
16			36^8	65%	3+2	144.	68.	36	35	2	1	2	0	1	6.	Slightly dusky. O² increased	16
17			36^8		3+2	136.	72.	36^4	—	2	1	2	0	0	5.	Good colour.	17
18			36^8		3+2	136	72.	36^8	—	2	0	2	0	0	4.	Colour improved.	18
19			36^8	62%	2+2.	140.	68.	36^6	—	2	0	2	0	0	4.	Dextrostix 45. Extremities blue.	19
20			36^8		2+2	144.	56	36^6	36	1	1	2	0	0	4.	Colour good. O² decreased.	20
21			36^8	56%	3	132.	64	36^8	—	1	1	2	0	0	4.	Irritable on handling.	21
22			36^8		3	144	64	36^9	—	0	1	2	0	0	3.	O² decreased. Red dile	22
23			36^8	40%	2	148.	62.	36^8	—	1	0	1	0	0	2.	removed.	23
24			36^8		2.	136.	58.	36^8	36^4	1	0	1	0	0	2.	Colour remaining good.	24

FIG. 14.

basic principles can be adapted according to the needs of most low birth weight infants.

NATURE OF FOOD
Full strength breast milk is of particular value to the very small or ill low birth weight infant during the first few weeks of life. This may be available from his mother or from the bank of pooled, pasteurized breast milk maintained in some large maternity units.

When breast milk is not available, half cream modified dried milk or evaporated milk products have to be used. Half cream modified dried milk products have the advantage that the protein content is greater than in breast milk. As the low birth weight infant requires up to 5g protein/kg/day, this requirement is virtually fulfilled by giving full strength half cream dried milk preparations. The electrolyte content is above that of breast milk and may give rise to oedema as the immature kidneys are unable to excrete excess salts. The concentration of the feed is governed by the infant's ability to digest and absorb the food, but full strength half cream milk feeds are introduced as soon as possible.

When fat tolerance has been achieved and the infant weighs 2kg or 5lb, full cream feeds may be introduced according to the infant's appetite, a 10% mixture being used.

For the large, immature infant of the diabetic mother, full cream modified cow's milk feeds are necessary from the second week.

When the low birth weight infant is nourished via the intravenous route, leavulose 20%, Aminosol and Intralipid may be used.

FEEDING REGIME FOR LOW BIRTH WEIGHT INFANTS
A low birth weight infant requires more fluid and kilocalories per kilogramme of body weight than does his full-term counterpart.

The full-term infant requires:

110kcal and 150ml/kg per day
(50kcal and 2½oz/lb per day)

The low birth weight infant requires:

130–150kcal and 200ml/kg per day
(60–70kcal and 3–3½oz/lb per day)

Infants who are premature by dates are fed according to their birth weight. The 'small-for-dates' infant who is less than 4/5ths of his expected weight for gestation is fed for his expected weight.

First feed: within 3–4 hours of birth. 24 hour volumes:

Day 1— 45ml/kg
Day 2— 60 ml/kg
Day 3— 80ml/kg
Day 4—105ml/kg

Day 5—130ml/kg
Day 6—140ml/kg
Day 7—150ml/kg
Day 8—160ml/kg
200ml/kg by day 14.

The first feed is of 5% dextrose. Subsequent feeds are of full strength milk mixture if tolerated, otherwise diluted according to tolerance. The fluid requirement for the day is divided into 7–22 parts, according to the size, condition and feed tolerance of the infant.

Those infants over 1·6kg or 3½lb can usually tolerate sufficient volume of feed for the daily requirements to be divided between 7 or 8 feeds, making 3 hourly feeding possible. Smaller infants require 2 hourly feeding, and hourly feeding is necessary to achieve fluid and food tolerance in the very immature infant. There is no place for demand feeding in the care of low birth weight infants.

METHOD

Breast. After a few initial tube or bottle feeds, an infant weighing 2kg or 4½lb or over may be strong enough to suck at the breast for all, or alternate feeds during the day. Alternatively, unless the infant is ill, bottle feeding is quickly established and weight gain is good.

Bottle. An infant weighing between 1·5kg and 2kg or 3½–4½lbs is usually able to suck and swallow, although he readily tires. Tube feeding may be initiated until his general condition is good and confirmation of his reflex control attained. A soft teat with a fairly large hole is necessary to avoid tiring. The smaller infant may be fed in his incubator or placed, warmly wrapped, on the nurse's knees. Constant reminding is necessary toward the end of the feed as the infant becomes drowsy, and gentle pressure of a finger placed under the chin will achieve this aim (FIG. 13, page 64). Use of a pipette, Belcroy feeder or spoon carries a greater risk of inhalation and unless used by experienced staff, these methods are best avoided.

Tube feeding. Because of the risk of inhaling vomitus, infants weighing less than 1·5kg or 3¼lb at birth or of less than thirty-four weeks gestation, are fed via a fine, indwelling polyvinyl naso-gastric tube, size 3·5F.G., allowing administration of frequent small feeds without undue disturbance of the infant. Passage of the tube requires expert care, but once in position it can be left for up to seven days before renewal is advisable.

Whichever method of feeding is adopted, disturbance following the feed should be reduced to a minimum. The mouth is inspected for evidence of monilial infection. The infant's napkin is changed and he is turned to the other side before feeding. The head of the cot, or incubator tray, is elevated slightly and maintained in that position for thirty minutes after feeding.

TABLE 11. Recognition, Prevention and Management of Complications to which the Low Birth Weight Infant is Prone.

Complication	Handicap	Clinical Manifestations	Prevention and/or Management
Prone to infection.	Inadequate maternal transfer of gamma globulins and anti-bodies. Poor manufacture of own antibodies.	Depends on site: Septicaemia— Lethargy Jaundice ↑ or ↓ temperature. Umbilical sepsis. Sticky eye. Skin lesions. Oral monilia. Diarrhoea etc.	Barrier nursing, Healthy staff. Infrequent gentle handling. Cleanliness with feeding. Prophylactic antibiotic therapy (if necessary). Early recognition and treatment.
Instability of body temperature.	Immature temperature-regulating centre. Insufficient energy reserves. Relatively large surface area. Lack of subcutaneous fat. Minimal muscular activity. Inadequate sweating mechanism.	Fluctuations in body temperature according to environment (poikilothermic). Tendency to become chilled. Easily overheated.	Maintenance of a warm stable environmental temperature. Conservation of heat. Exposure avoided. Adequate humidity to avoid heat loss.
Respiratory difficulties.	Immature or damaged respiratory centre. Lungs under developed and incompletely expanded (atelectasis). Soft pliable rib cage. Weak musculature of thorax. Reduced fibrinolysis (slow absorption of hyaline membrane). Cough reflex feeble or absent	Irregular respirations. Supraclavicular / Subcostal / Sternal / Intercostal } recession Tachypnoea. Inspiratory effort + + +. Expiratory grunt. Acidosis. = Danger of cerebral anoxaemia Aspiration pneumonia	Use of apnoea monitor. Cutaneous stimulation. Turned 2 hourly. Warmth. O_2 while cyanosed or Po_2 low. Humidity. Fluids + glucose. Alkalis. Antibiotics. Positive pressure ventilation. Care with feeding. Maintenance of a clear airway.

TABLE 11—continued

Complication	Handicap	Clinical Manifestations	Prevention and/or Management
Feeding difficulties.	Sucking Swallowing reflexes poor or Cough absent. Incompetent cardiac sphincter. Small stomach. Poorly developed musculature of alimentary tract. Fat poorly tolerated.	Regurgitation of food. Inability to fulfil energy demands of body. Slow weight gain. Abdominal distension and constipation. Abdominal distension. Diarrhoea and vomiting.	Small tube feeds at frequent intervals. Avoidance of excessive handling particularly after feeds. Feed adequate in carbohydrates and protein but low in fat content.
Hyper-bilirubinaemia.	Immature liver—lack of glucuronyl transferase causing inadequate clearance of bilirubin. Vitamin K intoxication. Haemolytic disease of the new-born. Infection.	Lethargy. Prolonged physiologial jaundice. Risk of kernicterus when serum bilirubin level exceeds 20 mg/100 ml. (See above)	Extra fluids to avoid haemoconcentration. Phototherapy. Exchange transfusion. Small doses only of Vitamin K_1. Exchange transfusion. (See above)

Anaemia.	1. *Early*—comparatively short life of erythrocytes.
	(70 instead of 120 days)
	Excessive breakdown over formation of red blood cells.
	2. *Late* (4 months +)
	Poor iron store.
	Rapid rate of growth.
	Aggravating factors:
	   Infection.
	   Haemorrhage.
		Pallor
		Lethargy
			1. Blood transfusion (packed cells).
			
			2. Oral iron supplements from 4 weeks onwards.
			Iron—
			   oral or intramuscular.
			   Folic acid.

Condition	Cause	Signs	Treatment
Haemorrhage.	Fragile capillaries. Immature liver—lack of prothrombin and essential globulins.	Cerebral haemorrhage: Wakeful. Restless. 'Cerebral' cry. Convulsions. Haemorrhagic disease of the newborn.	Care at delivery and subsequent handling. Sedation. Prophylactic Vitamin K_1. Fresh blood to replace loss.
Oedema.	Immature kidneys: Poor urine output. Poor urea and electrolyte clearance. Immature liver: Hypoproteinaemia. Aggravating factor: Chilling.	Generalised oedema. Diagnosed by weight gain, or weight loss following administration of diuretic.	Care with administration of electrolytic solution and in the use of modified cow's milk preparations. Adequate protein intake. Avoid chilling.
Hypoglycaemia.	Infants at particular risk: Dysmature infants due to poor glycogen store. Infants of diabetic mothers.	Jittery. Twitching—convulsions. Apnoeic attacks—cyanosis. Reluctance to feed.	Prevention: Dextrostix blood sugar estimates at frequent intervals. Initiation of early feeding. Chilling avoided. Treatment: Oral or intravenous dextrose 10% leavulose 20% etc. Steroids.
Hypocalcaemia.	Dysmature infants particularly at risk. Associated with increased phosphorus intake.	Tetany of the newborn: Irritability. Twitching. Convulsions.	Prevention: Modified cow's milk preparations avoided. Treatment: Intravenous calcium gluconate. Sedatives.
Retrolental fibroplasia.	Immature retina subjected to high concentration or prolonged administration of oxygen.		Oxygen given only when necessary and never above 40% concentration unless cyanosed or Po_2 level low.

Summary

Infants weighing 1·5kg or 3¼lb, or less—tube-fed 1 or 2 hourly.

Infants weighing 1·5–2kg or 3¼–4½lb—initially tube-fed 2–3 hourly. Bottle feeding quickly established.

Infants weighing 2kg or 4½lb, or more—bottle and/or breast-fed 3 hourly.

EXPECTED WEIGHT GAIN

After an initial weight loss of 10–15%, weight gain is slow, particularly in the very small infant who may take two to three weeks to regain his birth weight. This is followed by a relatively rapid rate of growth, emphasizing the need for additional kilocalories and protein and the necessity to introduce vitamins and mineral elements at an early age.

Weighing on alternate days, or twice weekly, is usually sufficient, the general condition of the infant being a good guide to satisfactory progress. Once the birth weight has been regained, an infant weighing 1·5kg or 2lb, or less, can be expected to gain approximately 15g or ½oz daily.

Between 1·5–2kg or 2½–3½lb, the daily expected weight gain is 15–25g. For the infant weighing over 2kg or 3½lb, the daily expected weight gain is 1oz or 30g.

The weight of a low birth weight infant usually exceeds 2·5kg or 5½lb by his expected day of delivery, and most are home by this date.

SUPPLEMENTS

Vitamin A, C and D supplements are commenced from the fourteenth day. One drop of concentrated multivitamin preparation is increased by one drop daily until the full requirement of 5 drops twice daily is reached.

Iron, as ferrous sulphate, or Colliron, is introduced on the twenty-first day and similarly increased until the full requirement is reached ten days later.

Subsequent Care of the Low Birth Weight Infant

The special care of a low birth weight infant does not end when he leaves the confines of a special care baby unit. Although in his early days he has benefited from the skilled nursing care given by specially trained staff, his mother should always have been made to feel a welcome visitor and an active participant in his love and care. Early establishment of a good mother–child relationship is desirable for subsequent security in the family unit.

Before his discharge home, the mother must feel competent in the care of her small child. Residence in the unit for a few days will allow her to gain confidence under supervision. The home conditions must be assessed before the infant is discharged, and adequate support from the premature baby nursing service (if the infant weighs less than 2·5kg (5½lb) on discharge) and a health visitor is ensured. The mother is encouraged to seek the advice given by the welfare services of her area and to fulfil the important 'follow-up' appointments to see the paediatrician. Low birth weight infants are more prone to gastro-intestinal and respiratory infection in the first year of life, so the necessary precautions must be observed.

In the absence of congenital malformation or cerebral damage, the low birth weight infant of five-years-of-age compares very favourably with full-term infants of similar genetic, social and environmental status. Those who were born with a defect, a low Apgar score, or suffered from an infection, anaemia, apnoeic attacks, hypoglycaemia or hypocalcaemia in the neonatal period are 'at risk' and are very carefully followed up. With an added disability to overcome, the comparison with their full-term counterparts is less favourable.

For Further Reading

CRAIG W. S. (1969). *Care of the Newly Born Infant.* 4th edition. E. & S. Livingstone, Edinburgh.
CROSSE V. M. (1966). *The Premature Infant.* 6th edition. J. & A. Churchill, London.

CHAPTER SIX

Meeting the Needs of the Sick Child

During this century, there has not only been a marked change in the pattern of childhood illness, but an enlightened approach to the child as a developing individual and the effect illness and admission to hospital have on both the child and his parents.

Fifty years ago, most of the paediatric hospital beds in this country were occupied by undernourished children from a poor social environment, suffering from such disease processes as gastro-enteritis, virulent infectious diseases, tuberculosis, rheumatic fever or rickets. Because of a vast improvement in living conditions and advancement in medical science, these conditions are rarely seen today, and there is less demand for paediatric beds. Instead, children are admitted to hospital for treatment of congenital abnormalities now amenable to life-saving surgery, metabolic disorders, malignant disease, injuries, accidental poisoning, mental subnormality, behaviour disorders, and many other conditions which were once considered to be beyond treatment, and in many instances caused death at an early age.

The work of Bowlby and Robertson on the effect separation and admission into hospital have on the child has shown that, to facilitate a speedy recovery from illness, a sick child should be nursed at home, or with his mother taking a large share in his care during his stay in hospital. Because hospital and illness involve an element of fear, admission to hospital appears to be potentially more detrimental to a young child's developing personality than any other common form of separation.

The report of the Platt Committee on 'The Welfare of Children in Hospital' (H.M.S.O. 1959) recommended that very young children should only be admitted to hospital when the necessary medical treatment they require cannot be given in any other way without real disadvantage.

While highly skilled medical treatment and nursing care are of utmost importance, it is essential that the atmosphere and facilities provided in a paediatric unit meet the child's psychological needs for love and security—by continuous or frequent contact with his mother, or mother substitute, and opportunities for supervised play.

The National Association for the Welfare of Children in Hospital began in 1961 as a small group of mothers who were concerned that, in spite of the recommendation made in the 1959 Platt Committee report, there was reluctance on the part of most hospital staffs to allow parents reasonable access to even quite small children. The Association has now expanded to include anyone interested in the well-being of sick children in its membership—doctors, nurses and social workers—and aims to promote the nursing of sick children at home whenever possible; to promote the welfare of sick children in hospital, and to publicise their special needs; to provide details of visiting and living-in facilities for mothers and to ensure that new paediatric units are designed with adequate accommodation for mothers to be with their children.

The secure five-year-old from a loving home environment is beginning to accept new situations with no undue anxiety and, if adequately and suitably prepared for his stay in hospital, he settles well. With increasing age, he is more able to comprehend what is going on around him. Time is becoming increasingly more meaningful. With assured frequent visits from his parents and contacts with familiar relatives and friends through letters, cards and parcels, he often enjoys the extra parental attention and spoiling associated with his stay in hospital and suffers no adverse effects from the separation. A less mature or insecure child of any age will experience greater difficulty in adapting to any new situation.

Alternatives to Hospital Admission

Many sick children are very satisfactorily cared for at home by their parents under the medical supervision of the family doctor. A mother is usually the best person to understand and tolerate the behaviour of her own child, well or sick. When the task becomes beyond her scope, additional support or alternative arrangements have to be made.

Home Care

The desirability of satisfactory home care depends on:
i the nature of the child's illness;
ii the social environment;
iii the ability of the mother to cope;
iv the availability of a suitable home nursing service, if necessary.

When the physical benefits of hospital care exceed the psychological advantages of home nursing, the child has to be admitted to hospital.

The city of Birmingham is fortunate in having a unique twenty-four hour children's home nursing service, allowing many severely handicapped children, and children suffering from acute infections, to be cared for in their own homes by their family doctor, with the valuable assistance of trained sick children's nurses. In addition, with the close co-operation of hospital paediatric units, many children requiring skilled nursing supervision are discharged home at an early date. The domestic assistance given by a home help will give the mother more time to devote to the care and welfare of her sick child. The success of such a scheme lies in close co-operation between the family doctor and his nurse colleagues, with the full support of the hospital specialist services as necessary. It is of great benefit to the psychological development of the young child during the vulnerable first four years of life, as well as being a more economic proposition.

Day Patient

Facilities for accommodating day patients are available in some paediatric units for carrying out special investigations and performing minor surgery. The length of stay is short and separation from mother avoided, causing minimal psychological disturbance to the child.

Overnight Admission

Similarly, for other surgery of a simple nature, the child's stay in hospital may be limited to overnight, as long as adequate medical and nursing follow-up can be carried out in a suitable home environment.

Effects of Admission to Hospital

The adverse effect which separation and fear, associated with admission to hospital, have on a sick child depend on his:
  i   age and emotional maturity;
  ii security in his home environment;
  iii previous traumatic experiences—if any;
  iv acceptance of treatment;
  v length of stay in hospital.

On the whole, infants under the age of four to six months settle happily, provided they are fed regularly, made comfortable and confidently handled. The six months to four years age group are particularly susceptible to psychological trauma, and their admission to hospital is avoided if at all possible. They are too young to understand explanations, but old enough to miss their familiar home surroundings. Some will make their objection to hospital known to all and are unconsolably miserable, while others—the so-called 'good toddlers'—show little emotion and remain quiet, withdrawn and apathetic, slowly storing up their aggressive feelings. Illness, particularly when associated with separation from home, frequently results in a degree of reversion to infantile behaviour. Wetting and soiling are common, and head banging, body rocking, nail-biting, nose-picking, thumb-sucking and masturbation may be seen in those withdrawing from the unfamiliar surroundings in which they have been abandoned or sent as a punishment—for this is as it appears to the toddler who is unable to understand why he has been rejected in this manner. This apparent rejection by his mother will create personality problems unless the child has frequent contact with those he has learned to love and trust in his familiar home environment.

Admission to Hospital

The Platt Committee report on 'The Welfare of Children in Hospital' recommended that children should be nursed in company with other children of the same age, in an environment where the special needs of sick children are appreciated and their behaviour understood and tolerated by staff specially trained in the care of sick children. The admission of children and adolescents to adult wards is not recommended, but quite a large proportion of sick children are still admitted for care in an adult specialist unit and many adolescents are admitted to adult wards because of the lack of alternative accommodation.

Unfortunately, because of the nature of their illness, many children have to be admitted to one of the few sick children's hospitals specializing in the care of this particular age group, many miles from home. Others may be admitted to children's wards or units attached to the local general hospital. The hospital is the child's temporary home and whether or not he is happy in it depends, to a large extent, on the ability of the staff to meet his total needs—physical, emotional, social, educational, as well as specific surgical and medical care.

A children's unit usually consists of a large area, preferably sub-divided, to accommodate small groups of children of different ages. A high proportion of single cubicles is necessary for use as:

1   Mother/child units.

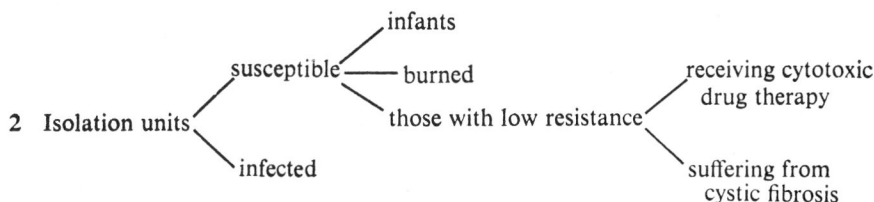

```
                            infants
             susceptible          burned              receiving cytotoxic
                                                       drug therapy
2  Isolation units                  those with low resistance
             infected                                  suffering from
                                                       cystic fibrosis
```

and for:

3   Ill children.
4   Adolescents.

In addition to the usual annexes associated with an adult ward, a separate play area and a feed kitchen are necessary. The unit is staffed by nurses who have acquired the skill, knowledge and expertise, preferably by training, and sometimes by experience, to reinforce their love for, and interest in, the care and welfare of sick children. Because of the training requirements laid down by the General Nursing Council, the student staff population of any ward is essentially a moving one, and a paediatric ward is no exception. Whenever possible, the child should be handled by as few people as practical. In this way he will get to know several people well instead of being vaguely familiar with all. Patient assignment rather than work assignment is ideal, giving the child a caring mother substitute in his own mother's absence.

Visiting

It is comparatively recent that parents have been given rightful access to their sick children, and, even today, less enlightened people still restrict visiting on the assumption that the presence of parents interrupts the ward routine, or that visiting upsets the children. It is inevitable for a small child to cry when his parents leave—this is only natural and of this the parents must be assured. It is far better for the child to see them and be upset than to suffer greater deprivation by parental absence.

Unrestricted visiting is a way in which separation in hospital has been made more bearable, both for the child and his parents. Parents are allowed to visit at any reasonable hour of the day to fit in with their family and work commitments. Father can visit on his way home from work instead of taking time off, and mother can give greater attention to the rest of the family when they are at home and visit her sick child while the family are at school. Rather than being a hindrance in the ward, the presence of mothers creates a more relaxed atphere. They can relieve the staff for other duties by feeding, washing and amusing their own child, and often reading to and amusing others whose mothers are unable to visit.

Parents must be made to feel wanted and that their presence in the ward is not resented. Just as we can quickly detect the attitude of relatives, so they can quickly detect our attitude towards them and their sick child.

Information should be made easy to obtain from a well-informed member of the staff. Some parents are afraid to ask because of appearing stupid, and others do not like to interrupt the busy sister or staff nurse from her nursing duties. Two-way communication is important and time and opportunity should be afforded by the ward staff.

Anxiety and feelings of guilt—usually unfounded—and resentment may sometimes be projected as a hostile attitude towards the hospital staff. Co-operation is lacking, and endless questions and complaints are made. How easy it is to label these parents as 'difficult'! They need understanding help from a sympathetic listener who can assist in the situation or guide them into appropriate channels of help.

Because of distance, family commitments, and economic reasons, some parents are not able to visit as often as they would like. They should not be made to feel they are neglecting their child, and financial assistance may be made available through the hospital medical social worker, if necessary. A small percentage of parents are too worried to visit for fear of what they will find. They, too, need sympathetic understanding, which possibly their more familiar family doctor is able to offer. Less responsible parents do not see the necessity for frequent visits. The more unsettled and difficult the home environment, the less likely the parents are to visit.

A hospital canteen and crèche for visitors' children are perhaps considerations for the future, for both would prove beneficial to visiting relatives.

Mother-Child Units

With the slow decline in the demand for paediatric beds, some hospitals have managed to adapt parts of their wards to provide units where a mother can live in a cubicle with her small child, taking a large share in his care. Where this facility is not available, alternative accommodation may be provided within the confines of the hospital to allow the mother to be with her child during the day, but sleep in her own room at night. As there is limited accommodation of this nature, priority is given to mothers of:

i   six month–four year age group;
ii   mentally subnormal of any age;
iii breast-fed infants;
iv   physically handicapped children for early discharge;
v   very ill children;
vi   those many miles from home.

This arrangement is of particular value in the settling-in period following sudden admission to hospital. It allows the child to become familiar with his new surroundings and to gain confidence in the people whom his mother trusts. Once a small child senses that his mother is satisfied with his care, he is more willing to co-operate with the medical and nursing staff, and more ready to tolerate short periods of maternal absence.

Preparation for Admission

Parents know the needs of their own child and it is they who can best prepare their child for a stay in hospital. They need guidance in this preparation, and most paediatric units circulate a national or locally produced leaflet giving up-to-date information. Where there is a language barrier, an appropriate translation should accompany the pictorial leaflet.

Parental worry and anxiety are quickly communicated to the child, and his confidence in hospital care depends on the degree of security he senses in his parents. It is important, therefore, that the parents are given advice and assurance during their visit to the out-patients department, or by their own family doctor or health visitor, so that they can give simple, truthful information to their child. Mass media, especially television, has done much to inform the public of life in hospital in general, and the leaflet will give particulars of local arrangements.

Emphasis on getting better is important so that the child is assured that this is the reason for his stay in hospital. Separation from home must be carefully explained, but the child assured that mummy and daddy will visit him every day (if this is true) and that he will be able to go home when the doctors and nurses have made him better. A favourite toy, labelled* with his name, or any other comforter, will give the child a tangible reminder of home in a situation divorced from all that is familiar. The parents are advised to include this in the small list of requirements necessary for their child's stay in hospital.

Reception

Admission to hospital is a routine procedure to the nursing staff of the admissions unit and the ward, but traumatic to the child and family concerned. First impressions go a long way, and a kind, understanding attitude will do much initially to establish parental confidence which is quickly reflected in the child. The formalities of admission should be quickly dispensed with, and the mother and child taken to the ward as soon as possible. Delay in the admission unit can be interpreted as inefficiency, and cause inconvenience to the family as well as increased apprehension in the child.

If this is the child's first admission to hospital, the doctor will record a full family history, including the health of both maternal and paternal families, and the health of the child's parents and siblings. The mother's obstetric history is often of great significance, and includes recording of the number of pregnancies and miscarriages, the place of delivery, period of gestation, complications of pregnancy and labour, and birth weight of her child to be admitted. A nutritional history is taken and the child's physical and mental achievements recorded. Illnesses requiring previous admission to hospital, allergies or drug reactions, and current medications are recorded. A careful history of the present illness is then obtained and the child examined.

EXAMINATION OF THE CHILD
While listening to the mother's story, the doctor observes the behaviour of the child—the position he adopts, his colour, facial expression, cry, movements and awareness. The routine adopted for examination of an adult and older child

* Marking ink should be used with caution—the label must be washed and ironed to prevent cutaneous absorption of the toxic content.

has to be modified according to the mental age of the child. For the infant and toddler, it is usually preferable that the mother stays with her child while the doctor makes his examination, but the doctor may prefer to postpone detailed examination until an older child is settled in his bed in the ward. Unnecessary exposure should be avoided at all ages and privacy is essential for the self-conscious older child.

Children cannot and will not be hurried. A quiet, gentle approach following a short chat or game help the doctor to establish rapport and to win the child's confidence. No amount of persuasion will convince a doubting toddler that active resistance makes the situation worse and restraint is nearly always necessary when the ears and throat are examined.

Examination may be confined to just one area of the body, but usually involves a full examination of every system and region of the body. Any instruments required for the examination should be kept out of sight until they are needed and it is sometimes an advantage to allow a child to handle an instrument and thus be assured of its harmless nature. The more distasteful or distressing procedures such as examination of the ears, nose, mouth and throat are left to the last.

It is important when admitting a child into any institution to ascertain from the parents what infectious diseases he has experienced and what artificial immunity he has received. Should a case of infectious disease occur in a ward, this information is of vital importance so that the appropriate precautions can be taken. Recent contact with an infectious illness may well postpone a child's stay in hospital, or the child may be admitted to an isolation unit until the incubation period has expired.

A note is made of the social conditions in which the child lives, i.e. the type of house, number of bedrooms, number of people sharing the accommodation, and the occupation of the father and mother. This information is not just a means of prying into the personal life of the family. It may well prove a guide to the future care of the child and give the staff a better insight into the child's home background which will influence his behaviour while in hospital. A simple questionnaire circulated to the parents will supply much of this information, prior to the child arriving in the admissions unit, and make his stay there as short as possible.

Once in the ward environment, the child, with his mother, is shown his bed and locker in which he can place his toys. Most children from the age of three years sleep in a low bed at home, and many from overcrowded living conditions share their bed with one or two siblings. The humiliation of having to sleep in a cot may be just too much for a four-year-old who may be only just managing to fight away his tears. Another child may wonder who, of the strange children around him, is going to share his bed. A thoughtful, understanding nurse can anticipate these little worries and reassure the child and his mother. In the bathroom he is bathed, if necessary, weighed and dressed in attractive day clothes of a suitable size, unless the hospital permits children to retain their own clearly labelled day and night clothes. An identification band, checked by his mother, is secured to his wrist. The hair is examined for lice. Throughout the procedures, his mother will remain with him and see him settled, preferably in the play area of the ward, before reassuring him of a visit later—if this is so. Children associate bed with sleep and unfortunately for some, bed in the daytime means punishment, so for routine admission to the ward, the child is best allowed up under supervision and dressed in suitable clothes for play.

The ward sister will want to see the mother for exchange of information and to reassure her of the staff's genuine interest in her child as an individual. First of all, she must confirm the child's name. Children often have a nickname or are known by their second name, which should be used. The child's feeding habits need to be discussed. If he is an infant, the quantity, quality and frequency of feeds must be known, and whether or not vitamin supplements or weaning diet have been started. For the toddler, the method of feeding needs to be established—many still enjoy a bottle last thing at night, even to the age of two years. A small child, particularly when insecure, derives much comfort from a dummy, and only a thoughtless nurse would deprive him of this pleasure. Some mothers are ashamed to admit that their small child is used to a dummy and unless asked directly, will not divulge this information. The child's toilet habits need to be discussed and any special names used by the child for the lavatory, pot, defaecation and micturition noted. Small children have likes and dislikes, real and imaginary fears, some have nightmares, and a few sleep-walk. Knowledge of all these points and any others will help the ward staff to understand their new charge.

The mother will be advised regarding visiting her child in hospital, and the medical social worker contacted if the family are in economic or social difficulty. Naturally, most mothers will want to spend as much time with their sick child as possible, but they must be encouraged not to forsake their other children completely in the process.

Telephone numbers are exchanged and the mother advised on convenient times to contact the ward staff. On infant's wards, feeding times are best avoided, and friends and relatives discouraged from making enquiries to the hospital at any time. They should be encouraged to obtain their information from the parents, as the parents may not wish personal information to be divulged to friends and neighbours. The nursing staff must observe the confidential nature of personal information.

The parents' wish regarding baptism of a small child must be known, and written consent for specific operations, tests and blood transfusions obtained.

Some parents travel many miles to bring their child into hospital. Their need for food and a drink should not be forgotten and they should be told where light refreshment or a meal can be obtained. A cup of tea made by the ward staff is much appreciated by the distressed parents of a very sick child.

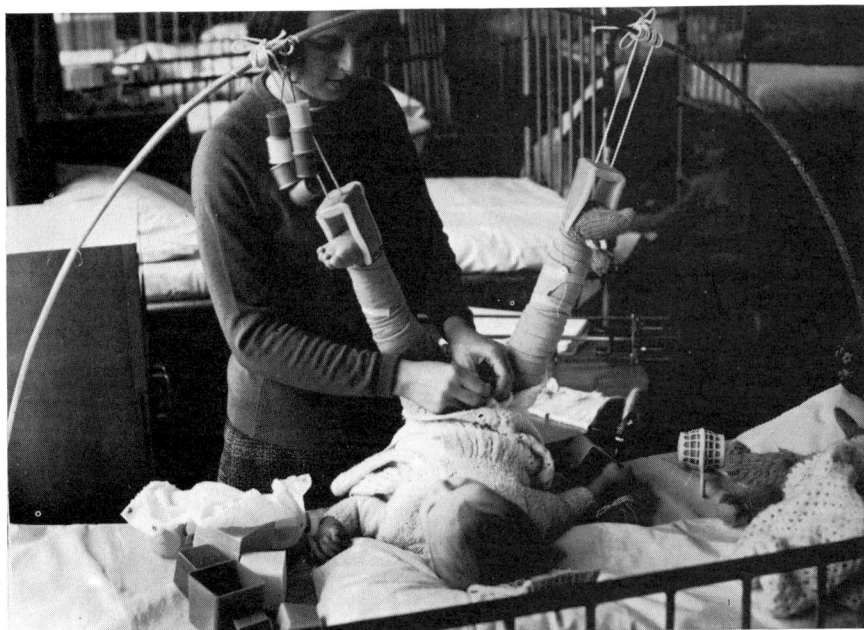

PLATE 5. 'Admission to hospital is more readily tolerated when mother is able to stay.'
At the age of ten months, Richard had to have treatment for his dislocated hip. His mother spent each day caring for his needs but went home to sleep at night. He experienced minimal ill effect from his admission to hospital.

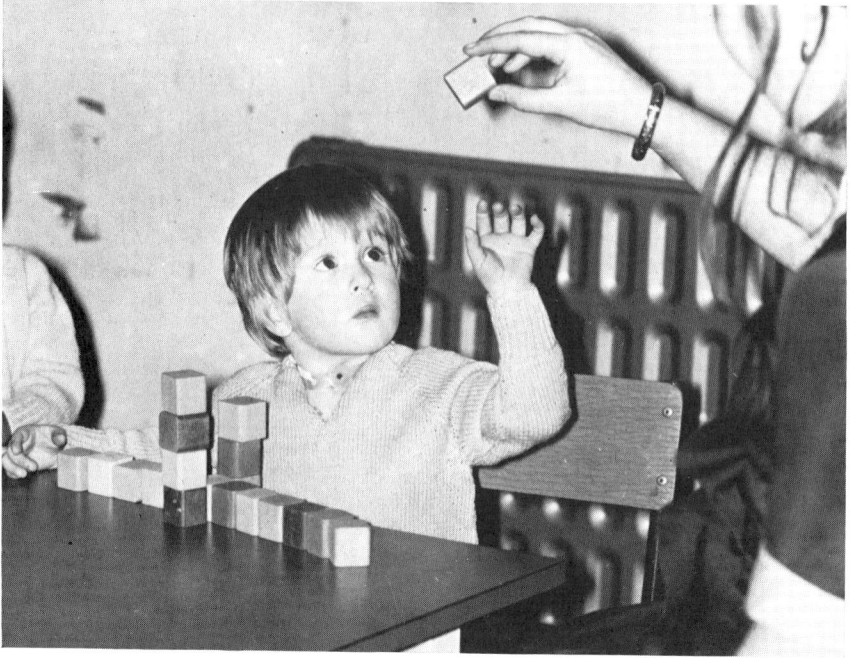

PLATE 6. Play in the Occupational Therapy Department.

Anthony has been in hospital for all of his two and a half years. At a time when he would normally have been starting to talk he was unable to do so, due to his tracheostomy. This led to constant frustration and consequent unacceptable behaviour in the ward.

Treatment aims to help him to overcome his frustrations and to direct his energies into more constructive play, to encourage normal learning patterns and socially acceptable behaviour and to help him gain self-esteem in his own achievements.

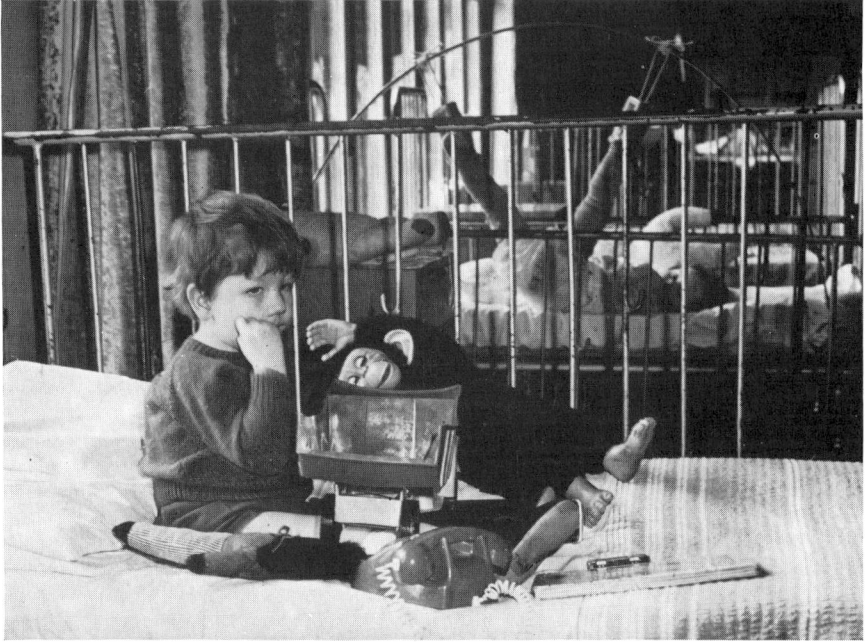

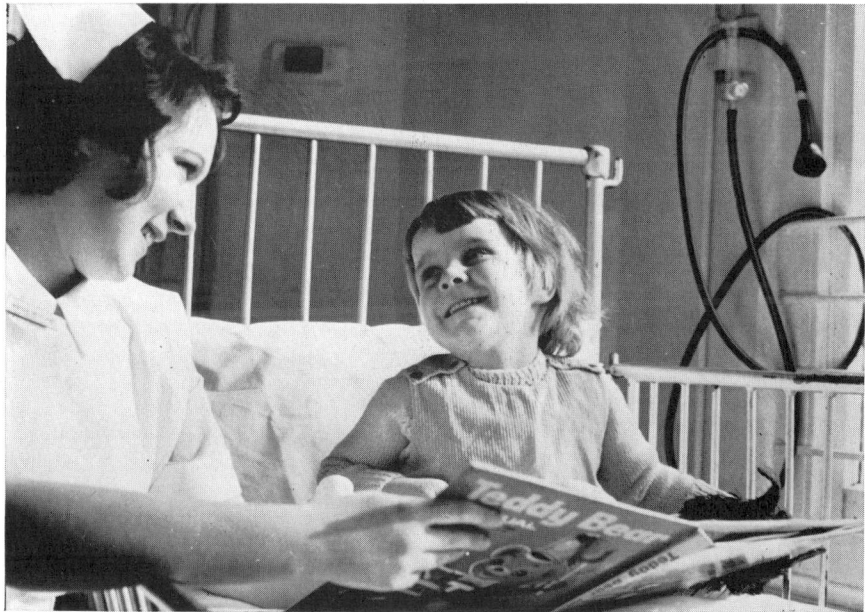

PLATE 7. Play in the wards.
(a) A plentiful supply of toys is not enough.
(b) Play is much more interesting when someone has time and thought to return.

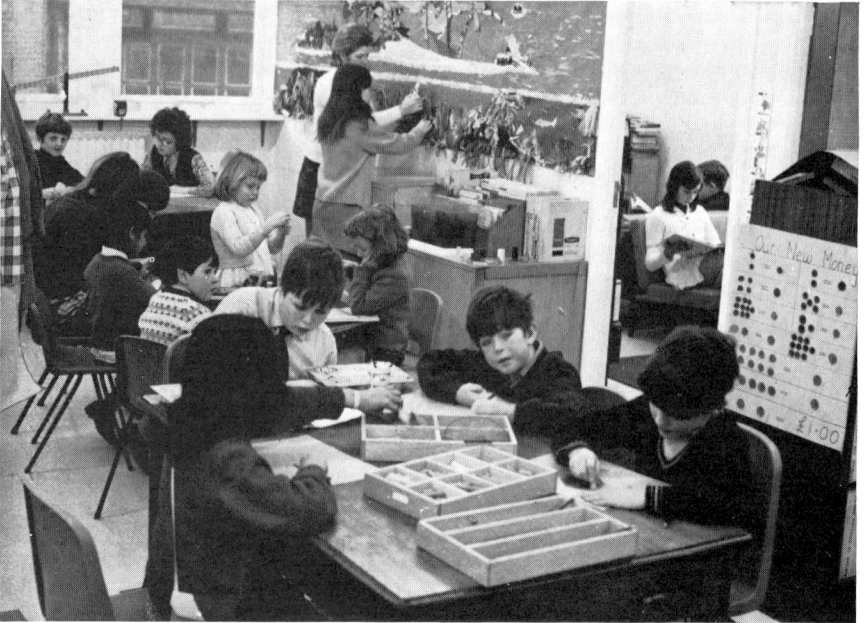

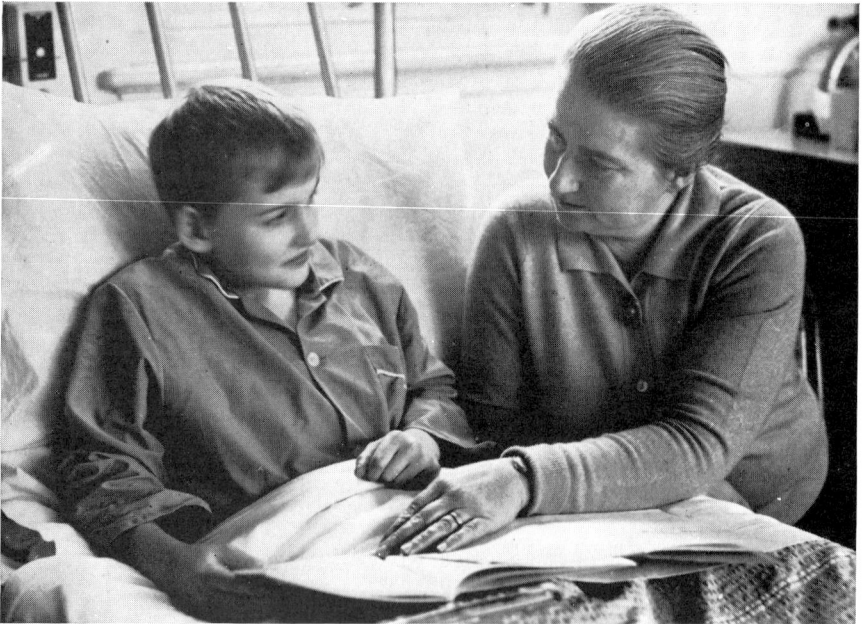

PLATE 8. Education.
Continuity of education is an important aspect in the care of children
in hospital. Those who are well enough go to the classrooms. Others,
like Keith, receive their instruction while confined to bed.

Recreation

Those who have a genuine interest in the welfare of sick children see play as an important part of their work. Any child is happier if occupied with an interesting task by someone who has the time and thought to return and encourage his activities. With the heavy work load on most children's wards, this important aspect of the child's care is frequently shelved by the nursing staff in favour of more technical duties, so that the apathetic behaviour of a small child lacking both suitable toys and adult attention is still seen. The provision of suitable play material is important, but not sufficient. Supervised play is desirable. The too few occupational therapists employed by the hospital authorities are usually fully occupied in giving individual supervision and are unable to give much time to group activities at ward level. The inclusion of 'playladies' or nursery nurses (who are trained in the special care of the under five age group and, therefore, particularly aware of the need for play) as an integral part of the ward team can help to fulfil the need for supervised play at ward level. Few children feel ill enough to want to be quiet and inactive for any length of time. Only the very sick child is content to clutch a favourite toy. The small child needs varied, supervised, messy play to vent his inner anxiety and gain relief from his 'bottled up' aggression. Dough, sand and water, paint and paper, give him this opportunity. For those confined to bed, waterproof protection of the bedclothes is necessary, and a firm cot or bed-table is required for writing and jigsaws. Objections to hospital treatment can be played out on a teddy or doll, under supervision.

As most children are up and about in the ward, a playroom or play area is an essential amenity in a children's ward. If partitioned off from the main ward area, the noise produced by happy children will not disturb the ill children confined to bed. A glass partition allows those confined to bed to watch the activities of the more boisterous, giving them encouragement to get well. A garden allows the children who are well enough to exercise their bodies in the fresh air and to release their surplus energy in organized ball games and other outdoor activities.

Domestic play gives the child a link with home, as well as sharing his play with others. Dolls, cots, prams, clothes, and facilities for pastry making, sweeping and dusting, washing and ironing, give him security in what is familiar. A story is a favourite pastime at all ages, especially if it is one with which the child is familiar. An ill child, unable to do anything creative, looks forward to storytime.

Most wards have a television set and a wireless, enabling the young patients to watch and listen to their favourite programmes.

A welcome visitor to the ward is the hospital chaplain who may well organize Sunday school or a service in the hospital chapel or on the wards. This the children thoroughly enjoy and it gives them a further link with the outside world.

Education

Continuity of education is important—a factor usually overlooked when a child is admitted to an adult ward. All large paediatric units, and some smaller units, have a special school administered by the local education authority, employing qualified teachers and nursery assistants. Much of its teaching is geared to the individual child rather than fitting the child into a rigid school programme. School hours are short—usually from 09.30 to 11.30 and 13.30 to 15.30 hours—and the children taught in a classroom, in groups in the wards, or as individuals. Teacher/parent/nurse co-operation is essential so that school hours remain undisturbed and the child not distracted unnecessarily from his lessons. Children often benefit from the individual tuition given at the hospital school, and on discharge home are able to take their normal place in an ordinary school.

Adolescent Units

The needs and interests of sick adolescent boys and girls differ from those of children and adults. They do not like being treated as children, but are frequently too boisterous to be happy in the quiet atmosphere of an adult ward.

The informal atmosphere of a small adolescent unit attached to a paediatric unit gives its occupants the necessary privacy and freedom to pursue their own special interests and education. They like to have pictures of their current 'pin-ups' displayed and to have the record player resounding 'pop' music—loud and clear. Frequently, adolescents like to help to care for and play with the small children on the ward, and many a happy, temporary friendship has been made in this way.

An adolescent's friends are almost as important to him as his parents and they should be allowed to visit, if this is requested.

For Further Reading

BOWLEY A. H. (1966). *The Psychological Care of the Child in Hospital.* E. & S. Livingstone, Edinburgh.
H.M.S.O. (1959). *The Welfare of Children in Hospital—Report of the Platt Committee.* London.
NOBLE E. (1967). *Play and the Sick Child,* 1st edition. Faber and Faber, London.
ROBERTSON J. (1970). *Young Children in Hospital.* 2nd edition. Tavistock Publications.
STACEY M. (1970). *Hospitals, Children and their Families—Report of a pilot study.* Routledge and Kegan Paul.

CHAPTER SEVEN

Basic Nursing Care

The content of Chapter 6 gives an insight into the ways in which the emotional, social and educational needs of the sick child can be met, thus reducing the adverse effects of separation from home. The content of this chapter is devoted to meeting the sick child's physical needs. The remainder of the book is concerned with the specific care and observation of children related to their surgical and medical needs.

Preparation for Procedures

A child's degree of co-operation depends on his trust in those caring for him. No one enjoys causing discomfort and distress to others, and particularly to the helpless child, but there are many occasions when in the interest of complete recovery, both are essential. Diagnostic and therapeutic procedures are endured with 'getting better and going home' in view, and should be carried out quickly and efficiently with the minimal amount of physical and psychological trauma. It is sometimes helpful if teddy undergoes the same treatment, although some children are loathe to let their favourite toy 'suffer'.

Careful preparation of the child is usually amply rewarded and throughout the text this is reiterated. Often gesture, manner and tone of voice mean far more to a young child than words of explanation. A simple, truthful explanation offered immediately prior to the procedure is usually accepted by an older child who should be assured of the nurse's presence throughout the procedure. Small children who are unable to understand and co-operate require a strong sedative to ensure that they are soundly asleep at the appointed time.

The unpredictable behaviour of the child demands the presence of two nurses for all procedures carried out by the nursing staff. One directs her undivided attention to the positioning, care and restraint of the child, while her colleague carries out the procedure. Blanket restraint may be necessary for a small infant (FIG. 15).

On completion of any unpleasant procedure, the child should be suitably

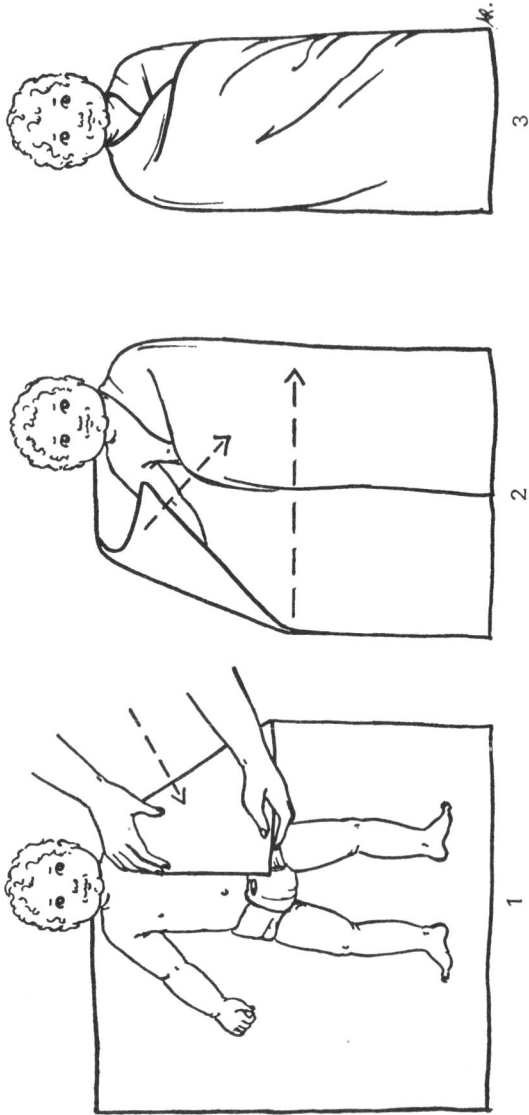

FIG. 15. Restraining a small child.

rewarded, both verbally and with extra love and attention. Comfort and praise should not be forgotten in the rush of the moment.

Fulfilling the Sick Child's Physical Needs

To a small child, a regular pattern of activity means security. A rigid ward routine not only ensures that everything is done, but that the child also knows what next to expect, and it should be an adaptation of what he has been used to at home.

The physical needs of the sick child are discussed under the following headings:
1   Comfort.
2   Rest and sleep.
3   Exercise.
4   Protection.
5   Nourishment.
6   Cleanliness.
7   Excretion.

Comfort

Few children are confined to bed for the full twenty-four hours so that both day and night clothes are necessary. The ward environment is usually warm enough for a thin nightdress or pyjamas to be adequate for the hours of sleep, and for light, practical, durable clothes to be worn during the day. All but the very ill are best dressed in a change of clothing during the day, the pyjama jacket being replaced by a vest, shirt and pullover, and the nightdress by a vest, dress and cardigan. For those who are able to be up, dungarees or cat-suits and jumpers are ideal for the toddlers, and the older children should be suitably dressed in well-fitting day clothes. Socks and shoes or slippers are necessary; a pair of well-fitting shoes being safer than slippers on the feet of a small child.

If a child is up for most of the day, then his bed requires making once only, first thing in the morning. His rest period can be taken on top of the bedclothes, or with the top bedclothes folded to the foot of the bed. A covering flannelette blanket ensures that he does not get chilled during this time. The whole length of an infant's or a toddler's cot should be protected with waterproof. If these precautions are taken, more time can then be devoted to the care of the children confined to bed. Their beds require re-making twice daily and the bedclothes, particularly the bottom sheet and drawsheet, changed and straightened as necessary between times. The pillows, too, require turning at frequent intervals; if the child has a high temperature, the waterproof protected pillows become hot, damp and uncomfortable. Light bedclothes only are necessary; one or two cotton blankets are usually sufficient. The weight of the bedclothes can be removed from the feet by the use of a bed-cradle.

POSITIONS USED IN NURSING

The following positions may be used for the comfort of the child and in the treatment of some conditions.

The upright position is used:

   i   when there is respiratory difficulty (dyspnoea);
  ii   following abdominal surgery;
 iii   in the treatment of hiatus hernia and achalasia of the cardia.

   Pillows should not be used during infancy and the use of soft pillows is best avoided during early childhood. The head and neck should be well supported, and the back straight to allow for full expansion of the chest during inspiration.

Methods

   i   With the use of pillows (and a back rest). This method is suitable for children over the age of about eighteen months. A pillow may be placed against the soles of the feet to prevent the child slipping out of position (FIG. 16);

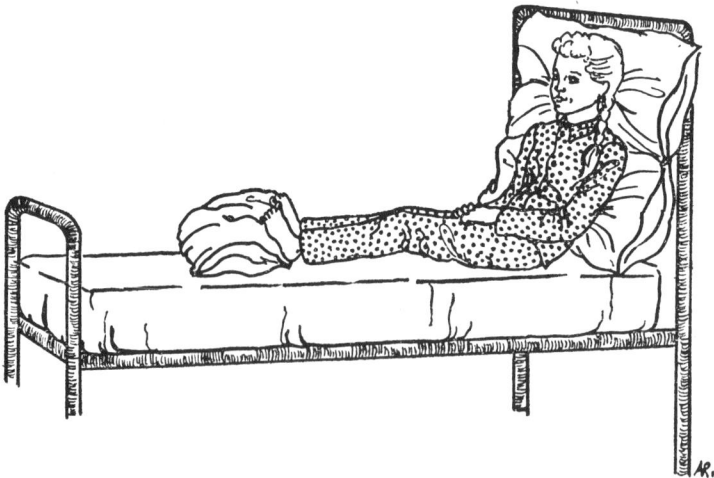

FIG. 16. Upright position.

   ii   Using a Safe Sitter chair. A safety harness secures the infant in an upright position. The buttocks and sacral area are sites of constant pressure and need frequent care (FIG. 5, page 38);
 iii   By elevation of the head of the cot or placing a firm pillow under the mattress. There is a tendency for an infant to slip beneath the bedclothes with the use of both of these methods;
  iv   By the use of an inclined bed and special harness. This is of particular value in the care of infants in cardiac failure.

The semi-recumbent position. This is a position commonly used during the day time. Two to three pillows are used to make the child comfortable on his back.

The recumbent or supine position. The child lies on his back with one pillow. This position is used:

i   for examination by the doctor;
ii for the removal of abdominal sutures.

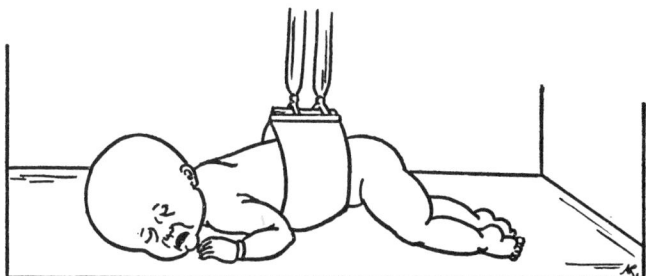

FIG. 17.

The prone position. This entails nursing the child in a face downwards position. This position is used if there is a defect, injury or burn of the back. Small, soft pillows placed under the chest, pelvis and ankles make this position more acceptable to the older child. A small child may have to be restrained to maintain the position. For infants with a spina bifida deformity, the prone position can be maintained with the use of a sling, and following repair of a myelomeningocele, this has the added advantage that some tension is taken off the lumbar-sacral suture line (FIG. 17). Infants with Pierre Robin syndrome involving a small receding chin (micrognathia), cleft palate and backward displacement of the tongue are frequently nursed in the prone position on a special frame to prevent the tongue obstructing the oro-pharynx.

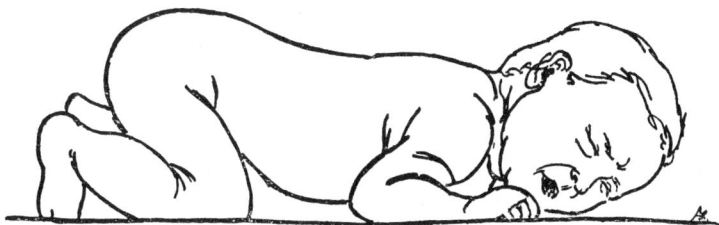

FIG. 18. Prone knee-chest position.

The prone knee-chest position. This position may be used to relieve a cyanotic attack in cyanotic congenital heart disease such as Fallot's tetralogy. (FIG. 18). *The three-quarters prone or semi-prone position.* Sometimes referred to as the post-tonsillectomy position, it is used to maintain a clear airway following tonsillectomy and in unconsciousness (FIG. 19).

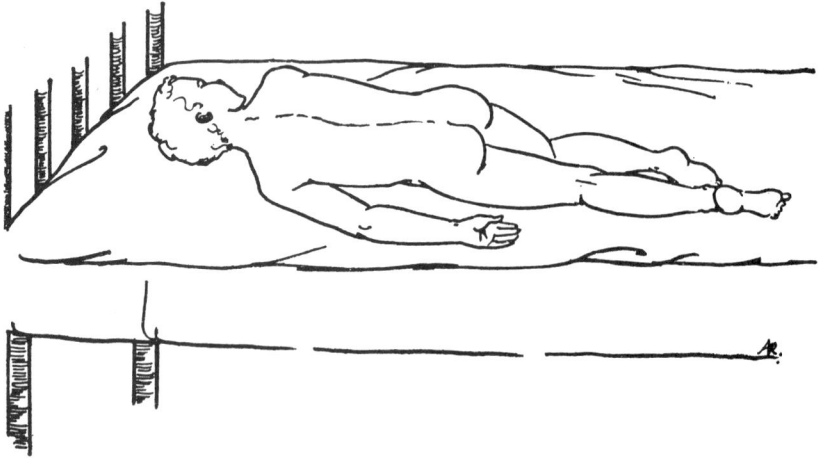

FIG. 19. Three-quarters prone, semi-prone or post-tonsillectomy position.

The lateral position. This is a position in common use for the following reasons:

 i It is the position in which most children sleep and in which small infants are nursed when awake and asleep;

 ii The left lateral position is used for rectal procedures;

 iii Unconscious patients are nursed in the left or right lateral or semi-prone position.

Care of Pressure Areas

Areas which are not designed to withstand pressure may become sore when a child is confined to bed for some length of time. This particularly applies to areas of the body where the skin covering a bony prominence is thin, e.g., the occiput, ears, scapulae, elbows, sacrum, hips, iliac crests, knees, heels, ankles and toes. The blood supply to the area is cut off, resulting in local death of the tissues. This is called a bed or pressure sore. The effects of pressure are made worse by moisture and friction.

Pressure sores are rarely seen in childhood, but may be seen complicating extreme debility or gross hydrocephalus. Children at particular risk include the emaciated, the unconscious, the paralyzed and those immobilized in splints or on traction. Obesity and incontinence intensify the risk.

PREVENTION OF PRESSURE SORES

1 Ensuring as far as possible that the child is given adequate nourishment to encourage the growth of healthy tissues.

2 Prevention and relief of pressure. Turning or changing the child's position every two to four hours will relieve the dependent areas of pressure. Pressure to local areas can be relieved by careful positioning of the limbs, with the use of waterproof protected sponge cushions, rings and pillows. A ripple-bed may be used, particularly if the child is heavy or very thin. A bed-cradle will relieve the weight of the bedclothes from the feet and legs and assist in the prevention of foot-drop.

3 Friction can be avoided by care with lifting and bedmaking, ensuring that the drawsheet is pulled taut and that toys, hair grips and crumbs are removed from the bed. Nurses should not wear watches and rings for any nursing procedures. Scratches made by these or long finger nails encourage breakdown of the skin.

4 Children who are incontinent require frequent washing and drying which deprive the skin of its normal oily protection. This should be replaced by massaging a small quantity of silicone or zinc and castor oil cream into the skin of the back and buttocks, twice a day.

Relief of Pain

Infants and young children are able to withstand some stressful situations which an adult finds intolerable. The absence of anxiety about themselves usually causes children to relax, thus reducing muscular pain and tension which are common in older children and adults. This does not suggest that children are without feeling, and every effort should be made to recognize a child's need for active relief of pain with analgesics. Discomfort due to constipation, a full bladder, an empty stomach, and excessive heat or chilling, should be similarly anticipated and relieved.

RELIEF OF LOCAL PAIN AND DISCOMFORT
Local application of cold, heat, and medicaments may be used to give relief of local symptoms.

COLD
When a cold object is applied to the skin, the superficial blood vessels respond by constricting. Application of cold may, therefore, be used for the following reasons:
  i To reduce congestion as in headache;
  ii To reduce swelling and tension due to extravasation of fluid, as in non-bacterial inflammation such as sprains and injuries to joints;
  iii To control capillary bleeding as in epistaxis and following dental surgery.

1 COLD COMPRESS
This may take the form of a double fold of old linen which is wrung out in iced water and applied to the affected area, for example, the forehead in headache.

To be effective, frequent renewal is necessary. Similarly, equal parts of water and methylated spirit or lead lotion (lotio plumbi) may be used to reduce the swelling and tension of sprains and other joint injuries.

2   ICE POULTICE

Proprietary packs of chemicals, 'dry ice', are available for applying cold to an area of the body. These are frozen in the ice box of a refrigerator and used as instructed by the manufacturer. The more traditional ice poultice may still be used with small chippings of ice contained in a small lint-lined plastic bag. The air is pressed out of the bag as the opening is sealed. If only a small poultice is required to control dental bleeding, the ice chippings may be conveniently contained in a finger cot.

HEAT

Local heat is applied to encourage local vasodilatation, thus increasing the blood supply to an area (hyperaemia), for the relief of pain and to localize suppuration.

Kaolin (Antiphlogistine) Poultice

Kaolin is a mixture of medicated clay and volatile oils which readily retains heat. For prolonged use it is changed every four to six hours.

REQUIREMENTS

Tin of kaolin.
Saucepan containing water.
Palette knife or metal spatula.
Poultice board.
Old linen or lint.
Gauze.
Cotton wool.
Bandage.
Scissors.
Warmed plates.

METHOD

The lid of the tin containing kaolin is loosened and the contents heated in a saucepan of boiling water. The clay is stirred with a metal spatula or palette knife so that it is heated evenly throughout. Care must be taken to ensure that the boiling water does not spill over into the tin of kaolin.

The old linen or lint is cut to the appropriate size and the heated kaolin is spread evenly to a depth of 1cm, leaving a margin of 2cm or so around the edge. A single layer of gauze is placed over the surface.

The poultice is placed flat between two warmed plates and taken to the child's bedside. The nurse checks the temperature of the poultice by placing it on her forearm and if it is not too hot, it is placed over the affected area and covered with a piece of cotton wool cut slightly larger than the poultice, and lightly bandaged in position.

Warmed olive oil may be used to clean the skin of dried kaolin when the poultice is removed.

MEDICAMENTS

Glycerin ichthammol is a mild antiseptic ointment used to relieve local inflammation, such as phlebitis, following intravenous therapy. The ointment is spread onto a piece of old linen or lint, using a spatula, and the application is placed over the affected area. Additional pieces of old linen or a layer of wool ensure that the substance does not stain the child's bed or personal clothing. The application is held in position with a cotton bandage or Netelast.

Rest and Sleep

The ward routine should allow ample time for rest and sleep, alternating with periods of activity and exercise. Younger children need ten to twelve hours of sleep at night as well as short naps during the morning and after lunch. Older children need less sleep during the night, but will usually fall asleep after lunch if given a peaceful and quiet environment. Nursing care and treatment should be organized so that long periods for undisturbed rest and sleep follow a period of intensive nursing care and treatment. An adequate fluid intake during the day avoids the necessity to wake a child at frequent intervals during the night. Essential care and treatment can usually be reduced to four hourly during the night unless the child is receiving intensive care.

At no other time does a small child miss his mother more than he does at 'tucking-up' time. Older children, too, like mother to be there to read a bedtime story or to listen to their prayers. In the absence of the mother, the nurse must take her place.

Most small children will fall asleep quite quickly after a long period of wakefulness. Following a wash and change, a warm drink and a cuddle, a toddler should be tucked up warmly and securely in his cot with his favourite toy within reach. If he should wake during the night, a change of napkin, a warm drink and a cuddle will usually suffice. A dose of chloral hydrate is no substitute for fulfilment of his physical and emotional needs, but if a small child is wakeful and fractious, the doctor may prescribe a sedative to encourage a normal rhythm of sleep. Unless uncomfortably wet, cold, hot, hungry or in pain, most small children are oblivious to noise once they have settled to sleep. Subdued lighting ensures that the children can be observed.

If settled too early in the evening, older children become restless and resentful.

Provided that the ill children are given opportunity for long hours of peaceful sleep, those who are not so ill appreciate time to watch television after the toddlers have gone to sleep. Children who are up and about can then visit the toilet and have a wash and clean their teeth after having their last warm drink. They, too, like to be tucked up with a little individual chat before settling down for the night. For those children confined to bed, a bedpan or urinal is given and the child is washed, his teeth cleaned and his hair brushed before being settled for the night. It should be ensured that he is comfortable in his bed. The pillows are 'puffed up', the drawsheet straightened and the bed freed from crumbs and toys. Rarely is a sedative necessary to encourage sleep.

For rest-time to prove beneficial, a calm ward atmosphere with minimal distraction is essential. If all the children are made to lie on their beds for an hour or so with a book, this gives opportunity for the small and ill children to go to sleep. During this time, those children admitted to hospital for treatment of a psychiatric disorder or for investigation may be given opportunity to vent their boisterous nature in a game of football outside.

Exercise

The physical complications of confinement to bed seen in adult patients are rarely seen in childhood, as only the extremely ill, unconscious and immobilized children remain still for any length of time. Boredom and frustration are likely when a child is deprived of exercise, and a child who has to spend a long time in bed needs to be occupied. Provided the ward is warm, an infant can be left free from restrictive bedclothes. Similarly, a toddler can exercise his body within the confines of his cot or a play-pen, and out in the open ward or a playroom while under constant supervision. Older children may need some encouragement to move, particularly following an abdominal operation, but early ambulation creates few problems in a paediatric unit. Provided that the children are suitably dressed, exercise in the fresh air is of benefit to most and essential for the more boisterous, physically fit children.

Remedial and preventive passive and active exercises are given by the physio-therapist and are discussed on page 406.

Protection

1   From infection (Chapter 8).
2   From injury.
Each year, substantial amounts of public money are claimed as compensation for an injury sustained during a stay in hospital. The care of a small child lacking in a sense of danger puts a big responsibility on the parents and an even bigger responsibility on those who have the care of other people's children.

The unpredictable behaviour of the young demands the presence of two nurses for all procedures carried out by the nursing staff, and errors related to the calculation and administration of the correct drug dosage are reduced if two nurses check and give all drugs.

As mentioned in the previous chapter, children should be allowed to be up and about whenever possible, rather than confined to bed. This places an increased responsibility on the ward team and emphasizes again the necessity for organized play activities in a play area in the ward. Each child should remain within the sight of a member of the staff at all times. To wander, apparently aimlessly, from one locker to another is the lot of many an adventurous toddler deprived of proper stimulation.

Accidental injury must be prevented at all costs, and a children's unit should be designed with the safety of the children in mind. Nothing should be left to chance, as little is beyond the scope of an adventurous toddler or a bored older child. All windows should be guarded and all doors giving access to stairs, fire escapes and balconies secured with high level locks or bolts. Similarly, the doors to rooms containing sterilizers and other potentially dangerous equipment should be kept closed when occupied, and locked when not in use. Doors designed to swing either way avoid the risk of pushing a door into the path of an oncoming child, and a glass panel allows the nurse to see that the path is clear before she opens the door. Radiators should be guarded to protect exploring fingers from burns.

Equipment left around the ward provides a new venture demanding exploration. Special care is necessary with electrical equipment and flexes should be short and unobtrusive. Drug cupboards should be kept locked, and all drugs—lotions, medicines and reagents—kept in their appropriate cupboards and not left out in the ward or annexes. Hot-water taps should be out of reach or controlled by a removable key.

Crockery should be of the unbreakable, non-chip variety to protect the child against sharp edges. Drinks and food should not be served to small children until they are of a suitable temperature to drink and eat. A hot plate could also cause an unnecessary injury, and knives and forks prove dangerous in the wrong hands. Food and sweets should be excluded from the children's lockers to prevent a child awaiting surgery being tempted, or tempting others, to indulge.

To avoid the risk of suffocation, thin plastic sheeting and bags should be excluded from paediatric units. The use of soft pillows should be confined to the older age group for the same reason. Safety-pins, hot-water bottles and other potentially dangerous objects should be treated with the respect they deserve.

Falls are reduced to a minimum if the floor is covered with a washable rather than a polished smooth surface, and if the children are dressed in clothes suitable for play and not long nightdresses and dressing gowns. Ill-fitting shoes and slippers also cause unnecessary clumsiness. A protective helmet, made-to-measure, may be worn by an epileptic or unsteady child to protect his head during a fall. The ward staff should take care that they do not trip on toys left around the floor.

Having freed the ward of all possible hazards and provided facilities for play, few children need punishment for misdeeds. Verbal correction is all that is necessary, and smacking children is strictly forbidden.

Should an accident involve one of the children, then this must be reported immediately and all the details recorded in writing. The child should be examined by the doctor and the necessary investigations and treatment carried out without delay. However trivial the nature of the accident, the parents should be told about it when they next visit.

The greatest responsibility related to the care of small children confined to bed is ensuring that the cot-sides are used correctly. Cot-sides are designed with the vertical bars close to prevent the child trapping his head or an extremity, and of adequate height to prevent him falling over the top. A stack of pillows, cot-tray or locker positioned by the cot-side reduces this height and increases the risk of injury from a fall.

It is imperative that cot-sides are not inadvertently left down, leaving the unattended child at grave risk. Most cot-sides have a locking device which should be secured into position each time the cot-side is put up. Unless two people are available for cot-making, the small child is best lifted from his cot. If this is not possible, then only one cot-side should be let down at any one time.

Diversional therapy is preferable to any form of restraint, but restrainers may have to be used when there is no other method of controlling the child while undergoing some form of treatment or investigation, or as a protective measure to prevent him injuring himself. Restrainers should never be used as a routine measure, and should only be used as the result of a deliberate decision of the ward sister, her deputy or a member of the medical staff who has been delegated this responsibility.*

BODY RESTRAINT

Improvised body restraint must never be used, e.g. a harness made from bandages. The restrainer should consist of a close-fitting bodice which fastens down the back and should be put on as part of the routine dressing procedure. Ties made of webbing or similar strong material attached to each side of the lower edge of the bodice are then secured to the cot-frame and underneath the mattress.

LOCAL RESTRAINT

Unless a child is able to understand that he must not, for example, remove his naso-gastric tube or scratch his eczematous skin, he must be restrained from the temptation.

Arm and hand restraint can be achieved in various ways, but the principles involved are common to all methods. Time and care are essential to ensure:

* Appendix to H.M. (66) 11 *Use of Restrainers for Children Nursed in Hospital.*

i   that all forms of restraint achieve their aim;

ii that unnecessary annoyance to the child is reduced to a minimum. Often restraint need only be worn at night when the child subconsciously interferes;

iii that all forms of restraint should be removed at least twice daily for inspection and cleansing of the area, and to exercise the limb while under supervision.

Elbow restraint. The extended elbows may be splinted as follows:

1   With protective padding and bandages. This method is suitable only for very small infants.

2   Wooden spatulae inserted into the slots in the sleeves of a well-fitting, purpose-made jacket.

3   Perspex cylinders secured to a specially designed jacket.

4   With plaster of Paris cylinders.

Elbow restraint allows the otherwise active child free movement of his hands, but inhibits interference with the face, scalp and neck. This method of restraint is ideal for children with a naso-gastric tube or scalp vein infusion in position, and following surgery to the lip and palate.

Hand restraint. On infrequent occasions it may be necessary to secure the child's hands away from the lower part of the body. If a small child has an intravenous infusion running into a vein in one arm, the opposite hand must often be restrained. For the child with exposed burns of the chest and abdomen, all four limbs may require restraint.

Hand restraint may be achieved as follows:

1   With protective padding and bandages. Clove hitch restraint is both simple and practical. Protective padding is applied to the wrist and a clove hitch is made over the padding. The ends of the bandage are then tied to an immovable horizontal bar of the cot. No other knot should be used as tension will cause tightening (FIG. 20).

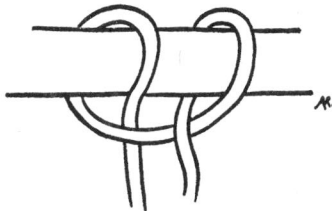

FIG. 20. Clove hitch for restraint.

2   Using Tubegauz. A short length of narrow Tubegauz is slipped over the wrist. A length of narrow adhesive tape is placed around the wrist over one end of the tubular bandage, and the length is drawn over the hand and secured to an immobile horizontal bar of the cot, allowing for a certain amount of freedom.

3   Using a specially designed wrist restrainer (FIG. 21).
4   Using cotton mittens. Cotton mittens may be made from two layers of Tubegauz secured at the wrist. Their use is confined to the younger age group and is not without its dangers (page 39).

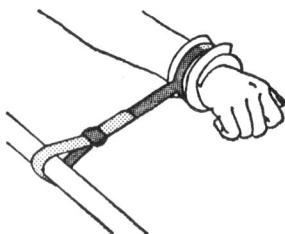

FIG. 21. Hand restraint using an Ace Limb Holder (Bacton, Dickinson U.K. Ltd.)

Leg restraint. One or both legs may have to be restrained for procedures associated with the lower half of the body. Leg restraint can be satisfactorily achieved using clove hitch or Tubegauz restraint as described above.

Nourishment

Meals in hospital follow the same pattern as those at home; the daily energy requirements being divided between three meals and one or two snacks, avoiding too long or too short a gap between any two of them. An adequate fluid intake must also be ensured:

	Toddlers	*Older Children*
06.30		A drink on waking
08.00	Breakfast	
10.00		A drink and biscuit
12.00		Dinner
14.00		A drink and fruit and/or sweets
17.00	Tea	Light tea
18.30	A bed-time drink	Supper
20.00		A bed-time drink

The content of meals and special diets is discussed in Chapter 10.

After visiting the lavatory and washing their hands, those children who are not confined to bed should be seated at a small table for their meals. All but the older children will need their food cut into small pieces, as few children are capable of manipulating a knife and fork for this purpose.

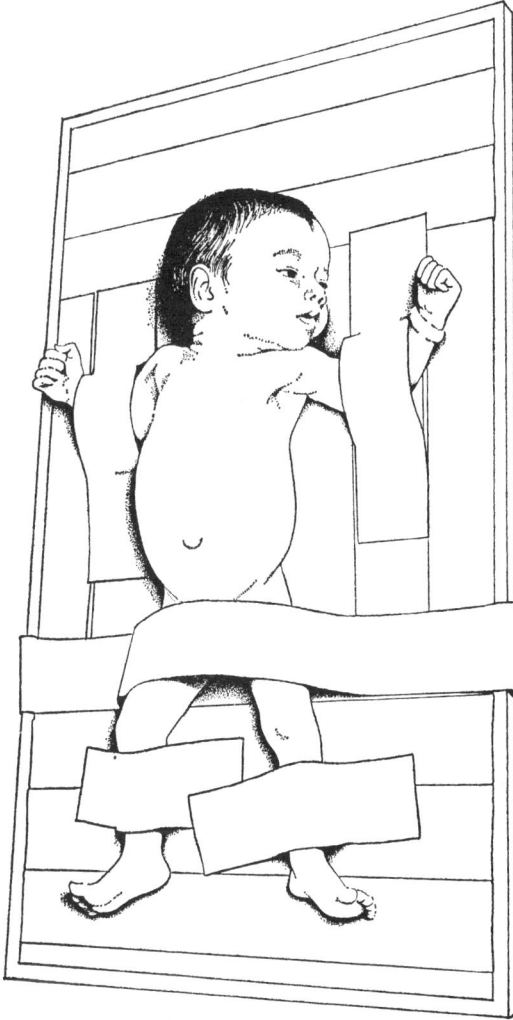

FIG. 22. Infant immobilizing board. (By kind permission of Down Bros. and Mayer and Phelps Ltd.)

Prior to each main meal, those children who are confined to bed should be offered a bedpan or urinal, or changed, their hands washed and toys put away. A bed-table or cot-tray is placed in position in front of an older child who is first made comfortable in a sitting position. A bib is fastened around the neck of a small child before he is seated on the nurse's knees or in a small chair with a tray attachment.

Immobilized and paralyzed children and those nursed at complete rest have to be fed while in their beds. The bedclothes are protected with a serviette before the nurse makes herself comfortable at the child's bedside to feed him from a spoon or fork. Fluids may be given through a Flexi-straw or from a teaspoon as few children find drinking from a feeding cup easy. Before leaving her patient, the nurse should ensure that all food and fluid have been swallowed.

Nutrition may have to be sustained by artificial means. The choice of method depends essentially on the disability to be overcome.

Artificial or Tube Feeding

INDICATIONS FOR ARTIFICIAL FEEDING
1   If the child is too immature, weak, ill or dyspnoeic to feed.
2   The unconscious child.
3   If difficulty is experienced with oral feeding due to gross mental retardation, micrognathia or inco-ordination of swallowing.
4   Refusal to eat—a very rare situation in childhood, but seen in anorexia nervosa in an older child.
5   To improve the kilocalorie and protein intake of a child experiencing difficulty in taking essential requirements.

METHODS USED IN ARTIFICIAL FEEDING
1   Intermittent feeding via an indwelling naso-gastric tube.
2   Continuous feeding via an indwelling naso-gastric tube.
3   Passage of an oro-gastric tube for each feed.
4   By gastrostomy tube.

GENERAL PRINCIPLES APPLIED TO ALL METHODS OF TUBE FEEDING
1   Only liquid or homogenized foods can be used.
2   When artificial feeding is prolonged, the content of the feed must meet the energy and fluid needs of the child.
3   An accurate fluid balance record is maintained.
4   The feed is given at body temperature and prepared at 38°C or 100°F.
5   Sterilized equipment is used for an infant. Clean equipment used for children is sterilized after use.
6   The feed is administered by gravity from a cylindrical funnel. Indiscriminate use of positive pressure created by a syringe can result in a powerful jet of fluid being directed through a fine tube on to the lining of the stomach, causing damage and subsequent ulceration. The method is therefore not recommended unless in experienced hands.
7   Care of the mouth is of utmost importance.
8   Medicines are given at the same time as the feed—usually beforehand, but this depends on the nature of the drug.
9   To prevent unnecessary disturbance of the child when the stomach is full, all nursing attention such as napkin changing, changing of position and oral toilet is carried out prior to feeding.

10   If the child is conscious, the meal is made to look and smell as appetizing as possible, thus encouraging the flow of digestive juices.

Naso-Gastric Intubation

This is a clean procedure using sterilized equipment for an infant.

REQUIREMENTS
Tray.
Pre-sterilized feeding tube:
   size 3·5, 6 or 9 F.G. (0, 2 or 4 E.G.) (infants)
   Levin's or Ryle's tube size 9–15 F.G. (4–8 E.G.) (children).
5ml syringe.
Spigot.
Blue litmus paper.
Container of warmed boiled water.
Non-allergic adhesive tape to secure tube in position.
Scissors.
Infant's teat in container.
Cotton wool balls for cleansing the nostrils.
Wrapping blanket.
Bib.

PREPARATION OF THE CHILD
A conscious child is told about the procedure and his co-operation sought. A small child is restrained in a wrapping blanket and supported on the nurse's knees. An unconscious child is placed in the lateral position with the head slightly raised The nurse washes and dries her hands.

METHOD
The nostrils are inspected and cleansed with small moistened pieces of cotton wool twisted into pledgets. The nostrils are used alternately when re-intubation is necessary.

The length of tube to be passed is estimated by measuring from the xiphisternum to the bridge of the nose and 6cm (2½ inches) added. The child should be lying down for this estimation to be accurate. An infant is then restrained in a treatment blanket and may be given an occluded sterile teat to suck to enable easier passage of the tube.

The end of the tube is moistened with water and passed along the floor of the nostril in a backwards and downwards direction into the pharynx. Oily lubricants are avoided in childhood as their inhalation could result in lipoid pneumonia. A co-operative, conscious child is asked to swallow at this point. The tube is advanced slowly and gently until the estimated required length of the tube is introduced. Should the child become cyanosed, the tube is withdrawn immediately. It is essential to localize the position of the end of the tube before any fluid is injected into its lumen. This is done by carrying out one or more of the following tests.

1   A syringe is attached to the tube and gentle negative pressure applied to withdraw a few millilitres of gastric fluid. If no fluid is withdrawn, the tube is passed a little further and aspiration repeated. If the end of the tube is in the stomach, the acid fluid aspirated will convert blue litmus paper to pink.

2   If there is still no aspirate, a little air is injected down the tube while the nurse listens for its entry into the stomach by holding the end of the stethoscope just below the xiphisternum.

3   A fine tube may become coiled in the pharynx. Examination of the mouth and throat with a good light will exclude this possibility.

4   If the free end of the tube is held under water and water is seen to flow into the tube on inspiration, or air bubbles through the water on expiration, the tube is in the air-passages and must be removed immediately. When satisfied that the end of the tube is in the stomach, the tube is attached to an immobile part of the face, avoiding placing the non-allergic adhesive tape too near the eyes or nostrils. A spigot is inserted to close the end of the tube.

The same fine polyvinyl or plastic naso-gastric tube can be left in position for one to two weeks without causing undue discomfort or irritation. Restraint of a small child and infant is essential. Frequent passage of a naso-gastric tube is not advisable and can be avoided if care is taken to ensure adequate splintage of the arms.

The normal secretions of the respiratory tract are swallowed during childhood as small children are unable to expectorate. Irritating secretions may be so excessive in inflammatory conditions of the respiratory tract as to cause gastritis and vomiting. Before naso-gastric tube feeding is instituted, these secretions should be removed by irrigating the stomach,via the feeding tube, using a syringe and a small quantity of boiled water.

Intermittent Feeding via an Indwelling Naso-Gastric Tube

REQUIREMENTS
Tray.
Container with warmed feed—temperature 38°C (100°F).
Food thermometer.
Measure containing 30ml warm boiled water.
5ml syringe.
Blue litmus paper.
Cylindrical funnel, length of tubing and graduated connection.
1 pair clip forceps.

Additional requirements:
Wrapping blanket (for infant).
Bib *or* serviette.
Tray of equipment for mouth care.

PREPARATION OF THE CHILD

Oral toilet is carried out. An infant's napkin is changed and an older child is made comfortable by offering a bedpan and changing his position in bed. Whenever possible, an infant should be warmly wrapped in a blanket and cuddled on the nurse's knees while being fed.

Immediately prior to feeding, the nurse washes and dries her hands.

METHOD

The spigot closing the naso-gastric tube is removed, the syringe attached and gentle negative pressure applied to withdraw a few millilitres of the gastric contents for litmus testing. This is a check to ensure that the end of the tube is still in the stomach and that the previous feed has passed into the duodenum. Any medicines are syringed slowly into the tube, followed immediately by the feed.

The temperature is checked by reading the food thermometer while it is still in the feed. Clip forceps are attached to the lower end of the tubing and the funnel is filled with feed. Air is expelled from the apparatus by releasing the clip and allowing some of the feed to return to the container. The flow of feed is interrupted by attaching the clip forceps and the graduated connection is then inserted into the feeding tube, the clip forceps released and the feed allowed to flow by gravity. The cylindrical funnel is held at an appropriate level to allow the feed to be administered over the following ten minutes. The contents of the funnel are replenished as necessary with the remainder of the feed which is left warming on the tray. When the feed reaches the junction of the funnel with the tubing, boiled water is added to clear the naso-gastric tube and to ensure that the feed is not retained in the tube; 1–5ml is sufficient in infancy and up to 30ml may be used in the older age groups. The graduated connection is disconnected from the feeding tube and the spigot inserted.

Unnecessary movement of the child is avoided. An infant is gently placed on his side in his cot and left undisturbed for at least half-an-hour.

The amount of fluid given is recorded on the fluid balance chart.

The equipment is rinsed in cold water, washed, rinsed and completely submerged in Milton 1:80, or boiled prior to re-use.

Continuous Gastric Infusion

If tolerance to intermittent naso-gastric tube feeding is poor, the fluid and energy requirement of the child may be administered by slowly dripping the feed into the stomach. This method may also be used to increase the daily intake of a child during the hours of sleep, when his intake would otherwise not meet his bodily demands.

REQUIREMENTS
As for naso-gastric intubation, and
Reservoir for feed
  i   Cylindrical funnel or
  ii glass infusion bottle and clip, rubber bung and 2 glass tubes—1 short, 1 long.
2 short lengths of tubing.
1 drip chamber.
1 graduated connection.
1 flow regulator.
Safety-pin.

Additional requirements:
  Infusion stand.

METHOD
The naso-gastric tube is passed as for naso-gastric intubation and the aspirate checked for acidity.

The apparatus is assembled, the reservoir suspended 30cm (12 inches) above the child's head and the air displaced by feed. The spigot closing ̦the naso-gastric tube is removed and the apparatus connected. The flow regulator is adjusted to allow the feed to drip slowly into the stomach. Drag on the tubing is prevented by using the safety-pin to secure the bed linen around the tubing.

Over-distension of the stomach and subsequent aspiration of the feed must be prevented at all costs. The reservoir should never contain a greater volume than the child's stomach will safely hold and the child should be kept under constant observation.

The apparatus is rinsed, washed and re-sterilized after each feed.

Intermittent Oro-Gastric Feeding

With the introduction of safe, non-irritating polyvinyl and plastic oesophageal tubes, intermittent passage of a tube for feeding purposes is now the exception rather than the rule. However, it is still the method of choice when it is considered unsafe to leave a naso-gastric tube in position or when regular artificial feeding is not necessary.

REQUIREMENTS
As for naso-gastric intubation and intermittent naso-gastric feeding.

As the tube is passed through the mouth, a larger tube of size 9–18 F.G. (4–10 E.G.) is required.

METHOD

The procedure is essentially as for naso-gastric intubation and feeding, with the following amendments.

The length of tube to be passed is measured from the xiphisternum to the bridge of the nose. As the tube is passed through the mouth, the additional 6cm (2½ inches) is not needed.

To pass the tube, the end is moistened and placed on the infant's tongue. While the infant sucks the tube, the nurse directs it firmly along the floor of the mouth into the oro-pharynx and advances it slowly and gently into the oeso-phagus and stomach for the assessed length. Retching can be reduced by the assisting nurse supporting the child's chin. The position of the tube is checked by testing a few millilitres of the aspirate with litmus paper and the tube is then held in position near the child's lips.

The procedure is continued as for naso-gastric feeding.

At the end of the feed, the tube is pinched firmly, while being withdrawn in one steady pull, to prevent fluid in the tube from being aspirated into the lungs.

Gastrostomy Feeding

A gastrostomy is an opening into the stomach through the abdominal wall, into which a self-retaining or Jacques catheter is inserted for 5 to 8cm (2–3 inches) and firmly secured with lengths of adhesive tape. It is imperative that the tube remains in the correct position. Should the tube come out, closure of the opening is rapid, making re-intubation difficult. If the tube is inserted too far, it may pass through the pyloric sphincter into the duodenum, or cause perforation of the stomach.

INDICATIONS FOR USE

1   For infants with oesophageal atresia requiring a temporary gastrostomy for feeding purposes, when the distance between the two ends of the oesophagus is too great to allow a primary anastamosis to be performed. The upper end of the oesophagus is brought onto the skin surface of the neck (oesophagostomy) to allow free drainage of swallowed saliva, oral fluids and weaning diet.

2   For children with an oesophageal stricture, due to ingestion of corrosive solution or fibrosis of an anastomosis.

3   For infants requiring prolonged artificial feeding. Prolonged naso-gastric intubation encourages incompetence of the cardiac sphincter muscle and ulcera-tion of the passage taken by the tube.

REQUIREMENTS

Tray.
Receiver to collect gastric residue.
10ml syringe to measure residue.

Cylindrical funnel, length of tubing and graduated connection.
Container with warmed feed—38°C (100°F).
Food thermometer.
Clip forceps.
Medicine glass containing 30ml boiled water.
Protection for the bed.

METHOD
The child is made comfortable in bed or sitting on a chair. An older child often enjoys assisting with his own feeding.

An infant would be changed and made comfortable to avoid too much movement after the feed has been given. If he is well enough, he may be wrapped in a blanket and sat on the nurse's knees while she gives him his feed. If the infant is to have a small quantity of fluid and diet by mouth, this may be given at the same time as the feed is given by the gastrostomy route. Oral 'feeding' will give the infant some satisfaction, as well as encourage natural cleansing of the mouth, stimulation of gastric juices and normal eating habits. A gallipot, or small receiver, is used to collect this 'feed'.

The dressing is checked to see that there is no leakage and that the tube is in position. The receiver is placed under the end of the gastrostomy tube and the spigot is removed. The gastric residue will drain into the receiver. This should be minimal in amount and will indicate that the tube is in the stomach and that the previous feed has been absorbed. Should the residue contain bile, duodenal intubation should be suspected and the matter reported. It may be necessary to measure and replace the residue.

The temperature of the feed is checked. The clip forceps are attached to the lower end of the tubing and the funnel is half-filled with feed. Air is expelled from the apparatus by releasing the clip and allowing some of the feed to run through into the container. The flow of feed is interrupted by attaching the clip forceps and the graduated connection is inserted into the open end of the gastrostomy tube. Any medicines are poured into the funnel at this stage. The funnel is held or secured at a height to allow the feed to run in slowly over the following ten minutes, the contents of the funnel being replenished with the remainder of the feed which is left warming. As crying and restlessness cause an increase in the intra-abdominal pressure, the feed will be forced back into the funnel. It is, therefore, advisable that the funnel is at no time more than half-full.

When all the feed has left the funnel, the tube is cleansed with a small quantity of boiled water. The tube is kinked, the connection removed and the spigot is securely replaced. Alternatively, the gastrostomy tube is left open to allow reflux of the gastric contents into the funnel and tubing which is secured 10cm or 4 inches above the infant's abdomen.

The dressing is re-checked, the tube and spigot tucked out of reach, and the infant made comfortable in bed.

CHANGING A GASTROSTOMY TUBE

A non-irritating polyvinyl, self-retaining balloon or Malecot catheter, or a Jacques catheter may be changed every two to three weeks as requested by the doctor. Rubber catheters require changing every forty-eight hours.

This procedure may be carried out by the doctor or by a member of the nursing staff just before the child is due to have a feed.

The balloon of a catheter is deflated and the gastrostomy tube withdrawn. This is quickly replaced by inserting the tip of the new catheter to 2·5–5cm (1–2 inches) beyond the last aperture or balloon bag, depending on the nature of the catheter and the size of the child. A balloon catheter is then inflated and the introducer of a Malecot catheter is withdrawn.

The catheter is secured firmly into position with lengths of narrow adhesive tape applied around the catheter and crossed over the abdominal wall.

Cleanliness

Most authorities ask that the child brings his own toilet requirements into hospital. Deficiencies should be made good from ward stock. Each child's locker should contain:

Toilet soap—preferably in a dish.
2 flannels—1 face, 1 body.
2 towels—1 face, 1 bath.
Tooth brush and paste.
Hair brush and comb.
Talcum powder and/or barrier cream.
Bath blanket—if confined to bed.

Care of the Skin

A daily bath is not only customary, but usually necessary for most children confined to hospital. This is given at any time during the day, with a preference for early morning for ill children confined to bed, and evening for children who are up for most of the day. The hands and face require a wash on waking and before going to bed, and the hands should be washed before meals and after visiting the lavatory or using a bedpan. The buttocks, external genitalia and groins of incontinent bigger children, toddlers and infants require washing at each change.

The child may be taken to the wash basin in the bathroom or have his wash while in bed. Supervision of all but the older child is essential.

Bathing in the Bathroom

Most children like having a bath, especially if given time to play in the water. To a few children a bath is a novelty and they may be somewhat apprehensive of the depth of water.

PREPARATION OF THE CHILD

The child is encouraged to visit the lavatory before having a bath. His toilet requirements are collected from his locker and taken to the bathroom and he is undressed as the bath water is run. His face is washed and dried at the wash basin.

METHOD

The bathroom windows are closed and the bath checked for cleanliness.

Cold water is run into the bath first, then hot water, mixing it to a temperature of 40°C or 105°F and to a suitable depth for the child. A bath thermometer is essential. Both taps are turned off before the child is gently lowered into the water with his back to the taps. When he has been washed and rinsed all over, a small child is lifted on to a raised, protected surface, or on to the nurse's protected knees. A bigger child stands on a bath mat. The child is wrapped in his bath towel while the whole body is dried. Special care is necessary to ensure that the axillae, groins, anal cleft and areas between the fingers and toes are thoroughly dry. A sprinkling of talcum powder is used, if desired, and the child dressed.

A small child should never be left in the bathroom alone and no child should be left with the bath ready for use. If the nurse is called away, she must find a substitute to stay in the bathroom, or take the child with her.

To avoid chilling, the child should return to the warm environment of the ward for the next half-an-hour. The bath is cleaned, the bathroom windows opened and the child's personal belongings are replaced in his locker. His wet bath towel is dried before folding and his flannels are best left exposed to dry in the air.

Bathing in Bed

If a child is unable to go to the bathroom for his bath, a bed bath is necessary. The procedure described below outlines the basic principles of this procedure. Modification is necessary to meet the needs of active toddlers and small infants. If the child is very ill, or a big child, two nurses are necessary for this procedure— one to wash and the other to dry and support the child.

REQUIREMENTS

In addition to the child's personal belongings listed above, the following are taken to his bedside:
Washing bowl of hand hot water.
Tooth beaker and receiver.
Clean bed linen.

Clean personal linen.
Soiled linen carrier.
All requirements for the procedure are placed either on a cleared locker-top, or on a small trolley.

PREPARATION OF THE CHILD
The child is prepared for the procedure in privacy, and the windows are closed. An opportunity is given for him to use a bedpan or urinal. The top bedclothes are stripped onto a chair, leaving him covered with the bath blanket. If possible, extra pillows are removed and the child is placed in a semi-recumbent position. Dyspnoeic children are left in an upright position and the procedure is modified to meet their particular need. The child is then undressed and his clothes are placed on the foot of the bed, or in the soiled linen carrier.

METHOD
Plenty of hand hot water is necessary, and changed whenever it becomes cool, soiled or excessively soapy. Chilling is avoided by exposing one small area at a time.

The face towel is placed under the chin and the face, neck and ears are washed and dried. Most children dislike having their faces washed with soap and this is best avoided.

The bath towel is placed under each arm in turn and the hands and arms are washed with a well soaped flannel, rinsed and dried.

The bath blanket is then folded to the level of the umbilicus to allow the exposed chest and axillae to be washed, rinsed and thoroughly dried. The chest is covered with the face towel and the abdomen and groins are exposed by folding down the bath blanket. Using the body flannel, the abdomen, groins and external genitalia are washed, rinsed and dried. The child is covered with the bath blanket while the water is changed. Protecting the bed with the large bath towel and exposing and elevating each leg and foot in turn, the extremities are washed, rinsed and dried. Great care is needed to dry the skin between the toes. The child is turned to one side and his back and buttocks are washed, rinsed and dried. The anal area is washed, rinsed and thoroughly dried. Talcum powder is applied to the skin of the back and barrier cream is applied to the buttocks if necessary. The bottom sheet and drawsheet are straightened or replaced by clean linen. The child is then turned on to his back and the bottom sheet and drawsheet are tucked in.

The bath completed, the child is dressed, finger and toe nails cut, the teeth brushed, and the hair combed into style.

The bath blanket is replaced by the top bedclothes, the pillows 'puffed up' and the child left comfortable and suitably occupied. His personal belongings are replaced in his locker and the communal equipment is cleaned and returned for further use.

Care of the Finger and Toe Nails

The finger and toe nails are trimmed and cleansed as necessary and the scissors disinfected after use. Each digit is held securely in one hand while the nail is trimmed—slightly rounded for finger nails and straight across for toe nails. To avoid accidents, the blades of the fine scissors should never be separated for a greater distance than is necessary. Trimmings should be carefully collected and disposed of.

The greatest care should be taken when cutting the nails of children with bleeding disorders.

Care of the Mouth

The healthy mouth is kept clean and fresh by:
   i   adequate nourishment to create healthy tissues;
  ii   an adequate fluid intake;
 iii   avoidance of excessive sugars;
  iv   mastication of hard foods;
   v   salivation;
  vi   cleaning the teeth at least twice daily;
 vii   regular visits to the dentist for check-ups.

ROUTINE CARE

The delicate lining of an infant's mouth will remain clean and moist without interference, provided the fluid intake is adequate.

Older children require tooth brush and paste for their twice daily oral toilet. The teeth should be cleaned using an up and down movement and instruction is given if the child is unfamiliar with the procedure. Small children need assistance and supervision to ensure that a correct technique is adopted.

If the child is not able to go to the bathroom, a beaker containing a mild antiseptic mouth-wash solution, such as Glycothymoline, and a receiver are taken to the bedside. The bed is protected with his face towel, and the child assisted with brushing his teeth and rinsing his mouth. Routine care should be given first thing in the morning and after all fluid and food have been given at night. To prevent dental caries, sweets are best avoided between meals.

Special Care of the Mouth

When it is impossible for the teeth to be cleaned in the usual way or when oral nourishment is not possible, the mouth needs special care to prevent infection and complications occurring.

As the result of ill health, the mouth becomes dry and unpleasant, resulting in a lack of appetite (anorexia) and a risk of infection. Special care of the mouth is carried out every three to four hours, usually when the patient is fed or when his four hourly observations are recorded.

Children at particular risk include those who are fed via the naso-gastric or parenteral routes, the unconscious, the debilitated and dyspnoeic children.

REQUIREMENTS

Tray
Sodium bicarbonate—1 teaspoon to 540ml.
Glycerine of thymol (Glycothymoline).
Glycerin.
White soft paraffin (White Vaseline).
Cotton wool balls.
Spencer Wells artery forceps.
Dissecting forceps.
Patient's face towel.
Receptacle for soiled swabs.

METHOD

The nurse washes and dries her hands. The bed is protected with the face towel, and a simple explanation is given. Following careful inspection, using a torch and spatula if necessary, the mouth is cleansed systematically, using cotton wool securely attached to clip forceps and each lotion in turn. To secure a piece of cotton wool onto clip forceps, the wool ball is unrolled and one end is placed between the partially separate serrated blades of the forceps. The wool is wrapped around the two blades and the free end is held between the two blades while the clip is closed. Care should be taken to see that the wool is securely attached to the forceps and that the pointed ends are adequately protected.

The swab is dipped into the lotion, making it moist. Excessive moisture may be inhaled; if insufficient moisture is used, wisps of cotton wool may be left on the rough, dry surface of an unhealthy tongue. Each swab is used once only, removed with dissecting forceps and placed in the receptacle for soiled swabs. The lotions are used as follows:

1 Sodium bicarbonate is effective for loosening mucus, but has an unpleasant taste not tolerated by young children and is best avoided.
2 Glycerin of thymol, a mild antiseptic, leaves a refreshing taste in the mouth.
3 Glycerin may be used on the tongue for its hygroscopic property.
4 Drying and cracking of the lips is prevented by smearing with a thin layer of white soft paraffin or other emollient.

A mouth-gag may be placed in position between the molar teeth of an unconscious child if the jaw is stiff, to allow for efficient oral care.

The individual tray should be renewed daily or more frequently as required.

For the special care of the mouth of an infant who is not fed orally, the tray should be prepared for each care, using sterile pre-packed cotton wool buds or other sterile soft material and boiled water.

Care of the Hair

Each child should have his own comb kept with his toilet requisites in his locker. The hair needs combing at least twice a day and long hair should be secured away from the face. Parental consent must be obtained before the hair is cut. Restless and febrile children nursed in the supine or recumbent position need special attention. More frequent combing is necessary, e.g. two hourly, to prevent the hair over the occipital region becoming tangled and matted.

Washing

Children confined to hospital for some weeks need to have their hair washed at weekly intervals. Most children can be taken to the bathroom for this purpose, but in some instances the requirements must be taken to the bedside and the hair washed with the child in bed. Adequate mackintosh protection for the child, the bed and the nurse is necessary. The hair should be rinsed well before being dried with a hair-drier.

Inspection of the Hair

On admission to hospital, and at regular intervals during a child's stay on the ward, the hair should be inspected for head lice or their eggs—nits. The infestation is the product of over-crowded, poor living conditions, but a child from the best of homes may have acquired the parasite.

REQUIREMENTS FOR INSPECTION
Tray
Medical wipes.
Bowl of mild antiseptic solution, e.g. aqueous solution of chlorhexidine 0·05%.
Receiver of disinfectant, e.g. aqueous solution of chlorhexidine 0·5%.
Child's own comb.
Tooth-comb.
Shoulder protection.

METHOD
Adequate privacy is afforded and a simple explanation is given to the child who may have experienced a similar inspection during a routine visit by the school nurse. The shoulders are protected. The scalp is inspected for scratches and sores, and the hair, particularly behind the ears and in the nape of the neck, is inspected for nits. The presence of glistening live nits near the scalp indicates

recent infestation. Empty shells appear dull and are further away from the scalp. Nits look not unlike dandruff, but can be readily distinguished by their resistance to removal.

To allow for easier combing, the tooth-comb is moistened with mild antiseptic solution and the hair combed systematically until the whole head has been inspected. In order to prevent scattering of the lice, each combing is collected into a medical wipe and inspected before submerging in the receiver containing disinfectant. On completion of the procedure, the combs are put to soak in disinfectant and any infestation is reported to sister.

Treatment of Infested Hair

REQUIREMENTS

As those listed above for inspection of the hair, together with
Insecticide:
  Lorexane 0·2% (I.C.I.) or
  Dicophane (D.D.T. Emulsion) 2%.

METHOD

The insecticide is diluted as required to give 30ml of the correct percentage concentration. A thin film is spread all over the hair, using medical wipes or cotton wool balls. The hair is left to dry. Covering the head is psychologically damaging and unnecessary. One treatment is usually sufficient as long as the hair is not washed for seven to ten days following application of Lorexane, or twenty-four hours following application of Dicophane.

Daily inspection using a fine tooth-comb is necessary to remove the recently hatched pediculi. Vinegar or 1% acetic acid will release the cement-like substance which secures the nits to the hair.

As infestation with lice is not usually confined to one member of the family, it is not sufficient to treat only the child. The public health department will co-operate to disinfest other members of the family, thus preventing re-infestation with each visit of the mother.

Excretion

Control of the bladder and bowel is achieved towards the middle of the second year of life when frequency and urgency of micturition are normal. Stressful situations cause regression to infantile behaviour, so that few small children confined to hospital can be relied on to stay dry and clean throughout the day and night.

A regular routine and good habits should be encouraged by offering toilet facilities at frequent, regular intervals, i.e. before and following meals and on waking and before going to bed. A small child should be sat on a warmed pot in a warm room, and an older child taken to or encouraged to visit the lavatory. For the children who are confined to bed, a pot, bedpan or urinal is taken to each child at these times and as requested between times. Accidental wetting or soiling of the bed cause considerable distress to an ill child and any request for a bedpan should be met without delay. Privacy should be afforded by the use of screens and the child should be supported in a suitable position to encourage elimination. It is frequently necessary for the nurse to stay with her patient while he uses a bedpan, and to cleanse the anal area following defaecation. The child is made comfortable and the covered bedpan is returned to the sluice for emptying, cleansing and disinfection. The nurse washes and dries her hands before attempting another job. If the child has attended to his own local toilet, his hands are washed and dried.

Constipation in childhood is usually due to poor bowel habits, but may be due to an insufficient fluid intake, anal pain or rectal paralysis. If aperients have failed to produce the necessary bowel action or are contra-indicated, a suppository or an enema may have to be given.

GENERAL PRINCIPLES APPLIED TO RECTAL PROCEDURES
1   Privacy should be afforded at all times.
2   A correct approach to the child is essential. A co-operative, relaxed child will feel some discomfort, but no actual pain, and of this he should be assured.
3   The presence of a second nurse is essential if the child is small, and desirable at other times.
4   Facilities for emptying the bladder should be offered before commencement.
5   The left lateral position, with the flexed lower limbs brought up to the chest and the buttocks drawn towards the edge of the mattress, is most convenient for rectal procedures. Waterproof protection is placed under the buttocks. The head is rested on one pillow, the top bedclothes are folded to the bottom of the bed and the child is protected with a treatment blanket, leaving only the anal area exposed.
6   A gloved finger, catheter or suppository require adequate lubrication with Vaseline or KY jelly prior to insertion into the rectum.
7   To avoid water intoxication, only isotonic solutions such as 0·9% sodium chloride are used for irrigation.
8   The solution is allowed to flow into the rectum by gravity, the funnel being raised or lowered to increase or decrease the rate of flow as necessary.
9   The solution is prepared at a temperature of 38°C or 100°F to be administered at body temperature.
10   Unless a retention enema has been administered, all solution used should be expelled or syphoned at the end of the procedure.
11   Inspection and recording of observations is important.

Suppositories

A suppository is a cone-shaped gelatinized preparation sometimes containing a medicament.

Reasons for giving a suppository:
1 To evacuate the bowel (glycerin and Dulcolax).
2 To administer a drug which is unpleasant to take orally (aminophylline).
3 In the relief of rectal or anal discomfort (Anusol).

REQUIREMENTS
Tray
Prescribed suppositories and prescription sheet.
Gallipot of warm water if they are glycerin.
Lubricant for other types.
Medical wipes.
Disposable glove.
Receptacle for used glove.

METHOD
The child is prepared and reassured as described in the preceding section. Using her gloved right hand, the nurse inserts the lubricated suppository through the anal sphincter to the length of her index finger. The anal area is cleansed and the glove and wipe are discarded. If there is a tendency for the suppository to be expelled, the buttocks may be held together for a few minutes. The child is left comfortable and occupied and reassured that a nurse is within his calling distance.

SPECIAL POINTS
Glycerin suppositories are lubricated by dipping the tip, only, in warm water. Their hygroscopic action proceeds as the gelatine melts and a bowel action can be expected twenty to thirty minutes later.

Dulcolax suppositories are potent and sometimes cause severe abdominal discomfort. Lubrication of the tip is necessary and the suppository is inserted so that it is in contact with the rectal mucosa. Local irritation produces additional mucus in the rectum and reflex evacuation of the bowel content five to ten minutes after insertion.

Suppositories containing drugs should not be rejected. Deep insertion is necessary and the child reassured that a bowel action is not necessary.

Enemas

An enema is an injection of fluid into the rectum for any of the following purposes:

1 CLEANSING
  i To evacuate the bowel
       soap and water (enema saponis).
       normal saline (simple enema).
       disposable chemical enema.
  ii To soften faeces
       olive oil;
       arachis oil.

2 THERAPEUTIC
  i To administer drugs
       basal anaesthesia
         thiopentone
         avertin.
       anti-inflammatory
         prednisone as Predsol.
  ii In the relief of intracranial pressure
       magnesium sulphate 25%.
  iii As a means of correcting mild dehydration
       0·9% sodium chloride.
  iv For the relief of abdominal distension
       oxbile
       turpentine.
  v In the hydrostatic reduction of intussusception
       barium sulphate.

3 DIAGNOSTIC
  To inject contrast medium prior to X-ray examination
  barium sulphate.

1 Evacuant Enemas

The administration of a traditional soap and water enema has been virtually superseded by the use of suppositories and disposable enemas.
  An evacuant enema may be used:
  i   in the relief of constipation;
  ii before giving a rectal or colonic washout;
  iii to empty the rectum prior to rectal examination, investigation or surgery.
  iv when rectal infusion is anticipated.

i Soap and water enema (enema saponis)

PRINCIPLE

The rectum is distended with 5% soap solution, causing reflex evacuation of the solid content of the bowel, together with the fluid. The quantity of fluid used is 30ml (1oz) per year of age.

REQUIREMENTS

Tray.

Measuring jug of solution—temperature 38°C or 100°F.

Lotion thermometer.

Funnel, length of tubing and connection.

Jacques catheter size 15–24 F.G. (8–14 E.G.)
    (size according to age).

Lubricant.

Medical wipes.

Waterproof protection for the bed.

Receptacle for soiled disposable equipment.

Receptacle for soiled non-disposable equipment.

Covered bedpan and toilet tissue.

METHOD

The child is reassured and prepared as described on page 124. The terminal 5–10cm (2–4 inches) of the catheter is lubricated and inserted 5–10cm through the anus into the rectum to release any flatus.

The temperature of the solution is checked by reading the lotion thermometer while it is still in the solution. The assembled apparatus is filled with the solution to displace the air, the tubing kinked and the connection inserted into the catheter. The solution is allowed to flow by gravity from the funnel into the rectum. As the fluid level falls, the funnel is replenished with a further supply from the jug until the full volume of solution has been given. Rapid administration will cause discomfort and distress and should be avoided.

The catheter is gently withdrawn through a medical wipe held over the anus and placed in the appropriate receptacle. The remaining apparatus is placed on the tray. The child is seated on a bedpan and supported in the sitting position to assist evacuation of the bowel content.

The anal area is cleansed with toilet tissue and the child is left comfortable and occupied in bed. A nurse should remain within calling distance, as frequently this procedure results in a desire to defaecate. If he is well enough, a visit to the lavatory may be sufficient to reassure the child, even if this is considered not to be necessary by the nurse.

The content of the bedpan is inspected before disposal and the result recorded. The catheter lumen is thoroughly cleansed by directing a jet of water through the eye and down the lumen prior to disinfection. The remaining apparatus is thoroughly washed and disinfected before re-use.

ii Simple enema

The requirements, preparation and procedure are as for a soap and water enema. 0·9% Sodium Chloride (one 5ml spoonful salt to 540ml water) is used instead of the 5% soap solution.

iii Disposable evacuant enema

PRINCIPLE
Up to 130ml of a hypertonic phosphate solution contained in a small plastic envelope is injected into the rectum through the ejecting nozzle. Irritation of the rectal mucosa promotes reflex evacuation of the bowel content. Its use is inadvisable for the younger age group. Up to 50% of the envelope content is used for a seven-year-old and 75% for a twelve-year-old child.

REQUIREMENTS
Tray.
Disposable enema.
Jug of warm water.
Lubricant.
Medical wipes.
Protection for the bed.
Receptacle for disposable articles.
Covered bedpan and toilet tissue.

METHOD
The child is reassured and positioned as described on page 124. The 'chill' is taken off the solution by standing the plastic envelope in a jug of warm water temperature 40°C or 105°F.

The instructions on the envelope should be read and understood. The cap is removed and the lubricated nozzle is gently inserted through the anal sphincter for 5–7cm or 2–3 inches. The plastic envelope is slowly rolled up to expel its content into the rectum, the nozzle is withdrawn and the envelope discarded.

Evacuation of the bowel content may be delayed for a few minutes. Further procedure and observation are as for soap and water enema.

2 Olive or Arachis Oil Enema

PRINCIPLE
Up to 180ml (60ml for three-year-old, 90ml for seven-year-old, 120ml for twelve-year-old) of warmed olive oil is slowly injected into the rectum, retained for

four to six hours and followed by a soap and water enema. It is used to soften the hard impacted faeces of severe constipation.

REQUIREMENTS
Tray.
Disposable pack
Funnel, tubing and connection.
Jug of warm water *or* Jug containing warm olive oil 37°C or 99°F.
Jacques catheter size 6 E.G. (12 F.G.).
Lubricant.
Medical wipes.
Protection for the bed.
Bed blocks.

METHOD
Preparation and reassurance of the child is as described on page 124. To facilitate retention, the foot of the bed is elevated on low bed blocks and the oil administered over a period of fifteen to twenty minutes. The catheter is then gently withdrawn.

The child remains in a supine or lateral position with suitable diversional therapy. It is sometimes more convenient to administer the oil last thing at night and the evacuant enema the following morning.

3. Retention Enema

i ANTI-INFLAMMATORY
Disposable packs containing 120–180ml of prednisone (Predsol) designed for self-administration by adults, lessen the local inflammatory process of ulcerative colitis. Warming the envelope is not desirable. It is usual to administer the enema slowly, immediately prior to bed-time so that retention is encouraged. This enema is a drug and therefore administered only on prescription by the medical staff.

ii MAGNESIUM SULPHATE ENEMA
The hygroscopic action of 25% magnesium sulphate is to draw water into the bowel. It is given to reduce intracranial pressure. The volume of fluid necessary is prescribed by the doctor. Retention for fifteen to thirty minutes is followed by evacuation of a watery stool. Its use has been virtually superseded by the use of intravenous mannitol 5%, 10%, 20% which increases the renal flow.

Manual Evacuation of Faeces

A rectal examination may confirm a diagnosis of faecal impaction which the doctor may require treated by manual evacuation. This procedure is used to relieve constipation in the paraplegic child with spina bifida.

Requirements are as for insertion of suppositories (page 125).

METHOD

The child is prepared and reassured as above. Using her gloved right hand, the nurse inserts her well-lubricated index finger into the rectum. The faecal mass is broken into small parts and extracted into a waiting receiver. The procedure is repeated until no faecoliths can be felt.

The anal area is cleansed and the child left comfortable and occupied.

For Further Reading

HECTOR W. (1970). *Modern Nursing—Theory and Practice*, 5th edition. William Heinemann (Medical Books) Ltd., London.

CHAPTER EIGHT

Isolation Nursing

Infection is the successful establishment and growth of pathogenic micro-organisms in the tissues of a susceptible person.

Many children are admitted to hospital with an infection. Others are particularly susceptible, e.g. infants, the debilitated, children suffering from extensive burns, and those receiving drugs that lower their resistance to infection, i.e. cytotoxic drugs, or mask signs and symptoms of prevailing infection, i.e. corticosteroids. Both infected and susceptible children require meticulous care to prevent dissemination of micro-organisms in the former group, and cross-infection (infection acquired during a stay in hospital) in susceptible children. A thorough understanding of the modes of transmission of micro-organisms is essential to the nurse caring for any sick person, and especially the young, as it is she who has the greatest opportunity to spread infection in the ward. The ultimate safety of the children in her care depends on her intelligent application of this knowledge in the ward situation.

Sources of Pathogenic Micro-Organisms

Man

Man is the main source of most infections that occur in the ward; patients, staff and visitors all being possible sources.

POTENTIAL PATHOGENIC MICRO-ORGANISMS

A newborn infant is a sterile creature who rapidly becomes contaminated with micro-organisms which take up residence on the skin, in the large intestine and in the orifices. These commensals, as they are called, form the normal flora of the body and live a parasitic relationship with man. Some perform a valuable function, as for example, production of vitamin K in the large intestine and hydrogen peroxide in the mouth, while others are potentially pathogenic. If a commensal moves from its normal habitat, infection may occur, e.g. large numbers of Escherichia coli (E. coli) inhabit the large intestine where most strains are completely harmless, but cause a severe urinary infection if introduced

131

into the bladder. Staphylococci on the intact skin are harmless, but cause auto-infection if the skin is broken, and wound infection if a patient's open wound is touched.

Commensals, then, are potentially pathogenic micro-organisms, and a nurse must be aware of their presence on the skin, and particularly its appendages such as the hair and nails, and in the nose, mouth and excreta.

PATHOGENIC MICRO-ORGANISMS

There is a concentrated source of pathogenic micro-organisms in a hospital ward where many of the children are suffering or recovering from diseases caused by micro-organisms.

A child may be suffering from an acute infection when the appropriate dis-charges from his body will be laden with pathogenic micro-organisms. Sputum and droplets originating from patients or staff suffering from a common cold, influenza or other respiratory infection will be highly infective and pathogenic micro-organisms will be readily disseminated unless suitable precautions are taken. The faeces excreted by children with infective gastro-enteritis, and the dressings removed from an infected wound require immediate and efficient disposal to keep the micro-organism count of the ward to a minimum. Children with chronic infections prove a continuous source of micro-organisms which may result in a more severe infection in a debilitated child.

During the incubation period of some of the common infectious diseases of childhood, the concentration of micro-organisms in discharges—usually drop-lets—is very high. As signs and symptoms of the infection are exhibited later, this innocent child may be the means of passing the infection to other susceptible children.

Pathogenic micro-organisms may be carried by a child or a member of the staff who is well and completely unaware of their presence. This group of people are referred to as symptomless carriers and are particularly dangerous in their innocence. A convalescing child may still excrete micro-organisms of his earlier infection for some time after losing his signs and symptoms. This type of carrier is referred to as a convalescent carrier.

To summarize, human sources of pathogenic micro-organisms are found in the following situations:
1 The child suffering from acute or chronic infection.
2 During the latter days of the incubation period of an infection.
3 Patients and staff who are
     i symptomless carriers;
    ii convalescent carriers.

Nature

Soil, particularly if heavily manured, contains large numbers of micro-organisms which are pathogenic to man. The spore-forming Clostridia group responsible for tetanus and gas gangrene remain dormant in the soil, and cause severe, if not fatal, illness should they gain entry and multiply in favourable conditions in the body. Proteus and Pseudomonas micro-organisms also originate from the soil as well as the large intestine of man and animals.

Animals

On the whole, each animal species has its own group of infective agents, but some micro-organisms with a source in animals may also cause infection in man. Bovine tuberculosis, for example, used to be common before the days of pasteurization of milk. Some gastro-intestinal infections are of animal source, e.g. Salmonella. The plasmodium of malaria has two hosts—man and the mosquito—both essential for its existence and multiplication.

Transmission of Micro-Organisms from their Source to a Susceptible Patient

Micro-organisms vary in their ability to live away from a suitable environment. On the whole, pathogenic micro-organisms in man thrive in a warm, moist environment where food is plentiful and where the optimum temperature is that of the body. Some micro-organisms, however, are able to resist adverse conditions by forming a resistant coat. In this spore-form, they can live for many months and are resistant to boiling, and some disinfectants.

There are three possible groups of infection in a paediatric unit—respiratory, gastro-intestinal and wound. (See Chapter 13 for wound infection).

In each instance the following must be considered:
1 Control of the source of infection.
2 A break in the line of transmission.
3 Protection of the susceptible child.

Transmission of Respiratory Infections

Respiratory infections are very common indeed, micro-organisms being projected from the respiratory tract during ordinary speaking, coughing and sneezing. As the infection is spread mainly by airborne transmission, a solid barrier must be put between the infected child and the next. Children with respiratory infections should, therefore, be nursed in isolation in separate cubicles, well-ventilated to the exterior and not to a communal corridor. The dust of the area must be kept under control to prevent air-currents disseminating the micro-organisms.

It is advisable for those attending the sick child to wear a mask. If it is the nurse who is the sufferer of an upper respiratory tract infection, then she should be omitted from the care of ill and small infants. When attending to other patients, a mask is worn to prevent dissemination of her droplets. The mask should be changed every hour as it soon becomes moist and inefficient.

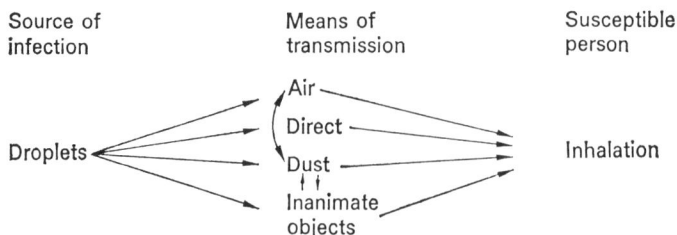

FIG. 23. Transmission of respiratory infections.

An older child should be encouraged to cough and sneeze into a paper hand-kerchief which is immediately disposed of in a covered receptacle for subsequent incineration. This aspect of health education is, unfortunately, not practised even by some members of the adult population.

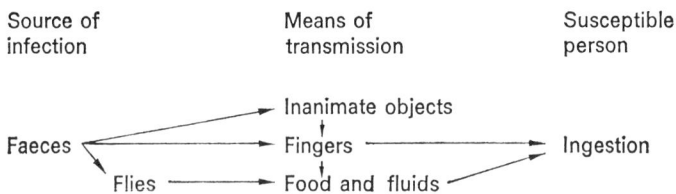

FIG. 24. Transmission of gastro-intestinal infections.

Transmission of Gastro-Intestinal Infections

Gastro-intestinal disorders in early childhood are particularly dangerous and may lead to a widespread outbreak with mortality unless prevented or adequately controlled.

Faeces is the source of infection, so that the special care of sufferers is concerned with efficient disposal of excreta and napkins, and careful handwashing after napkin changing, collecting a used bedpan, and before handling food. Flies are not usually a problem in the hospital environment, but is should be remembered that they frequent both faeces and food. Faeces, flies, fingers and food all need special care to prevent and control gastro-intestinal infection. Provided a good technique is used, an adult or older child may safely be barrier nursed in a corner of a large ward when suffering from a gastro-intestinal infection. The standard of personal hygiene of small children, however, is rarely of a sufficiently high level to allow this means of isolation.

In addition to the usual means of transmission, enteropathogenic E. coli infections of the gastro-intestinal tract are spread by airborne transmission. These micro-organisms can be grown from the dust of a cubicle housing an infant sufferer. Additional precautions must, therefore, be taken to prevent air and dust-borne dissemination of the micro-organisms.

In a large paediatric unit there is usually a high concentration of ill, often low birth weight infants suffering from major congenital disabilities, when superimposed infection may well reduce their chance of survival. To prevent introduction of infection into such a unit, suspected infant carriers are excluded until a negative stool or rectal swab is reported. Routine weekly stool specimens from all infants are examined for pathogenic micro-organisms. In the event of an outbreak of infective diarrhoea, stool specimens from infants and staff are examined to find the source, and the affected infant is transferred to an infectious diseases ward.

Principles of Isolation Nursing

All isolation or barrier nursing techniques have a certain amount in common and are adapted to meet the needs of individual patients.

An isolation technique is effective in preventing cross-infection only if every member of the hospital team coming into contact with the child and his immediate environment observe the rules twenty-four hours of the day, seven days of the week. Remember: 'a chain is only as strong as its weakest link'.

There are two main reasons for isolating a child from other patients:
1 He may be suffering from an infection, and require isolation to prevent dissemination of micro-organisms.
2 He may be susceptible to infection, and need protection from infection from other children and the hospital environment.

The essential difference in the isolation technique adopted in these two situations is that the contaminated equipment taken out of the isolated environment of an infectious child must be incinerated or disinfected, whereas only clean equipment, free from pathogenic micro-organisms, may be taken into the cubicle of a susceptible child.

Staffing an Isolation Unit

There is an obvious need for a high staff–patient ratio to fulfil the demands of isolation nursing. Patient assignment is ideal, thus limiting the number of people entering the isolation area, and giving the child a mother substitute whom he can get to know and trust.

Hospital personnel must be adequately protected by active artificial immunity against the more severe airborne infections. Where a high standard of personal hygiene and a careful isolation technique are practised, infections of gastro-intestinal origin should not be contracted by the staff.

A nurse has a responsibility to her patient. Any skin lesion, diarrhoea or upper respiratory tract infection should be reported, as these could readily be transmitted to a susceptible child, with serious consequences.

Accommodation and Requirements

Most purpose-built paediatric units consist of a high proportion of single cubicles to allow infected or susceptible children to be isolated from other children. Good observation of the child from the corridor and other cubicles should be made possible by the liberal use of clear glass, with screening provided as necessary. This also has the advantage that it allows the child, whose own physical activity is restricted, to watch the activities of the small world around him. Children are essentially gregarious and find lack of companionship in a single room lonely and frustrating. Every effort should be made to give an isolated child the extra love and attention he needs so badly. Parents should be encouraged to visit. The majority of parents quickly master the technique of hand washing and use of gowns.

A liberal supply of toys should be available in the area as an infectious, but otherwise reasonably well child may be bored and tempted to mischief. Paper and toys of no great financial or sentimental value can be incinerated after use, and others terminally disinfected by boiling, immersion in disinfectant (e.g. Savlon 1 in 200 for 1 hour), or disinfected in a formalin cabinet, as appropriate.

Micro-organisms thrive in a warm, moist, dark environment. The cubicle should therefore be light, draught-free, but well-ventilated to the exterior and not to a communal corridor, and dust kept in abeyance. Swing doors are ideal to allow free access into and out of the cubicle without contaminating the hands. Special care and thought are required if door latches have to be handled. Cubicle doors should always be kept closed to prevent cross-ventilation.

As far as possible, each cubicle should be completely self-contained, using disposable equipment where available. Other equipment will require disinfecting before further use by other patients.

The equipment includes:

A wash basin with elbow or foot operated taps, liquid soap dispenser, paper towels and receptacle for used towels.

The usual simple, easy to clean furniture—cot or bed, locker, nursing chair and one other, or two stacking chairs, child's small chair and table, screen and other furniture, as demanded.

Requirements for personal cleanliness and nursing care, including a bath thermometer.

Small supply of clean bed and personal linen, non-porous bags, medical wipes, as necessary.

Clinical thermometer, pulsometer, throat-torch, spatula, tape measure, sphygmomanometer cuff, aural speculae, as required.

Cutlery and crockery for an older child, container of Milton 1 in 80 and bottle
brush standing in Savlon 1 in 200 for care and disinfection of infant's feeding
bottles.

Three covered, lined receptacles for:
  i   napkins;
  ii soiled linen;
  iii burnable rubbish.

Cleaning equipment—damp dusters, mop, etc.

Gowns: two for nursing staff and two for visitors (hanging on separate hangers
or hooks).

Records and charts are best kept outside the isolation area and regarded as
clean. If frequent recordings have to be made, the appropriate chart and
ballpoint pen are included in the self-contained isolation area.

Communal equipment, such as a weighing machine, must be carefully protected from contamination when used in the cubicle. A second, 'clean' nurse
weighs the infant while the gowned cubicle nurse attends to his needs.

Domestic Management of the Area

Ideally, each isolation area should be self-contained with equipment for cleaning
purposes, and the domestic staff must be carefully initiated into its use and the
need for special care. Dust should be kept under control by the use of a vacuum
cleaner incorporating a disinfecting filter, and damp-dusting of all surfaces.

It may be desirable for the nurse caring for the occupant to carry out the
necessary cleaning of the cubicle.

Hand Washing

Elbow or foot operated mixing taps, an endless supply of paper towels and anti-
bacterial washing soap, soap leaves or cream are essential inside the isolation
area.

The hands should be washed and dried well:
1   Before putting on a protective gown.
2   During the patient's care, as demanded.
3   On completion of the procedure and before removing the gown.
4   Before leaving the isolation area—washed at the basin inside the area and
dried on a clean towel outside the area (not possible when the door knob must
be handled); OR before leaving the isolation area and again outside the isolation
area.

Careful drying with paper towels and a hot air hand-drier and the additional
use of chlorhexidine hand cream help to prevent the frequently washed hands
from becoming sore.

Use of Masks

Masks are worn:

    i to protect a particularly susceptible patient from droplets expelled by the nurse;

    ii to give relative protection to the nurse from a heavy discharge of airborne micro-organisms projected from the patient.

A clean, disposable mask should be put on before entry into the isolation area. If boilable cotton masks are worn, an impervious layer of cellophane is put between the cotton layers. Handled only by its strings, the mask is placed securely in position, completely covering the nose and mouth. At no time should the mask be touched before it is removed or exchanged for a clean one. Only the strings should be handled as it is removed for disposal and subsequent incineration (or laundering, if cotton). The hands should then be washed and dried.

Moist, soiled masks are not only ineffective but potentially dangerous. When in continuous use, paper masks should be changed every hour.

Use of Gowns

Protective gowns should be worn by all personnel for all procedures involving attention to the child or disturbance of his bedclothes.

Gowns may be disposable or made of boilable cotton and should bear a familiar marking to distinguish the contaminated outside from the 'clean' inside. Three-quarter length sleeves allow for adequate washing and drying of the hands and forearms and protection of the elbow when nursing an infant. Tapes at the neck and in the side seams at waist level are used to secure the gown in position. Ideally, a clean gown should be worn for each visit to the patient and in any case, gowns should be changed daily and when wet or soiled. At least two gowns are necessary for each isolated child, with additional gowns provided for relatives. Each gown should be hung on a coat hanger or by loops inside the isolation area with the 'clean' inside of the gown completely out of sight. Unless a clean gown is used each time, the outside of the gown is considered contaminated.

Hand Washing and Gowning Routine (FIG. 25)

A clean mask is put on if necessary before entering the isolation area.

The cubicle is checked to see that all the immediate requirements are available.

The hands are washed and dried.

Using the right hand, the 'clean' coat hanger is taken from its hook and the left arm slipped into the gown sleeve.

The coat hanger is then taken into the left hand, the right arm slipped into its sleeve and the coat hanger returned to its hook.

The tapes at the neck and waist are fastened so that the gown covers the back of the uniform completely.

The necessary attention is given to the child.

On completion, the nurse unfastens the tapes securing her gown before washing and drying her hands.

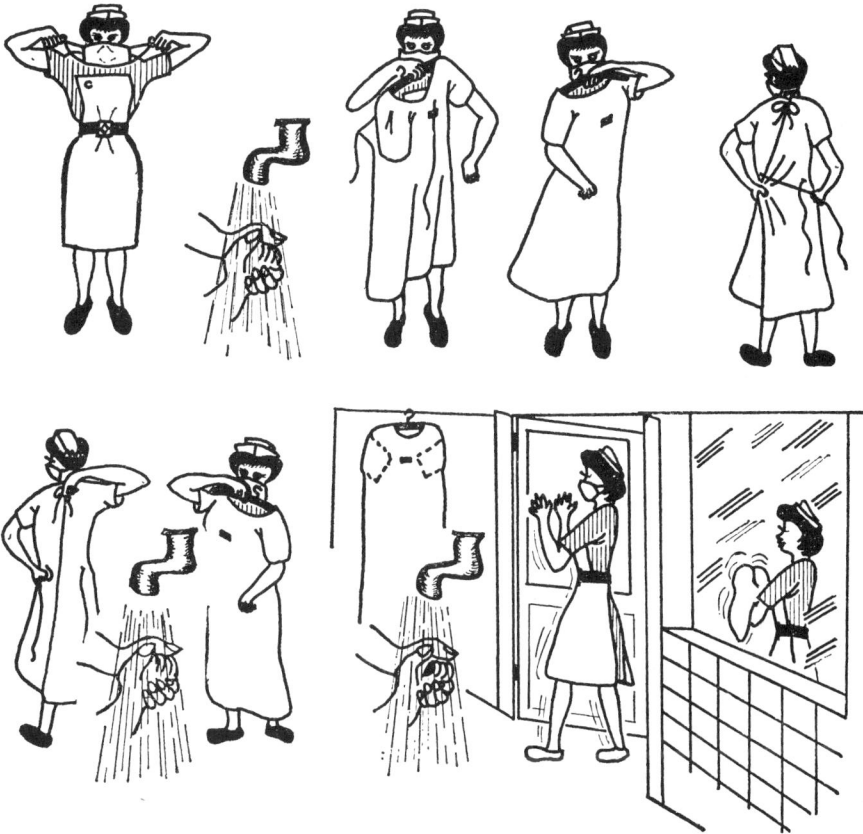

FIG. 25. Barrier nursing—hand washing and gowning technique.

The coat hanger, held in the right hand, is introduced into the left sleeve and the left arm withdrawn.

Similarly, the right arm is withdrawn. The gown is hung up and arranged so that the 'clean' inside is out of sight.

The hands are washed and excess moisture shaken off, taking care not to contaminate the uniform.

Passing through the swing door, the nurse dries her hands on a clean towel outside the isolation area, removes her mask, and washes and dries her hands.

Alternatively (when a door handle has to be turned), the hands are washed and dried inside the cubicle before leaving, and again outside the cubicle after removing the mask.

Food, and Serving Meals

A gowned nurse prepares the child's meal tray from crockery and cutlery in the area, and collects the food served at the cubicle door.

Uneaten food is scraped into an impervious bag for incineration—not for the pig bucket.

Unless disposable equipment is used, or communal ward sterilization of utensils practised, the crockery and cutlery are washed at the sink and dried on paper towels for re-use by the child.

Disposable plates, cups and cutlery are put into the impervious bag with uneaten food, the top screwed and the bag collected for incineration in a second impervious container brought to the cubicle door.

Infant Feeding

The infant's feed, collected in the usual way, is placed on the flat surface of a locker or table out of reach of an active infant.

The teat container is placed by the feed, the lid removed (inside of lid uppermost on the table) and the protective cap is removed from the bottle.

The nurse then washes and dries her hands well and before touching anything else, takes the teat from the container and secures it in position on the feeding bottle.

The protective gown is then put on.

An infant who may be taken from his cot for feeding is sat on a small waterproof square and napkin to prevent contamination of the nurse's protective gown and underlying uniform dress.

On completion of the feed, the bottle and teat are washed and rinsed with running water, using a bottle brush, the teat is returned to its container of Milton 1 in 80 and the bottle and plastic receptacle used for warming the feed are immersed in Milton 1 in 80 for $1\frac{1}{2}$ hours before removal from the area. As Milton solution corrodes metal, Savlon 1 in 200 may be substituted for the Milton solution when the equipment is immersed for $1\frac{1}{2}$ hours before being removed from the area.

If disposable bottles and teats are used, these are placed in a non-porous bag and incinerated.

Disposal of Excreta

USE OF NAPKINS

When the infection is of gastro-intestinal origin, soiled napkins are a potent source of micro-organisms, and their adequate disposal must be faultless.

Both boilable cotton and disposable napkins are in use.

If cotton napkins are used, these are best placed in a special polythene bag carrying an alginate thread and closed with an elastic band. The sealed bag is then placed in a clean, distinctively marked laundry bag, brought to the cubicle door, in which the napkins are dispatched to the laundry. Adopting this method of disposal, the napkins are not handled again until laundered, when the alginate thread dissolves, allowing the foul napkin to escape into the hot sodium bicarbonate solution, untouched by hand. On no account should sluicing of soiled napkins be undertaken by the nursing staff or in the ward environment.

Disposable napkins may be preferred. Following use, these should be placed in a strong impervious bag, the neck screwed, collected in a clean container at the cubicle door and immediately disposed of by incineration. The container, unless a disposable, second impervious bag, is then disinfected.

BEDPANS

Similarly, when the infection is of gastro-intestinal origin, great care must be taken in the disposal of faeces and the disinfection of bedpans.

The bedpan may be kept in the cubicle and returned there after emptying and disinfecting in the usual way. Alternatively, a bedpan may be collected from the ward supply and emptied, cleaned and disinfected in an efficient bedpan 'sterilizer' after use, and returned to the ward supply.

Attending to the child's toilet needs entails leaving the isolation area with a heavily contaminated piece of equipment. Great care must be taken to see that one hand is kept clean to allow uncontaminated articles to be handled and that nothing touches the covered bedpan. The hands must then be thoroughly washed and dried before handling the bedpan on completion of the cleansing and disinfecting cycle.

If the child has a severe gastro-intestinal infection, or sewage disposal in the area is not considered adequate to exclude pathogenic micro-organisms from the sewage effluent, the faeces may be covered with a disinfectant, e.g. Izal 1 in 10 for 1 hour prior to disposal. The bedpan is then disinfected in the usual way.

Disposal of Linen

Wet or foul linen may be disposed of and laundered as for napkins. Dry linen is placed in a lined pedal bin and collected at the cubicle door in a clean bag used especially for infected linen. When the soiled linen is inside, the bag is fastened and dispatched to the laundry.

When the hospital linen is laundered away from hospital control, prior disinfection of infected linen may be requested. Closed containers of Sudol 1% may be used for soaking the linen for one hour.

Terminal Disinfection

The disposable equipment is incinerated and the non-disposable equipment disinfected by boiling or immersion in a suitable disinfectant, e.g. Savlon 1 in 100 for one hour. All linen, including cotton blankets, is sent to the laundry in the recognized manner for infected linen. The furniture, walls and floor are thoroughly washed with soap and water and the room is left to air.

Soap, water, fresh-air and sunshine do much to eliminate micro-organisms, but when the child has suffered a virulent infection, the cubicle may be disinfected with formaldehyde gas. All equipment used in the area is spread over the surfaces, and cupboard doors and boxes are opened so that the gas can penetrate. The windows are closed and sealed, as are all connections to other cubicles, the corridor and the exterior. The cubicle is then sprayed with formalin and the door sealed from the outside. No gas should percolate into the remainder of the ward.

Twelve to twenty-four hours later, the room is unsealed, aired and thoroughly cleaned, as above, the equipment is washed and put into general circulation and the linen sent to the laundry.

For Further Reading

GIBSON M. and MANN T. P. 'Barrier Nursing for Sick Children,' *Nursing Times*, 24.9.65. and 1.10.65.

CHAPTER NINE

Observation–Its Importance and Significance

One of the qualities of a good nurse is that she should be observant. This applies particularly to the nurse caring for sick children. A small child is unable to communicate the way he feels and his symptoms may be masked by the emotional upset of admission to hospital.

A child's response to illness is different from that of adults. In childhood, there is often a dramatic response to treatment. The reverse also applies; deterioration in a child's condition can be unbelievably rapid to the nurse who has only experienced the care of sick adults.

From the content of Chapter 1, it is apparent that healthy children of the same age vary in physical, mental, social and emotional development, this being dependent on their innate potential influenced by their immediate environment. Behaviour of one age group is considered abnormal in another—it is not expected, for example, that a healthy five-year-old has the temper tantrums common in the two-year-old. To recognize an abnormal situation, it is essential that a nurse caring for sick children is conversant with the growth and development of healthy children, as well as normal physiological functioning.

General Observations

BEHAVIOUR OF THE CHILD
Healthy children are rarely still for any length of time during the day and sleep soundly at night.
Excessive activity or restlessness. These symptoms may be observed as normal or as the result of physical illness or emotional disturbance due to:
  i   excitement;
  ii an itch;
  iii a full bladder;
  iv a cough;

  v cerebral anoxaemia (lack of oxygen to the brain) and irritation;
  vi pain—seen as head-rolling or pulling of the ears in otitis media, and rapid flexion of the knees to the abdomen in intestinal colic;
  vii a psychological disorder—'over-active';
  viii hypoglycaemia.

Hypoglycaemia. The causes, manifestations and treatment of hypoglycaemia of the newborn are discussed in Chapter 5.

A low blood sugar level in the older age group is a complication of insulin therapy used in the control of diabetes mellitus. There is an imbalance in the amount of insulin administered for metabolism of the carbohydrate content of the diet; too much insulin or exercise having been taken for the amount of carbo-hydrate ingested.

As the blood sugar level falls, so the child rapidly shows signs and symptoms of hypoglycaemia. Irritability and irrational behaviour are early signs. The skin is moist and sweating and an older child may complain of lethargy, hunger and a feeling of faintness. No time should be lost in administering two rounded teaspoons of glucose in water (10g glucose) to a diabetic child found in this state, as twitching, convulsions and coma quickly ensue. If the child has already lost consciousness, the doctor must be informed immediately and an injection tray prepared for the administration of intravenous 50% dextrose or intramuscular glucagon.

A subsequent Dextrostix or laboratory estimation of the blood sugar level will confirm the diagnosis, if necessary, a urine test for sugar being a less accurate guide.

Drowsiness and lethargy. This may be due to excessive fatigue and lack of sleep in an otherwise healthy child. An ill child is frequently lethargic and limp to handle, these often being early signs that a child is not well. In the carefree childhood years, sleeplessness (insomnia) is rare. Increasing drowsiness may be a sign that a brain-injured child is deteriorating (see conscious level).

Crying. The only method an infant has of expressing his grievances to the outside world is by crying. His cry may be due to discomfort from an empty stomach, wind, or a wet napkin, or just because he needs company. With experience, a nurse can tell whether an infant is cross or really in pain. An angry infant will usually stop crying if he is picked up or just spoken to. If he is not pacified by attention, then this is a sure sign that he is not well. If the child is suffering from cerebral irritation, the cry may be shrill.

Position. Children adopt unusual positions when experiencing discomfort, and often this observation can guide a doctor in his diagnosis.
1 The child suffering from photophobia (dislike of light), due to local inflammation of the eyes or cerebral irritation, as in meningitis, will turn his head from the light or bury his head under the bedclothes.
2 The child with constant abdominal pain lies curled up in bed. When the pain is intermittent and sharp (colic), rapid flexion of the knees is seen.

3   Head retraction and arching of the back (opisthotonos) are seen when the muscles of the vertebral column are contracted.

4   A squatting position is adopted by small children with severe cyanotic heart disease.

5   A dyspnoeic child may kneel, his body and arms thrown up over his pillows to increase the capacity of the thoracic cavity.

Conscious Level

A conscious child is aware of his surroundings, alert and orientated.

Consciousness is lost and gained in four stages:

1   Normal consciousness—the child is alert and aware of his environment.

2   Confused—the child is drowsy and irritable when disturbed, and an older child will talk if only to say 'stop it'.

3   Stupor—the child can be temporarily roused following infliction of painful stimuli, but will not speak or respond to the spoken word.

4   Coma—the child is unconscious and makes no physical or verbal response to painful stimuli.

Loss of consciousness may be due to anaesthesia, diabetic coma, poisoning due to barbiturates, a severe head injury or other intra-cranial disorder, such as a cerebral tumour. Following a head injury, the conscious level may be assessed and recorded at quarter or half-hourly intervals. To make an accurate assessment, the child must be roused to his highest level of consciousness by adequate verbal and physical stimulation (FIG. 27).

Convulsions

Convulsions or fits are a fairly common symptom of disease in childhood, about 6% of the population experiencing at least one during their childhood years. This is thought to be due to instability of the immature nervous system during the early years of life, giving a low threshold for irritability.

Convulsions vary in cause and severity. The main causes of convulsions in the newborn period are cerebral defect, anoxaemia or haemorrhage, generalized infection, hypoglycaemia and hypocalcaemia and are all observed as local or generalized twitchings of the limbs and face. Febrile convulsions due to a sudden rise in body temperature, often heralding the onset of an infective illness, are the main cause of convulsions seen in the older infant and pre-school child (six months to five years age group). Over the age of five years, the most common cause is epilepsy. Both febrile and grand mal epileptiform convulsions are characterized by rapidly alternating contraction and relaxation of the skeletal muscles of a digit, limb, limbs, one side of the body or the body generally, and are usually accompanied by incontinence and a period of unconsciousness. A warning cry may be given by an epileptic child. Petit mal type epilepsy is characterized by brief, transient lapses of consciousness, accompanied by a 'vacant' expression.

Infants under the age of one year may experience frequent lightning fits, salaam attacks or infantile spasms. These fits are characterized by frequent transient muscular spasms, accompanied by a cry. With flexion of the trunk, the head and arms are flung downwards in a salaam. The attacks are usually associated with mental subnormality.

Breath-holding attacks in the frustrated toddler may cause transient unconsciousness, cyanosis and some localized twitching.

The nurse should note and record the following observations when witnessing a convulsion:

1 The time, therefore maintaining a record of the frequency of convulsions.
2 The duration of the convulsion.
3 Any warning given to the child or staff. An older child may experience a sensation, or a younger child may cry out.
4 The type and distribution of the convulsive movements:
      i The parts of the body affected;
     ii Continuous muscular contraction (tonus);
    iii Spasmodic irregular movements due to alternating contraction and relaxation of the muscles (clonus);
     iv Deviation or rolling of the eyeballs.
5 Any incontinence during the convulsion.
6 The level of consciousness during and after the fit.

While the child is under constant observation for the duration of the fit, he is protected from harm by being turned on to one side to allow saliva and mucus to drain from the mouth. Harmful objects are moved away from the immediate vicinity of the convulsing body, and a wooden wedge or other soft, rigid object is placed between the child's molar teeth to prevent painful damage to the tongue.

Pupil Reactions

The pupils are usually of equal size and react to light by constricting. When the

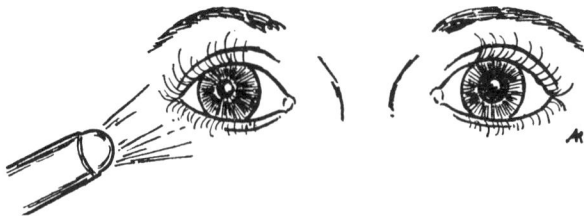

FIG. 26. Testing a pupil's reaction to light. Note the position of the torch. Compare the size of the pupils.

NURSING REPORT ON A PATIENT WITH DISTURBANCE OF CONSCIOUSNESS

NAME JANE WHITE.   AGE 5 YRS.   DATE FEB. 1971.   WARD 7.

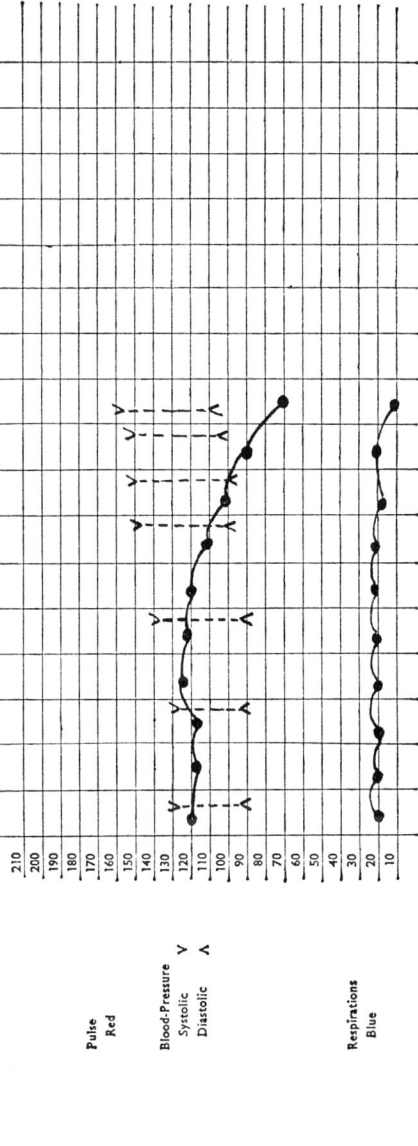

Fig. 27. (These observations, i.e. a fall in the pulse rate, a rise in the blood pressure and a deterioration in the conscious level are highly suggestive of a rapid rise in the intracranial pressure, possibly due to an extra-dural (middle meningeal artery) haemorrhage, if the child had sustained a head-injury. A doctor should have been informed at 11.30 hours.)

brain is under pressure, damaged or diseased, there may be inequality in the size of the pupils and failure of one or both to react to light.

The eyelids are opened and the size and equality of the pupils noted. A small torch with an adequate light is then shone indirectly (from one side) on to one eye to check that the pupil has its normal brisk response to light. The other eye is then examined in the same manner. The result is recorded and any deviation from the normal for the child is reported (FIG 27).

Skin

The healthy, intact skin forms a protective barrier between the external environment and the underlying structures of the body. The skin of a healthy child is pink, warm, dry and supple. When bathing a child on admission, and during his subsequent care in hospital, the nurse can learn a great deal about the child's condition.

Cleanliness of the child will indicate the general standard of parental care he has received.

Colour. i *Pallor*—the colour of the skin and mucous membranes give some indication of the amount and quality of the blood in the superficial blood vessels, but is a poor guide in the assessment of general health. In shock following haemorrhage, the blood vessels of the skin constrict to conserve the blood for supplying vital structures with oxygen and nourishment. The anaemic child will appear pale, due to a reduction in the circulating oxyhaemoglobin which gives the blood its normal rich red colouring.

ii *Cyanosis* is blueness of the skin due to an increased amount of reduced (de-oxygenated) haemoglobin in circulation. Diseases of the heart and lungs cause central cyanosis when the skin of the whole body has a blue tinge. Peripheral cyanosis is more common and occurs when there is stagnation of venous blood in the extremities, causing the hands and feet to be blue and cold.

iii *Jaundice* is the result of excess bilirubin in the blood due to immaturity of the liver (physiological jaundice), profound infection in the newborn, excessive breakdown of red blood cells (haemolytic jaundice) and disease of the liver or biliary system. Jaundice may be associated with excretion of pale stools.

The skin of a dehydrated child is dry and has lost its normal elastic recoil. Recent loss of weight shows as loose folds of inelastic skin.

A hot, moist skin, due to the presence of excess sweat is seen when the body is overheated, following exercise or over-clothing, and when the temperature is raised due to the presence of infection, or following brain damage or surgery. *A cold, clammy skin* is felt in hypoglycaemia and in states of stress, such as peripheral circulatory failure, due to gross fluid, electrolyte and blood loss.

Rashes or eruptions vary in type, e.g. superficial patchy redness (erythematous), discoloured patches (macular), small solid elevations (pimples) (papular), blisters (vesicular), or pimples containing pus (pustular) and distribution, i.e. localized when one area is affected, or generalized when the rash is present over the whole body.

Haemorrhages seen as petechiae (purple spots—small effusions of blood under the epidermis) are usually associated with a deficiency of one of the factors essential for the formation of a blood clot and may be localized or generally distributed.

Bruises are common in childhood due to the usual childhood falls. Any excessive bruising or bruising in unusual areas should be reported. These could be the result of a blood disorder or ill treatment.

A dry, scaly skin is seen in children suffering from eczema and other skin disorders (page 329).

Coughing and Sputum

COUGH

A cough is a necessary reflex action to protect the air passages from entry of foreign material and to expel sputum from the air passages. It is a very common symptom in childhood with its associated high incidence of respiratory tract infections.

Small children are unable to cough up (expectorate) the secretions of the respiratory tract directed into the throat by the ciliated epithelial lining of the trachea, so they are swallowed.

The time coughing occurs, and the type of cough, should be noted:

Time. For example, whether the child is awakened by an attack of coughing, or if there is any relationship between a coughing attack and the intake of food.

Type. Early inflammatory conditions of the upper respiratory tract produce a dry cough. Fumes and food irritate the upper respiratory tract to give a non-productive cough.

A productive cough is a later sign of inflammation of the air passages, or may be due to bronchiectasis, or post-nasal discharge from infected air sinuses irritating the upper respiratory passages.

Characteristics. In some conditions, children experience fits of coughing which can be utterly exhausting. The classical example is the paroxysmal coughing of whooping cough (pertussis) which often terminates in the exhausted child vomiting.

A harsh, rasping, dry cough of rapid onset is usually associated with acute inflammation of the larynx and trachea.

A stridulous cough, and stridor heard on inspiration, is an indication of partial obstruction of the air passages. This may be congenital, or may be due to local inflammation or the presence of a foreign body. These children require constant observation to detect immediately any deterioration in their condition, i.e. a rise in the pulse rate, restlessness associated with increasing dyspnoea and deterioration in colour.

A wheezing cough is the result of spasm of the smooth muscle of the bronchioles and is commonly due to asthma.

SPUTUM

Sputum is the material produced by the respiratory passages during coughing.

Mucus. In the healthy child, a small quantity of mucus is produced, and in inflammatory conditions of the respiratory tract this is produced in excess.

Mucopus. As micro-organisms intervene, the sputum becomes cloudy to form mucopus.

Pus. In the rare conditions, bronchiectasis and lung abscess, pus is expectorated.

Blood. The expectoration of bright red, frothy blood (haemoptysis) is rare in childhood. Streaks of blood, however, may be seen in the sputum produced by a child with a severe inflammatory condition of the air passages, or following traumatic aspiration of the upper respiratory passages.

Watery sputum. When pulmonary hypertension is present, as in children with heart failure or a heart defect allowing blood to flow from the left side of the heart to the right, watery fluid accumulates in the lungs which must be aspirated or expectorated.

Micturition and Urine

The daily urine output varies with age from small amounts of dilute urine passed at frequent intervals in the newborn, to larger quantities of more concentrated urine passed less frequently in older children.

Control of the bladder is achieved towards the middle of the second year of life when frequency and urgency of micturition are normal, but accidents occur even in the home environment. It is usually some months, and possibly several years later that a child can be relied on to be dry on waking.

Incontinence of urine is common amongst young children in hospital. Before the child has learned to control the natural reflex, incontinence is quite normal and to be expected. When out of his familiar surroundings and routine, a small child may regress to infantile behaviour. He should be sat on a pot or the lavatory at frequent, regular intervals to encourage a regular routine and good habits. Damage or disease of the spinal cord and some disorders of the bladder cause incontinence of urine. Dribbling incontinence is often the result of an incompetent sphincter muscle, or it may be due to overflow of urine from an over-distended bladder. When retention of urine with overflow is suspected, the bladder can be palpated above the symphysis pubis.

Retention of urine—urine is produced by the kidneys but is abnormally retained in the bladder, due to damage to the nerves controlling bladder function, the presence of urethral valves or to psychological reasons.

Suppression of urine—urine is not being produced by the kidneys which may be diseased or suffering from an inadequate blood supply. The child therefore suffers from *anuria*.

Oliguria—is a reduction in the normal urine output for the child and is usually caused by renal damage or a grossly diminished fluid intake or excessive loss.

Polyuria—is an increase in the amount of urine passed, due to an excessive fluid intake or diabetes mellitus or diabetes insipidus.

Frequency of micturition is common in small children until full bladder control is established, and is a means of seeking attention. As the bladder is capable of retaining a limited amount of urine, frequency is also associated with polyuria. Inflammation of the bladder—cystitis—will cause frequency and dysuria.

Dysuria—(pain on micturition) is usually associated with a local condition such as ammoniacal dermatitis, meatal ulcer or excoriation of the vulva.

The nurse should note particularly any frequency or urgency of micturition and any pain experienced by the child.

By maintaining a strict fluid balance chart, the twenty-four hour urine output can be compared with the fluid intake for the same period. The characteristics of normal urine and tests for abnormalities are given in Chapter 21.

Defaecation and Stools

Meconium, the dark green tenacious first stools of the newborn, passed within the first twenty-four hours of life, consist of swallowed liquor, lanugo, bile, epithelial cells and mucus. With the introduction to artificial milk feeds, the stools gradually change to a pale yellow-grey colour of semi-formed consistency, passed five or six times daily. The stools of breast-fed infants are less frequent, sometimes two or three a week and are loose and mustard-orange in colour. With the introduction to mixed feeding, the stools become less frequent—one to two daily—formed, and adopt a characteristic odour and brown colour.

DEFAECATION

Bowel training is begun at an early age. Usually by the age of eighteen months, defaecation is under the control of the will. Regular functioning of the bowel, twice daily, daily or alternate days, depends on:
  i   habit training;
  ii diet and fluid intake;
  iii exercise.

Some children may experience difficulty when expected to use a bedpan. If at all possible, a child should be allowed to go to the lavatory for this purpose. A newly potty-trained toddler may revert to infantile behaviour as part of the regressive effects of separation from his mother. Frequent attention at regular intervals is necessary to encourage a good routine and clean habits in such a child.

The frequency of defaecation and consistency of stools should be noted, i.e. whether watery, loose, frothy, undigested, formed or constipated.

Constipation is the infrequent passage of hard, dry stools. Causes of constipation include poor bowel training, insufficient fluid intake and anal pain.

Diarrhoea is the frequent passage of loose, fluid stools and is associated with a wide variety of conditions. An excessive sugar intake, malabsorption, gastro-enteritis and parenteral infections (infections outside the alimentary tract) are some of the causes of diarrhoea in infancy. The usual causes in older children are of local, infective or inflammatory origin, or associated with oral administration of wide spectrum antibiotics.

ABNORMALITIES OF STOOLS

1   Black, dry stools are seen following the ingestion of iron.

2   Black, tarry stools (melaena) contain digested blood.

3   Fresh blood is seen on the stools in dysentery, colitis, intussusception and local anal lesions such as anal fissure.

4   Pale, bulky offensive stools, due to the presence of excess fat (steatorrhoea) are passed by children suffering from coeliac disease, cystic fibrosis, giardiasis and disaccharide intolerance.

5   Pale, putty coloured, dry stools are the result of failure of bile pigments to reach the alimentary tract and are seen in children with infective hepatitis and congenital obliteration of the bile duct.

6   Frothy, yellow stools occur when the carbohydrate intake is excessive.

7   Green, sour smelling, fluid stools are seen in children with gastro-enteritis.

8   Small green constipated stools are a sign of starvation.

9   Excessive mucus is seen where there is an inflammatory condition of the colon.

10   Foreign bodies inadvertently ingested are usually excreted in the stools.

11   The stools should be carefully inspected for internal parasites, such as threadworms and tape worm segments and head, if intestinal infestation is suspected.

Immediate recording of bowel actions in childhood is very important—a small child is unable to speak for himself, and an older child may give a positive answer once he has experienced the consequences of saying 'no'. A description of the stool should be made on the fluid balance chart during infancy. When the stool is loose or offensive, it should be saved for inspection and a specimen sent to the laboratory for examination.

Vomiting and Vomitus

VOMITING

Vomiting is a reflex action common in childhood. The cause may be associated with a mechanical or infective disorder, irritation of the alimentary tract, or may originate in the brain.

If the stomach is overdistended or irritated, it will reject its contents. Mechanical or paralytic intestinal obstruction interrupts the normal passage of food and digestive secretions which are vomited. The vomiting centre in the medulla oblongata is irritated by some drugs, a raised intracranial pressure, inflammation, or a marked rise in the hydrogen ion concentration of the blood (acidosis) causing the child to vomit.

Vomiting often accompanies a chest infection and is frequently associated with coughing in small children who are unable to expectorate the secretions from the respiratory tract. This mucus is swallowed, and is rejected by the stomach because of its irritating effect.

The time vomiting occurs in relation to food and pain should be noted. Knowledge of the way in which the vomit is ejected will also help the doctor in making a diagnosis.

Usually, vomiting requires considerable effort and is exhausting, especially to an already weakened child.

Little effort is required to expel the rejected contents of the stomach in, for example, a child with intestinal obstruction or hiatus hernia. Forceful and projectile vomiting is seen in an infant suffering from pyloric stenosis.

A reassuring hand on the brow or just the presence of a nurse at the bedside will help to make this unpleasant, and often frightening experience to the child more tolerable. A mouth-wash will improve the taste in the mouth after the vomiting attack, and sponging of the face is comforting.

VOMITUS

The amount of fluid vomited should be measured or its volume assessed, and the content inspected before both observations are recorded on the child's fluid balance chart. Repeated attacks of vomiting readily cause dehydration, especially in the young child.

The content of the vomit varies with the type of food ingested and the cause of the vomiting:

1   If the food has not reached the stomach, it is returned completely undigested, as seen in children with hiatus hernia and achalasia of the cardia.

2   The presence of partly-digested food or curdled milk indicates that the food has been mixed with hydrochloric acid in the stomach.

3   Vomit containing bile is green, as the golden coloured intestinal secretions have been mixed with hydrochloric acid. Bile is seen in the vomit of children, other than those suffering from intestinal obstruction.

4   Fresh blood may be vomited (haematemesis) as the result of gastric irritation due to aspirin ingestion, in oesophageal varices, and if blood from the nose or throat has been swallowed. When blood has been partly digested, the vomit appears as coffee-grounds.

5   In response to chemical or infective irritation of the gastric mucosa, excessive

amounts of mucus are produced which will be seen in the vomit of children suffering from gastritis.

Reporting and Recording Observations

Each hospital adopts its own routine for reporting and choice of charts for recording observations, and every nurse should make herself familiar with both. Any deviation from the normal should be reported and recorded on the appropriate chart.

The intervals between recordings of clinical observations vary with the severity of the child's illness and the likelihood of the occurrence of complications.

Most children in hospital have their temperature, pulse and respiration rates recorded at least once daily. Children admitted in an emergency usually require the three recordings to be made at four-hourly intervals. The pulse rate may be recorded as frequently as at quarter or half-hourly intervals following operation or injury.

Recording the blood pressure of infants is beyond the scope of the average paediatric nurse. The older child may have his blood pressure recorded daily, four-hourly, or hourly, depending on the reason for making the observation.

A strict fluid balance chart is maintained for ill children and all infants admitted to hospital. The fluid intake recorded is the amount of fluid actually taken. If it is important that an accurate recording of the urine output of a small child is to be made, a urine collection bag is used. Normally, it is sufficient to note the number of times the infant is wet or soiled.

Special charts for recording the progress of a child with head injuries, diabetes or convulsions, are used as appropriate.

Weight

All children should be accurately weighed on admission and at intervals during their stay in hospital. Drug dosage, fluid requirement and energy needs all depend on the child's weight. The child should be weighed at the same time in relation to food, and wearing the same amount of clothing, or nude. Older children unable to balance on the platform of the scales may be nursed by an adult whose weight is subtracted from the total figure.

Children suffering from diseases of the heart or kidneys and those receiving corticosteroid therapy may be weighed daily to assess fluid retention. All other infants are weighed on alternate days or twice a week, and children less frequently.

Height and Length

The height of some children is measured routinely on admission. If the surface area of the child is to be assessed (page 447), this measurement is essential. Until a child is old enough to co-operate by standing straight and still against a ruler, it is more accurate for the measurement to be made with him lying supine on a flat surface.

Head Circumference

The head circumference of an infant is measured at birth and at intervals to assess normal progress, deviation from the normal, and to ascertain the progress of a child following a drainage operation for hydrocephalus. The tape-measure is placed around the occipito-frontal circumference.

Temperature

Mammals maintain a fairly constant body temperature in spite of the changing temperature of their environment. The temperature-regulating centre in the hypothalamus is not fully developed in the first years of life, so that young children, and especially infants, are prone to extremes of body temperature if overheated or chilled.

The range of normal body temperature is 36·3°–37·2°C (97·4°–99°F). The standard clinical thermometer is calibrated to record a temperature within the range of 35°–43°C or 95°–110°F to the nearest 0·2°C or °F. A subnormal thermometer with a range of 25°–40°C or 80°–110°F should be used when hypothermia (a temperature below 35°C or 95°F) is suspected, and for recording the temperature of all newborn, low birth weight and ill infants. To avoid failure to recognize early hypothermia when the mercury does not rise to 35°C or 95°F on a standard clinical thermometer after the appropriate length of time, the infant's temperature must be recorded again, using a subnormal thermometer.

VARIATIONS IN BODY TEMPERATURE
Normal range = 36·3°–37·2°C (97·4°–99°F). A variation of 6°C or 10°F on either side of the normal range, unless instituted under controlled conditions, is usually incompatible with life.

Pyrexia = a temperature above 37·2°C (99°F)

Low pyrexia = 37·2°–38·4°C (99°–101°F)

Moderate pyrexia = 38·4°–39·5°C (101°–103°F)

High pyrexia = 39·5°–40·6°C (103°–105°F)

Hyperpyrexia = above 40·6°C (105°F)

Hypothermia = below 35°C (95°F)

In a healthy child there is a rise in temperature of 0·6°C (1°F) during the day. Excitement, exertion and ingestion of hot foods cause the temperature to rise.

Infection is the main reason for the body temperature to rise, as in febrile conditions the temperature-regulating 'thermostat' is set higher. Dehydration may also result in very high temperatures being recorded in the newborn period. Following extensive surgery or trauma, a rise in body temperature is seen, due to the absorption of blood. Even children are capable of malingering. Vigorous rubbing of the thermometer bulb will cause the mercury to rise very quickly, e.g. 5°C in ten seconds!

Recording the Temperature

The temperature recorded depends on the part of the body used to take the temperature:
1 Axilla or groin—0·6°C (1°F) below oral recording.
2 Mouth—0·6°C (1°F) below rectal recording.
3 Rectum—1°C (2°F) above skin recording
            0·6°C (1°F) above oral recording.

To obtain a satisfactory record of the child's progress, the temperature must be recorded at the same site each time. Oral temperatures should not be recorded in any patient who is unco-operative, restless or unconscious. This includes the majority of children who come into hospital. When caring for a group of children of a wide age range, a ruling should be made to avoid confusion:
Examples
1 Rectal temperature recording for the first twelve months of life (infants suffering with enteritis excepted). Skin (axillary) temperature recording after the first year of life, unless otherwise instructed.
2 Rectal temperature recording for the first twelve months. Skin temperature recorded for the next nine years; oral temperature recorded after the age of ten years.

REQUIREMENTS
Clinical thermometer, standard and/or subnormal, standing in a container of
    mild antiseptic such as aqueous solution of chlorhexidine 0·05%.
Swab—wool or tissue.
Watch with second hand, or pulsometer for counting the pulse and respiration
    rates.
Child's temperature record.
Lubricant, e.g. Vaseline, for rectal recording.

METHOD
1 Skin—the axilla or groin is freed from clothing, moisture and talcum powder.
2 Mouth—ensure that the child has not had a hot drink within the previous fifteen minutes.

3   Rectum—the anal area is cleansed and the bed or nurse's knees protected.

The thermometer is taken from its container and the bulb wiped and inspected for damage. If the level of mercury is above 35°C (95°F), the thermometer is grasped firmly and with two or three sharp flicks of the wrist, the level of mercury is shaken to below 35°C (95°F).

1   *Skin*—the thermometer is placed in the axilla or groin, ensuring that the two skin surfaces meet around the thermometer. The child is held for three minutes, during which time the pulse and respiration rates can be counted.

2   *Mouth*—the thermometer bulb is placed under the tongue at the side of the mouth and the child is asked to close his lips, but not his teeth. It is left in this position for two minutes, during which time the pulse and respiration rates can be counted.

3   *Rectum*—the thermometer bulb is lubricated with a small quantity of Vaseline or other non-irritating lubricant. With a bigger child in the left lateral position, and an infant held firmly by the feet on his back, the lubricated thermometer is inserted 2·5cm (1 inch) into the rectum and held in place for one minute.

After the appropriate length of time, the thermometer is removed from the site, wiped with the swab and the mercury level read. The mercury is then shaken down and the thermometer replaced in its holder.

The child is dressed as required and the thermometer reading is recorded on the patient's chart. Any gross discrepancy on previous recordings should be reported immediately.

When the child no longer requires the use of his thermometer, it is washed well with cool, soapy water, rinsed and immersed in a suitable disinfectant, e.g. chlorhexidine 0·5% in spirit for one hour.

TEMPERATURE MONITORING

To prevent disturbance of a child requiring frequent recording of body temperature, an electronic recorder may be used. The suitably lubricated thermister is inserted into either the mid-oesophagus or rectum and attached by a flex to the recorder. At the turn of a switch, the child's body temperature is shown on an illuminated dial.

Pulse

Each beat of the pulse represents one cardiac cycle. As the left ventricle forces its contained blood into the systemic arteries, the wave of increased pressure can be felt where an artery over-rides a bone. The pulse rate is the number of times the pressure in the artery impinges on the palpating finger-tips.

SITES USED FOR LOCATING THE PULSE

1   The radial artery may be felt where it over-rides the radius at the anterior lateral aspect of the wrist.

2   Over the temporal bone, just in front of the ear—this is a good site to use when undue disturbance of the child is to be avoided.

3   The pulse rate can be counted at the anterior fontanelle in a small infant.

VARIATIONS IN PULSE

When recording the pulse, not only is the pulse rate counted but the rhythm and volume are noted.

Rate—the pulse rate varies with age, being rapid at birth and gradually slowing with progression of years. Excitement, fear, restlessness, exertion and crying all increase the heart rate and, therefore, the pulse rate. It is reasonable for the pulse of infants and toddlers to be recorded before being disturbed for taking the temperature. An abnormal increase in the heart rate (tachycardia) occurs with fever, following a brisk haemorrhage, and following administration of some drugs. The pulse rate is slow during sleep, rest and relaxation. An abnormal fall in the pulse rate (bradycardia) is often indicative of a raised intracranial pressure, due to haemorrhage, a tumour or hydrocephalus. The pulse and respiration rates are usually in a 4:1 ratio. With every 0·6°C (1°F) rise in temperature, the pulse increases approximately 10 beats/minute.

Rhythm—the normal pulse has a regular rhythm. This may vary slightly in the young child when the pulse rate increases during inspiration and has a tendency to slow during expiration. This normal phenomenon is called sinus arrhythmia. Other arrhythmias (irregularities of heart beat or pulse) may be felt as missed or extra beats or coupling of the beats. Any abnormality of rhythm should be reported immediately.

Volume—the blood vessels of children are more readily compressed by heavy palpation than those of adults, and particularly the elderly. A pulse of poor volume is often the result of shock, haemorrhage or other conditions causing circulatory collapse.

RECORDING THE PULSE RATE

For older children, the pulse rate is usually counted while the thermometer is recording the temperature. The pulse rate of smaller children is best recorded before taking down the cot-side and disturbing the child. If this is not possible then a toddler's attention can be distracted by a toy or the nurse's watch.

As exercise increases the pulse rate, the child should have been resting quietly for five minutes following excitement or exertion. The arm is allowed to rest or is flexed over the chest, the pulse located, and gentle pressure applied with one or two fingertips over the route taken by the artery. With the watch held in the free hand, the pulse rate is counted and the rhythm and tension noted. If there is irregularity of the pulse, it is counted for a full minute. The pulse may be counted for half-a-minute in other circumstances and the result multiplied by two.

The pulse rate per minute is recorded on the appropriate chart and any undue rise or fall in the rate or irregularity is reported.

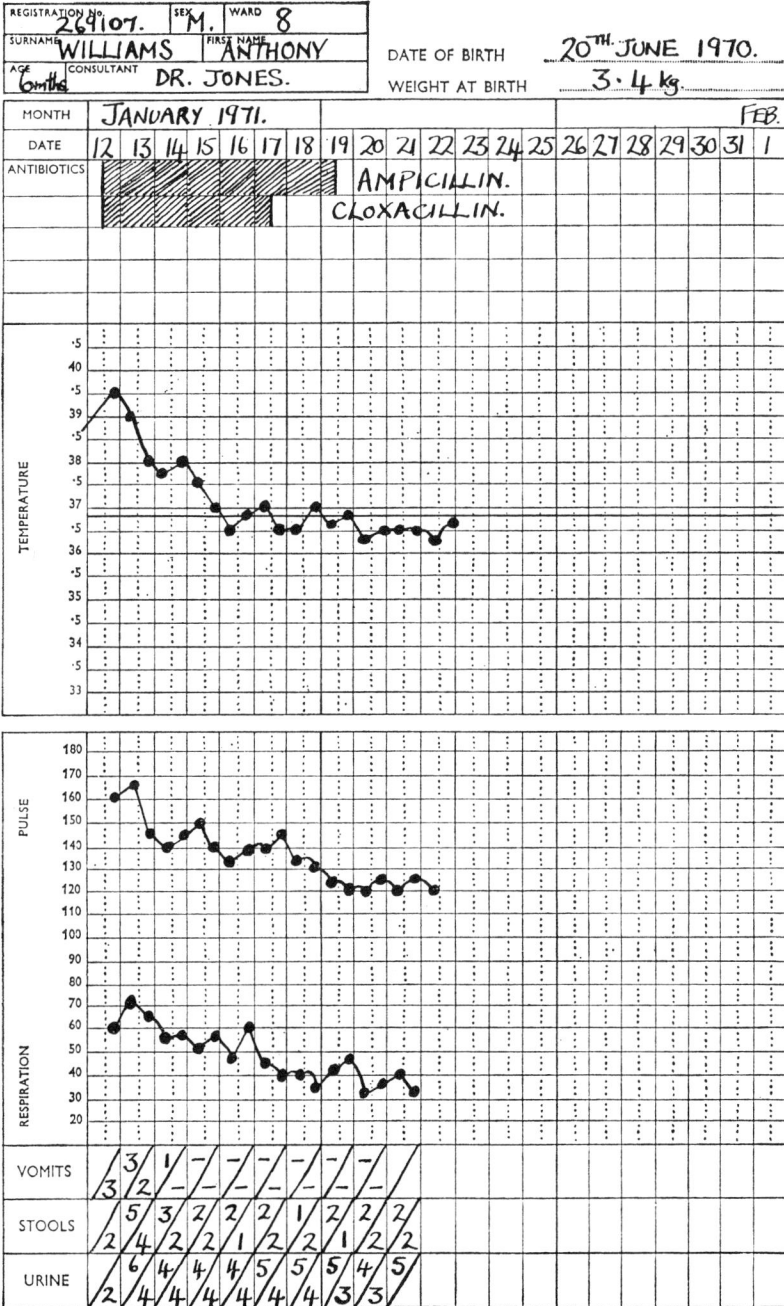

REGISTRATION No. 269107.	SEX M.	WARD 8		
SURNAME WILLIAMS	FIRST NAME ANTHONY		DATE OF BIRTH	20TH. JUNE 1970.
AGE 6mths	CONSULTANT DR. JONES.		WEIGHT AT BIRTH	3·4 kg.

MONTH	JANUARY 1971.	FEB.

DATE	12	13	14	15	16	17	18	19	20	21	22	23	24	25	26	27	28	29	30	31	1

ANTIBIOTICS

AMPICILLIN.

CLOXACILLIN.

TEMPERATURE

PULSE

RESPIRATION

VOMITS	3/3	1/2	−/−	−/−	−/−	−/−	−/−	−/−	−/−												
STOOLS	5/2	3/4	2/2	2/2	2/1	1/2	2/2	2/1	2/2												
URINE	6/2	4/4	4/4	4/4	5/4	5/4	5/4	4/3	5/3												

FIG. 28.

SLEEPING PULSE

It is sometimes necessary to record the pulse rate of a child during the hours of sleep. Normally, the pulse rate of a sleeping child is lower than that recorded when awake. In rheumatic fever with associated carditis, the sleeping pulse rate is raised out of all proportion to the degree of pyrexia and an assessment of the child's progress can be made by nightly recording of this observation.

The sleeping pulse is usually recorded in a different colour on the child's chart.

Apex Beat

The apex beat may be recorded:
i   when difficulty is encountered recording the pulse rate in the usual way, e.g. a rate of 180 or more/minute;
ii when there is a discrepancy between the rate of the heart and the palpable pulse (a pulse deficit).

REQUIREMENTS

Stethoscope.
Watch with second hand.
Second nurse if a discrepancy is suspected.

METHOD

The position of the apex of the heart varies with age and the size of the heart, but can readily be located by placing a warmed hand on the left side of the chest (right side in dextrocardia) over and just below the nipple-line. The warmed stethoscope is placed over the site where the apex of the heart can be felt hitting the chest wall. Two sounds will be heard; a dull 'lubb' as the inlet (tricuspid and mitral) valves close, followed by a shorter, sharp 'dup' as the outlet (aortic and pulmonary) valves close. Each 'lubb-dup' represents one cardiac cycle and is counted as one beat.

If the rate of the apex beat is to be compared with the pulse rate, then the second nurse locates the radial pulse and each nurse counts at her own site simultaneously for the same one minute, using the same watch. Both figures are recorded on the chart, one above the other, the apex beat recording usually being made with a different colour.

Blood Pressure

Blood pressure is the force which blood exerts on the walls of blood vessels, and varies in the different vessels, i.e. higher in the arteries than the veins.

FACTORS ESSENTIAL FOR THE REGULATION AND MAINTENANCE OF BLOOD PRESSURE

1 The output of the heart which depends on:
    i   the output of blood per contraction;
    ii the rate of the heart;
    iii the venous return.

2 The peripheral resistance—the resistance in the walls of the arterioles to the flow of blood from the arteries.

3 The elasticity in the walls of the arteries.

4 The viscosity of the blood—this is increased by over-production of red blood cells (polycythaemia).

5 The total quantity of blood in circulation. Following an acute, severe haemorrhage, the blood pressure will fall.

1 SYSTEMIC ARTERIAL PRESSURE

When blood pressure is recorded, it is usually the arterial blood pressure that is being measured, i.e. the pressure of the blood in the artery when the heart is contracting (systolic blood pressure) and during relaxation of the heart muscle (diastolic blood pressure). The difference between the two pressures is called the pulse pressure.

Variations in Blood Pressure. Emotion causes the blood pressure to rise. A pathological increase in the arterial blood pressure (hypertension) causes additional strain on the heart, and increases the risk of cerebral vascular accident. These complications are rare in childhood. Hypotension (a decrease in arterial blood pressure) results in an inadequate supply of oxygen reaching the brain, causing a syncope or faint.

REQUIREMENTS FOR RECORDING ARTERIAL BLOOD PRESSURE

Sphygmomanometer with cuff of appropriate size.
Stethoscope.

    A cuff of suitable size is chosen, the width of which should not exceed two-thirds of the length of the child's upper arm as the accuracy of the reading is related to the size of the cuff used. The same cuff should be used for all recordings.

METHOD

The child should be calm and quiet. It is pointless struggling to record the blood pressure of a fractious child. The arm is slipped out of its sleeve and the cuff, with the tubing towards the child's head, is wrapped evenly around the upper part of the arm, and the end tucked in. The arm is straightened and the brachial artery located towards the medial side of the anterior aspect of the elbow joint (the antecubital fossa). The cuff tubing is attached to the sphygmomanometer, the valve on the compression bulb is closed and air is pumped into the cuff until the pulsating brachial artery, and consequently the radial pulse, can no longer be felt. The pressure in the cuff is then raised a further 20mm Hg.

With the diaphragm of the stethoscope over the brachial artery, the air is slowly released from the cuff by gradually opening the valve on the compression bulb. The nurse watches the column of mercury in the sphygmomanometer and listens for the sharp tapping on the stethoscope as the blood begins to flow through the previously occluded brachial artery. The level of the mercury read at the point where these regular tapping sounds are first heard, is the systolic pressure.

The slow release of air from the cuff is continued until the regular, sharp tapping sounds are replaced by softer, blowing sounds. At the change of sounds, the level of mercury is again noted as this is the diastolic pressure. If it has not been possible to make an accurate recording, all the air is released from the cuff to prevent venous congestion in the extremity before attempting another reading.

The blood pressure is recorded on the appropriate chart and expressed as

$$\frac{\text{systolic blood pressure}}{\text{diastolic blood pressure}}$$

TABLE 12. Normal Range of Pulse, Respiration and Blood Pressure.
(See Table 2 for range during infancy.)

Age in years	Pulse rate per minute	Respiration: rate per minute	Blood Pressure mm Hg
3–6	100–90	30–20	100–110/60–70
7–10	100–80	24–20	100–120/60–80
1–14	90–70	20	110–120/70–80

2 CENTRAL VENOUS PRESSURE (C.V.P.)

This observation is confined to the experienced staff of an intensive therapy unit where frequent estimation of the central venous pressure is a routine procedure following major heart surgery and severe injuries.

The central venous pressure represents what is left of the systemic arterial pressure after the blood has traversed the arterioles, capillaries and venules. A reduced blood volume (hypovolaemia) will give a low recording. A failing or inefficient heart, or pressure on the heart from without, i.e. tamponade, causes the central venous pressure to rise.

Venous pressure cannot be measured in the same way as arterial blood pressure. A vena cava is cannulated via one of the large veins—the jugular or the femoral vein—and patency is maintained by a slow saline infusion. A mark is made over the sternal angle on which a centimetre ruler is placed vertically.

The child is nursed supine for this observation. The nurse washes and dries her hands, discontinues and disconnects the intravenous infusion and holds the venous catheter vertically above the mark on the sternum. The saline level in the catheter will fall until central venous pressure exceeds the pressure exerted by the column of saline. The ruler is placed on the sternal angle and the column of fluid is measured at its lowest level as it oscillates in the catheter.

The catheter is refilled by lowering the open end over a receptacle until all air is displaced and its blood content is dripping freely. It is then reconnected to the recipient set or syringed and flushed through with a small quantity of saline before readjusting the infusion to the prescribed rate.

Alternatively, a manometer may be used to take the recording. This is attached to the second arm of a two-way tap positioned between the recipient set and the intravenous catheter.

The normal range of central venous pressure is 7–10cm of saline (or 5–8mm Hg). Recordings below 5 and above 12cm of saline are considered abnormal.

Electrocardiogram (ECG) in Assessing Cardiac Function

The regular rhythmic contraction of heart muscle is spontaneously initiated by the pacemaker of the heart—the sino-atrial node—situated at the junction of the superior vena cava with the right atrium. Innervation of the sino-atrial node with fibres of the autonomic nervous system allows the heart rate to be adjusted according to the needs of the body.

The impulse passes over the atria, causing both to contract simultaneously. Following a short delay at the atrio-ventricular node, it passes to the bundle of His, and into branches of special Purkinje fibres on either side of the interventricular septum. Spontaneous contraction of both ventricles results. These waves of excitation (causing contraction) and recovery (causing relaxation) involve the movement of electrically charged atoms or ions, sodium (Na^+), potassium (K^+) and calcium (Ca^{++}), and give rise to changing electrical fields which can be detected by carefully positioned electrodes on the resting body surface.

An electrocardiogram is a graphic representation of the electrical changes associated with contraction and relaxation of heart muscle. The normal electrocardiograph (ECG) deflections are designated by the letters PQRST.

An electrocardiogram is recorded by direct writing or on an oscilloscope to

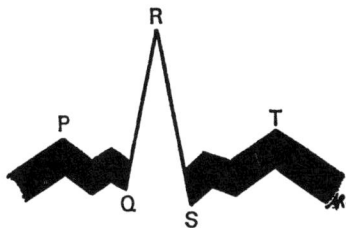

FIG. 29. The normal electrocardiogram. The P wave represents atrial systole (contraction). The QRS complex represents ventricular systole. The T wave represents the recovery phase following ventricular contraction.

aid in the diagnosis of a cardiac disorder. Continuous monitoring of the electrical activities of the heart is used increasingly to detect a sudden arrhythmia. Electrode jelly is applied to the dry skin to reduce resistance between the body surface and the metal monitoring electrodes and to prevent damage to the skin surface. The electrodes should be suitably positioned to allow for nursing care to be carried out and should be removed, the area cleansed, and further electrode jelly applied every four hours. Absence of electrode jelly, loose connections at the electrodes, and movement of the child cause inaccurate tracings to be recorded.

Respiration

Involuntary respiration adopts a regular rhythm in older children and adults, but during the first months of life it is perfectly normal for an infant to breathe at irregular intervals with short periods of apnoea.

VARIATIONS OF RESPIRATION

As with the pulse, when counting the respiration rate, other points should be observed. The rhythm of breathing, depth of each inspiration and any visual or audible distress experienced by the child must all be assessed.

Rate—the respiratory rate varies with age. It is increased in exercise and excitement and decreased during rest, sleep and relaxation. The presence of infection increases the body's need for oxygen; an increased respiration rate (tachypnoea) is therefore seen in febrile conditions. Local conditions of the chest increase the respiration rate even further. A slowing of the respiration rate is often the result of a raised intracranial pressure.

Rhythm—the normal rhythm of respiration is interrupted when the older child is aware that his respiration rate is being counted. It is a good idea, therefore, to continue to hold the child's wrist with the arm flexed over his chest while counting the rise and fall of the chest. Cheyne-Stokes respirations consist of a temporary cessation of breathing (apnoea), followed by respirations which increase in depth to a maximum. This type of respiration is rarely seen except in terminal illness and in an immature infant.

Depth—if breathing is painful, inspiration is rapid and shallow. If the need of the body for oxygen is great or if there is an excess of carbon dioxide in the blood, then the respirations will be deep (hyperpnoea).

Distress—or difficulty with breathing (dyspnoea) may be seen and/or heard. Normally, breathing is carried out by contraction and relaxation of the diaphragm and intercostal muscles. If difficulty is encountered, additional muscles are used. The rib-cage of the infant is soft and pliable. Difficulty with breathing is seen as intercostal, subcostal and sternal recession. In older children, the muscles of the shoulders may be used to try and increase the capacity of the chest. This particularly applies in asthma. The nostrils are seen to blow in and out when the child is distressed.

The occurrence of any audible sound in relation to inspiration and expiration should be noted, e.g. a wheeze may be inspiratory due to partial obstruction of the air-passages or expiratory, as in asthma. Grunting, sighing, yawning are further examples.

RECORDING THE RESPIRATION RATE
The rise and fall of the child's chest can be felt or seen and counted, i.e. zero, 1, 2, 3 etc., for a full minute without the child being aware of what the nurse is doing.

For Further Reading

CHAMBERLAIN E. N. and OGILVIE C. M. (1967). *Symptoms and Signs in Clinical Medicine*, 8th edition. John Wright and Sons Ltd., Bristol.

CHAPTER TEN

Diet in Health and Disease

In this chapter a brief outline of the science of nutrition is given, together with the application of this science to the planning of meals (dietetics) for healthy and sick children.

A Balanced Diet

A well-balanced diet is essential for good health and well-being at all ages, and should be sufficient both in quality and quantity.

QUALITY OF DIET	QUANTITY OF DIET
For growth and repair:	*For energy production:*
Proteins	Carbohydrates⎫ (according to
Mineral elements	Fats ⎭ energy expenditure)
For protection:	
Mineral elements	Proteins
Vitamins	

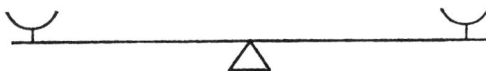

Nutrients

Carbohydrates

Carbohydrates are made up of carbon, hydrogen and oxygen. They are taken in the diet as starches (polysaccharides) and sugars (disaccharides) and broken down into their appropriate simple sugars (monosaccharides) by mechanical and chemical action in the alimentary tract.

DIGESTION OF CARBOHYDRATES

Polysaccharides	*Disaccharides*	*Monosaccharides*

Starch ⎫
Dextrins ⎬ ⟶ Maltose ⟶ Glucose + Glucose
Glycogen ⎭   Lactose ⟶ Glucose + Galactose
      Sucrose ⟶ Glucose + Fructose

Enzyme action: Salivary and   Maltase ⎫
   Pancreatic Amylase   Lactase ⎬ respectively from succus entericus
                         Sucrase ⎭

CHIEF SOURCES OF CARBOHYDRATES IN THE DIET
Starches—bread, flour and other cereals, potatoes.
Sugars—cane, preserves and lactose (milk sugar).

DIETARY REQUIREMENT
Dietary requirement is according to need and depends on the energy expenditure.
Usually 50–60% of the energy requirement is taken in the form of carbohydrate.

FUNCTIONS OF CARBOHYDRATE
The function of carbohydrate in the body is for the production of heat and energy which results from oxidation of glucose in the tissues.

$$C_6H_{12}O_6 + 6O_2 \longrightarrow 6H_2O + 6CO_2 \begin{cases} \longrightarrow \text{heat} \\ \longrightarrow \text{energy} \end{cases}$$

Each gramme of carbohydrate produces approximately 4kcal when oxidized in the body (1oz = 28·35g or approximately 30g).

An excessive carbohydrate intake is a very common dietary fault as it is comparatively cheap and palatable. When pocket money is liberal, kilocalories in the form of sweets and 'pop' are often taken in excess, producing obesity and dental caries.

During illness and starvation, the carbohydrate intake is often below the needs of the body. Firstly, the limited glycogen store is used to maintain the blood sugar within the normal range of 80–120mg/100ml; then the fat deposits are used. Ketones, the end products of the inadequate breakdown of fat, are found in excess in the blood and excreted by the kidneys.

Fats

Fats, like carbohydrates, contain carbon, hydrogen and oxygen in their molecules, but in different proportions. They are taken into the body as saturated or unsaturated fats, emulsified by the action of bile salts and broken down to fatty acids and glycerol by lipase.

DIGESTION OF FATS

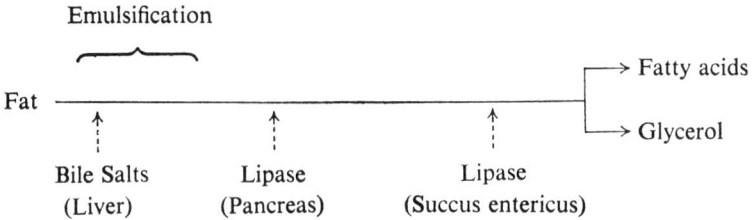

Emulsification

Fat ⟶⟶⟶⟶⟶⟶⟶⟶⟶⟶⟶⟶ ⟶ Fatty acids
⟶ Glycerol

Bile Salts   Lipase   Lipase
(Liver)   (Pancreas)   (Succus entericus)

Chief sources of fat in the diet. Fats are of animal or vegetable origin and are taken as meat, fat, butter and oils.

DIETARY REQUIREMENT

Fats can be synthesized in the body from carbohydrates and proteins. One gramme of fat produces 9kcal when oxidized in the body. Fat is therefore a convenient means of giving food of high energy value. Approximately 25–40% of the energy requirement is usually taken in the form of fat, but this is interchangeable with carbohydrates.

FUNCTIONS OF FAT IN THE BODY

1   A source of heat and energy.
2   To supply adequate amounts of the fat soluble vitamins A, D, E and K.
3   Fat is a 'protein sparer'. When given with protein, it allows the protein to be used for growth and repair as it supplies the needs of the body for heat and energy.

Protein

In addition to carbon, hydrogen and oxygen, protein contains nitrogen in its molecule and is an essential constituent of animal and plant protoplasm.

Proteins are made up of a chain of amino acids. Unlike polysaccharides which consist of a chain of like molecules (glucose), proteins consist of a chain of varying combinations of the twenty-four different known amino acids. In childhood, ten of these amino acids are essential, i.e. they must be taken in the diet as they cannot be synthesized in the body. These are arginine, histidine, isoleucine, leucine, lysine, methionine, phenylalanine, threonine, tryptophan and valine.

DIGESTION OF PROTEINS

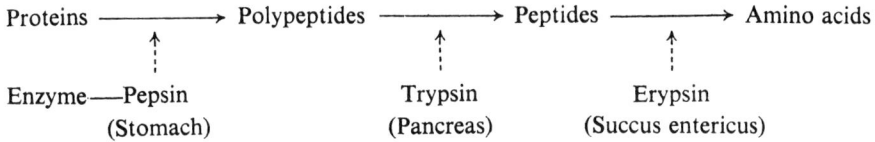

Proteins ⟶ Polypeptides ⟶ Peptides ⟶ Amino acids

Enzyme——Pepsin   Trypsin   Erypsin
        (Stomach)   (Pancreas)   (Succus entericus)

Chief sources of protein in the diet. First class proteins. Proteins obtained from animal source, i.e. meat, eggs, milk and cheese are called first class proteins because of the availability of essential amino acids in their substance. Second class proteins of vegetable origin are eaten as bread, flour and other cereals, nuts and pulses, and are deficient in one or more of the essential amino acids.

DIETARY REQUIREMENT

10% of the energy requirement should be in the form of protein which should be distributed throughout the main meals of the day as it cannot be stored in the body.

FUNCTION OF PROTEIN IN THE BODY

1   Growth and repair of tissues.
2   Essential for the formation of enzymes, hormones, plasma proteins, haemoglobin, etc.
3   As a source of energy.

One gramme of protein produces approximately 4kcal when oxidized in the body. When taken in excess of body need, or in the absence of adequate carbohydrate or fat, the protein undergoes the process of deamination in the liver, when the nitrogenous portion is converted to urea and excreted by the kidneys. The carbon, hydrogen and oxygen are retained for storage as a potential source of heat and energy. It is important, therefore, for a meal to include sufficient carbohydrate and/or fat to 'spare' the protein.

Energy Value of Nutrients

Carbohydrates, fats and proteins all produce energy when oxidized in the body:

    1 gramme of carbohydrate produces approximately 4kcal*
    1 gramme of fat produces approximately 9kcal
    1 gramme of protein produces approximately 4kcal

* A kilocalorie (kcal) is the amount of heat required to raise 1 kilogramme of water through 1°C.

Main sources of energy foods in the diet. Bread, flour and other cereals, fats, dairy produce, sugar and preserves provide the main sources of energy foods in the diet.

Energy is required by the body for:

1   Basal metabolism. Basal metabolism is the amount of energy required by an individual while the body is at rest and without food; in other words, the energy required to fulfil the requirements of the vital processes of the body. Basal metabolism is lowest at birth, but rises to a peak during the early years of childhood ($30kcal/m^2/hr$ at birth, $53kcal/m^2/hr$ at one year).

2   Everyday activities.

3   Muscular work.

The amount of energy used by different individuals of different age groups depends on the total living tissue in the body. This is proportional to the surface area of the body. (Surface area is dependent on weight and height of the individual.) Children need less kilocalories than adults as they are smaller in size, but as the child has a greater surface area in relation to his weight than the adult, his energy requirement is proportionately greater.

Mineral Elements

Mineral elements are distributed throughout a wide range of foods and are, therefore, present in a good all-round diet. When planning a diet, only the calcium and iron content of the diet must be considered.

Mineral Element.	*Function in the Body*
Calcium	Clotting of blood, muscular activity.
Magnesium	Constituents of bone.
Phosphorus	
Sulphur	Constituents of body cells — essential in metabolic processes.
Manganese	
Iron	Production of haemoglobin.
Sodium	
Potassium	Constituents of body fluids.
Chloride	
Iodine	For adequate thyroid activity.
Copper	For formation of haemoglobin.
Cobalt	For correct formation of red blood cells.

CALCIUM

An adequate intake of calcium and phosphorus is essential for the correct formation of bones and teeth, the clotting process of blood and functioning of muscles.

Bones act as a reservoir for calcium and phosphorus. To maintain the blood calcium level of 9–11·5mg/100ml, parathormone (the hormone produced by the parathyroid glands) mobilizes calcium and phosphorus from bone and teeth if dietary calcium is inadequate.

Chief sources of calcium in the diet. Foods high in calcium content are cheese and milk. A pint of milk taken daily supplies a large percentage of the body's need for calcium. Flour is fortified with calcium carbonate.

The presence of fat in the intestine prevents adequate absorption of calcium from the gut. Phosphorus is widely distributed, making deficiency rare.

IRON

About three-quarters of the iron in the body is found in the blood. Iron deficiency anaemia is common in low birth weight infants and is a common nutritional disorder, particularly in the early years of life. Milk is deficient in iron, and early weaning on to iron-containing foods, e.g. fortified cereals, egg yolk and puréed meat, will help to overcome this shortage.

Chief sources of iron in the diet. Eggs, meat, cereals, potatoes, green vegetables and flour. Liver is particularly rich in iron.

Vitamins

Vitamins are essential nutrients as they cannot be synthesized in the body. Their functions vary, but they are mainly concerned with the prevention of ill-health.

Most of the vitamins are provided in a well-balanced diet, but care must be taken to ensure that the full range of vitamins are represented.

Vitamins A, D, E and K are fat soluble vitamins. This means that they are found exclusively in the fatty part of animal and vegetable foods and can only be absorbed from the small intestine when there is correct absorption of fats.

Vitamin B complex and vitamin C are water soluble and their absorption is less complex.

Fat Soluble Vitamins

VITAMIN A

Vitamin A is of particular importance in childhood as it is essential for growth. It is also essential for the formation of visual purple in the rods of the retina to allow for night vision. The epithelial surfaces—the skin and the mucous membranes—require vitamin A to prevent hardening and to resist infection. Small quantities of vitamin A can be stored in the liver.

Chief sources of vitamin A in the diet. Vitamin A is found occurring naturally in eggs, dairy produce, fish oils and liver. Margarine is fortified with vitamin A and is an excellent source. Precursors of vitamin A are found in carotene of carrots and other root and green vegetables.

VITAMIN D

Like vitamin A, vitamin D is of considerable importance during the years of growth and development as it is essential for the absorption and laying down of calcium and phosphorus in the bones and teeth. Deficiency of this vitamin leads to the development of rickets. For this reason, vitamin preparations should be given during early childhood to supplement the vitamin D content of milk. Many of the proprietary milk preparations and baby cereals are fortified with vitamin D.

Chief sources of vitamin D in the diet. Dairy produce, eggs, fish, fat and margarine. In addition, vitamin D is produced in the body by the action of ultra-violet light on the sterols in the skin.

VITAMIN K

Vitamin K is essential for the formation of prothrombin, which is a necessary protein required in the clotting of shed blood. Dietary deficiency is rare, but cow's milk is lacking in vitamin K. Vitamin K is synthesized by the commensals of the large intestine, but as the large intestine of the newborn infant is sterile, there is a tendency for bleeding to occur as the prothrombin level in the blood is low.

Water Soluble Vitamins

VITAMIN B COMPLEX

Vitamins of the B group are required in small quantities, and are widely distributed in a well-balanced diet. Below are tabled some of the more important in this group.

Vitamin	Main source in the diet	Function in the body.
Thiamine (B1)	Bread flour, meat, potatoes, other vegetables.	Carbohydrate metabolism. Growth. Prevention of beri-beri.
Riboflavine (B2)	Dairy produce, meat (destroyed by sunlight).	Growth. Prevention of lesions of the epithelial tissues.
Nicotinic Acid (B3)	Meat, bread, flour and other cereals, potatoes.	Growth. Prevention of pellargra.
Folic acid	Liver and leafy vegetables. Synthesized in large intestine.	Formation of red blood cells.
(B12)	Milk, meat, eggs and fish, liver— excellent source. Synthesized in large intestine.	Formation of red blood cells.

Vitamin C (Ascorbic Acid)

Vitamin C occurs almost exclusively in fresh vegatables and citrus fruits. It is readily destroyed by heat, therefore raw, rather than cooked, vegetables are a better source of vitamin C.

Vitamin C is essential for growth, correct formation of connective tissue, promotion of healing and the prevention of scurvy. Scurvy in infants is characterized by an increased permeability of capillaries, causing painful sub-periosteal bleeding.

Chief sources of vitamin C in the diet. Potatoes, green vegetables, fresh citrus fruit. Milk is not a dependable source of vitamin C. Juices of high vitamin C content such as orange juice, blackcurrant juice and rose-hip syrup may be given to artificially-fed infants. Alternatively, the vitamin may be given as ascorbic acid tablets or in a multivitamin preparation.

Feeding Healthy Children

As children have small stomachs and a comparatively large energy requirement, nutrients need to be given every three to four hours. The daily requirements are best distributed in the form of three meals and one or two snacks in twenty-four hours.

Good eating habits should be established from an early age, with meals being served at regular intervals and eating between meals discouraged. Sweets are best given at the end of a meal, rather than between meals, to prevent appetite for protein foods being curbed. Small children find security in a rigid routine. They like to have their own tableware with a picture to see as their dish or cup is emptied.

Adequate time should be allowed to ensure that meal-times have as little distraction as possible, even if this means that they have to be adjusted according to the television programme of the day.

Food should be served attractively in suitably sized helpings for the different age groups. A second helping may always be given, whereas an overloaded plate will discourage most children from eating their meals.

Food should be of suitable texture according to the age of the child. During the weaning period, puréed foods are given to accustom the infant to less liquid nourishment. Gradually, mashed and minced foods replace the puréed food so that the infant is encouraged to masticate. During the pre-school years, the child learns to eat foods which require considerable chewing to help initially with teething and to encourage a good blood supply to the gums and teeth. Spicy foods and foods with strong flavours are best avoided in early childhood, but may be introduced as tastes for the different foods are acquired.

TABLE 13. Approximate Daily Dietary Needs.

Age	Fluid ml/kg	Kilocalories per kg	Protein g/kg	Calcium mg/day	Iron mg/day
0–1	150	120–105	2·8	600	6
1–2	100	105	2·6	500	7
2–3	100	100	2·5	500	7
3–5	90	95	2·4	500	8
5–7	90	90	2·2	500	8
7–9	80	85	2·1	500	10
Boys					
9–12	70	75	2	700	13
12–15	60	60	1·3	700	14
15–18	60	50	1·2	600	15
Girls					
9–12	70	70	1·7	700	13
12–15	60	50	1·2	700	14
15–18	60	40	1	600	15

Based on the Report of the Panel on Recommended Daily Allowances of Nutrients for the United Kingdom. H.M.S.O. 1969.

The Essentials of an Adequate Diet in Childhood

1   Foods required for building purposes should be well represented. These include protein (half of which should be from animal source), calcium, vitamin D and iron.

2   The protective foods in the form of vitamins and mineral elements should all be included.

3   Appetite determines how much energy food is required. Children are very active, requiring a greater number of kilocalories in proportion to their size. Their comparatively large appetites are not an indication of greed, but a true reflection of their need for energy-producing foods. Fat and carbohydrates are, therefore, given to fulfil this requirement.

4   Food given to children of the various age groups should be palatable and popular.

FOOD GROUPS

Milk Group. Milk—1 pint daily in childhood.

  Supplies: protein, calcium and riboflavine.

Meat Group. This group includes meat, fish, poultry, cheese and eggs.

  Supplies: protein, vitamin B and iron, vitamins A and D in fatty fish. Iodine in sea fish.

Fruit and vegetable group. Supplies: vitamin C in varying quantities, vitamin A as carotene, and roughage (indigestible fibre).

Cereal Group. Bread, breakfast cereals, flour, etc., are included in this group.
   Supplies: energy, protein, iron, vitamin B complex.
Fat Group. This includes dairy produce, and oils of vegetable origin.
   Supplies: energy and vitamins A and D.
Summary. Broadly speaking, foods from the above groups should be included
in the daily diet:
   1 pint of milk.
   2–3 helpings from the meat group.
   3–4 helpings from the fruit and vegetable group.
   Energy producing foods from the cereal and fat groups according to appetite.
   Fluid intake according to age and needs of the child.
   In addition, vitamin supplements should be given daily up to the age of two
      years.

A Suitable Day's Menu for the Pre-School Child

Breakfast:	Cereals.
	Egg, bacon or sausage.
	Bread or toast.
	Butter.
	Milk to drink.
Mid-morning:	Orange juice or milk.
	Biscuit.
Dinner:	Meat, fish or cheese.
	Potatoes.
	Second vegetable.
	Milk pudding, fruit and custard, etc.
Tea:	(Egg, cheese, fish) Marmite.
	Bread.
	Butter.
	Milk to drink.
	Jelly, apple or orange.
	Biscuit or small cake.
Bedtime:	Milk.

A Suitable Day's Menu for the School Child

Breakfast:	Cereal or porridge.
	Egg, bacon or fish.
	Toast and marmalade or Marmite.
	Tea, coffee or milk to drink.

Mid-morning: School milk (if under seven-years-of-age).

Dinner: Meat, fish, egg or cheese.
              Potatoes.
              Second vegetable, or salad.
              Milk or steamed pudding, pastry or stewed fruit and custard.

High tea: Cheese, egg or meat dishes, e.g. macaroni cheese, egg on toast,
                  salads, etc.
              Fruit, stewed or fresh.
              Cake or biscuits.
              Tea or milk to drink.

Bed-time: Milk as cocoa, Bournvita, Horlicks, etc.

School dinners are planned to supply the child with one good meal a day and must include at least 20g of protein. This is to safeguard the nutrition of children from the lower income groups.

Feeding Sick Children

Most children are fond of their food and eat well. Unless attention-seeking, reluctance to eat or feed is usually an early sign that a child is unwell. Feeding a sick child can prove difficult, especially if he is away from his familiar home environment. Every effort should be made to give him what he fancies and it is usually an advantage for his mother to be present at meal-times.

During the acute stage of an illness, it is impossible to supply a child's full energy requirements, but a normal fluid intake must be maintained by one or another route. Malnutrition will in itself hinder recovery, so it is essential that the child's energy needs are met as soon as possible. Tolerance to the food rather than full nutrition is the aim in the early days of recovery. If only small quantities can be taken at one time, full fluid intake must be ensured by giving frequent drinks, preferably during the day, so that adequate rest and sleep can be assured at night.

If an adequate fluid intake cannot be maintained by the oral route, a naso-gastric tube may be passed and the fluid administered intermittently or dripped into the stomach. Alternatively, the rectal or subcutaneous routes may be used, but in severe dehydration, all fluids are given intravenously.

Fluid Diet

A fluid diet is essential for all infants and for children in the following categories:
  i   those who are ill and weak with no appetite;

ii those who cannot chew or digest;
iii those who require tube feeding;
iv those who are unable to take sufficient nourishment as solid food because of difficulty or pain when swallowing (dysphagia).

CLEAR FLUIDS

5% sugar in N/5 saline producing 20kcal/100ml is offered at frequent intervals to sustain the fluid, but not the energy requirement of an ill infant.

For older children, water is made more interesting and acceptable with the addition of fruit juices and glucose. Kilocalories are best given in the form of glucose as sugar is sweet and nauseating in large amounts. Energy foods are necessary to prevent ketosis developing in a febrile child. One heaped teaspoon of glucose produces 20kcal and is acceptable if dissolved in 30ml of flavoured water. Ribena, in addition to producing 36kcal/15ml of concentrate, is a rich source of vitamin C. When the fluid intake must be restricted, fruit flavoured Hycal (Beecham) proves an excellent source of carbohydrate energy—1 bottle (180ml) producing 424 kilocalories.

As the condition of an infant inproves, the 5% sugar in N/5 saline feeds are gradually strengthened daily or on alternate days with half or full cream milk mixtures, prepared as quarter-strength (3%), half-strength (6%), three-quarters strength (9%), full-strength (12·5%) feeds. The period of time between feeds is gradually increased until the infant is back to his usual feeding regime. Mixed feeding is introduced as the infant's condition improves.

As the condition of an older child improves, the clear fluids are substituted for milk drinks and gradually a light, nourishing diet is introduced.

FULL-FLUID DIET (SUITABLE FOR TUBE FEEDING)

The preparation of fluid diets has been made easy by the introduction of proprietary preparations, some of which are complete foods, e.g. Complan (Glaxo), while others fulfil a need for additional protein, e.g. Casilan (Glaxo). A variety of fluids should be given to prevent gastro-intestinal upsets. The child's fluid and energy requirement can be met by using a complete food such as Complan, or by homogenizing and liquidizing selected foods contained in a normal diet, e.g. milk, eggs, cream, glucose, strained meats, etc. Tube feeds should be strained to remove lumps.

The two examples given below are suitable for an eight-year-old-boy weighing 25kg.

With reference to TABLE 13:

$$\text{Fluid requirement} = 80\text{ml} \times 25 = 2000\text{ml}$$
$$\text{Energy requirement} = 85\text{kcal} \times 25 = 2125\text{kcal}$$
$$\text{Protein requirement} = 2 \cdot 1\text{g} \times 25 = 52 \cdot 5\text{g}$$

Example 1.

Constituent	Amount g	Protein g	Fat g	Carbohydrate g	Kilocalories
Cow's milk	500	17·5	22	22·5	325
Complan	150	46	22	66	675
Prosparol	60	—	30	—	270
Caloreen	120	—	—	120	480
Water to	1800				
6 feeds each of 300 ml		63·5	74	208·5	1750
Ribena	30	—	—	18	72
Water to	200				
1 feed of 200 ml		63·5	74	226·5	1822

Example 2.

Constituent	Amount g	Protein g	Fat g	Carbohydrate g	Kilocalories
Cow's milk	600	21	26·5	27	390
Eggs (3)	6	21	21	—	270
Dried skimmed milk	90	30	—	45	300
Prosparol	60	—	30	—	270
Caloreen	120	—	—	120	480
Water to	1600				
5 feeds each of 320 ml		72	77·5	192	1710
Ribena	60	—	—	36	137
Water to	400				
2 feeds of 200 ml		72	77·5	228	1847

The energy value of these examples is divided approximately as follows:

Protein provides	14–16% of the energy intake.
Fat provides	34–38% of the energy intake.
Carbohydrate provides	48–52% of the energy intake.

SUPPLEMENTARY FLUID FEEDS

Following a debilitating illness or operation, the child's need for protein is particularly great. Such a child may be given nourishing drinks containing protein to supplement the normal ward diet. These should be offered at frequent intervals during the day at times which will not curb his appetite for the three main meals and should be made palatable and acceptable to the 'food faddy' convalescent child.

A 20% solution of Complan with added glucose (1 teaspoon/150ml), prepared as directed on the package, supplies approximately 6g protein and 100kcal/100ml and is acceptable if suitably flavoured. A high protein milk shake or egg flip may be given as a mid-morning or bed-time drink, or to replace an occasional main meal.

High Protein Milk Shake (1 × 150 ml shake)

Constituent	Amount g	Protein g	Fat g	Carbohydrate g	Kilocalories
Cow's milk (5 oz)	150	5	6·6	6·8	98
Casilan (2 teasp)	10	9	0·2	—	45
Glucose (1 teasp.)	5	—	—	5	20
Milk shake syrup to taste					
		14	6·8	11·8	163

METHOD
The dry ingredients are mixed to a paste with a small quantity of milk and whisked until smooth. The remaining milk is then slowly stirred in. Flavouring and colouring, or milk shake syrup, is added. An ice cream may be added just before serving. These additives increase the energy value of the shake.

High Protein Egg Flip

Constituent	Amount g	Protein g	Fat g	Carbohydrate g	Kilocalories
1 Egg	60	7	7	—	90
Milk (4 oz)	120	4·2	5·2	5·4	78
Casilan (1 teasp)	5	4·5	0·1	—	23
Glucose (3 teasp)	15	—	—	15	45
Flavouring to taste					
		15·7	12·3	20·4	236

METHOD
The egg, glucose and Casilan are whisked together while the milk is brought to the boil. When settled, the boiled milk is poured on the mixture, while stirring. Flavouring and colouring may be added to taste and the mixture strained before serving either hot or cold.

SOFT DIET
A soft diet consists of a normal diet modified in texture, and is used during the months of weaning and in conditions where mastication is contra-indicated, or swallowing difficult.

Therapeutic Diets

Diets used in the treatment of children must satisfy all the nutritional requirements of the child so far discussed, except when contra-indicated by the child's
illness.

HIGH PROTEIN DIET

A high protein diet is often ordered to give the patient additional nitrogen for
body building and tissue repair. In disease, and following injury or surgery, the
protein intake should be increased to counteract the increased protein loss. A
high protein diet is also indicated in the following situations:
1   Malnutrition.
2   Burns—to replace protein lost from burned area.
3   Nephrotic syndrome—to replace protein lost in urine.
    (+low salt diet)
4   Ulcerative colitis.
    (+low residue diet)
    The aim is to give the child one-and-a-half to twice (or even a greater quantity)
the normal requirement of protein. Children may find difficulty taking the diet,
and protein can conveniently be given by adding high protein content powders
to milk and milk dishes. Sufficient carbohydrate and fat should be given to
prevent the protein being used for the production of heat and energy (page 169).

Protein content of some foods

Milk	3·5g/100ml	0·9g/oz
Complan	31 g/100g	8·8g/oz
Casilan	90 g/100g	26 g/oz
Prosol	63 g/100g	17·8g/oz
Skimmed milk powder	35 g/100g	9·8g/oz
Egg	7 g/egg	7 g/egg
Carnation breakfast food	28·3g/100g	8·5g/oz

LOW PROTEIN DIET

A low protein diet is required for two main reasons:
1   When the failing kidneys are unable to excrete the nitrogenous end products
of protein metabolism. In patients with acute glomerular nephritis and renal
failure, a low protein diet will allow the kidneys to rest and prevent accumulation
of urea in the blood.
2   The liver is the only organ in the body where deamination of protein and
production of urea take place. Patients suffering from disease of the liver therefore require a low protein diet.

The aim of this diet is to keep the patient in nitrogen balance, i.e. the nitrogen intake must be equivalent to the nitrogen output. A minimum amount of protein is given to compensate for endogenous nitrogen metabolism (the metabolism of nitrogenous substances which arises from within the cells of the body)—equivalent to 20g protein/day.

A diet high in carbohydrate content is given for its protein-sparing effect.

MODIFIED GIOVANNETTI DIET

This diet provides the daily requirements of essential amino acids except methionine (which is given as an oral supplement) to a child suffering from chronic renal failure. The protein intake reduced to as little as 10g is taken in the form of milk, eggs, vegetables and fruit. Flour, meat, fish and cheese are strictly forbidden. An adequate energy intake in the form of Hycal or Caloreen is necessary to minimize the breakdown of proteins built within the body (catabolism of endogenous protein). Hyperkalaemia and hypernatraemia are controlled by reducing the potassium and sodium content of the diet respectively. Oral iron and vitamin supplements are necessary. Fluid intake may have to be restricted.

LOW SALT DIET

Dietary salt may be restricted when there is oedema or ascites present, as in:
  i   congestive heart failure;
 ii   kidney disorders, e.g. nephrotic syndrome;
iii   cirrhosis of the liver with ascites.

Salt may be restricted from the diet in two main ways:
1   No added salt to the food, and foods of high salt content such as tinned meats and fish, ham, cheese and Marmite are restricted.
2   Foods of low salt content, including most breakfast cereals, confectionery and chocolate, are excluded in addition to (1), and Edosol (Trufood) is substituted for milk.

For children suffering from kidney disorders such as nephrotic syndrome, a diet high in protein but low in salt content may be prescribed.

LOW KILOCALORIE DIET FOR OBESITY

Obesity is a problem of our affluent society. Many children are overweight due to over-indulgence of high carbohydrate foods often dating back to infancy. This may be due to emotional insecurity, poor eating habits or just sheer greed. Prevention of obesity is far better than trying to reduce the weight of an obese child.

The aim of the low kilocalorie diet is to give less energy foods than the normal daily requirement for the child, so that the remainder of the energy is obtained from the breakdown of the fat deposits in the body. Eating habits should be improved and eating between the three main meals and two snacks a day discouraged. Sweet foods are best avoided to wean the child from foods of high energy value.

To lose weight, the energy value of the food eaten is reduced without decreasing body activity. Alternatively, the activity of the individual may be increased without additional kilocalories being taken—a more difficult situation to fulfil, particularly in childhood where self-discipline is not established.

Foods forbidden: sugar, biscuits, cakes, pastries, puddings made with flour or suet, all fried foods, cereals, thickened gravy and soups, sweets, chocolate, ice cream, fruit squashes and 'pop'.

Other foods of high energy value such as bread and potatoes may be taken in limited quantities, i.e. 90g (3oz) of bread and 60g (2oz) of potato daily.

DIET IN DIABETES MELLITUS

Insulin produced by the islets of Langerhans in the pancreas is essential for absorption of glucose into the cells and for the conversion of glucose into glycogen (animal starch). Adrenaline, growth hormone, glucocorticoids and glucagon antagonize the action of insulin, causing mobilization of glucose from the glycogen stores to increase the blood sugar level.

In diabetes mellitus there is insufficient insulin to metabolize the carbohydrate intake. The blood sugar level exceeds the renal threshhold of 180ml/100ml and sugar is excreted in the urine (glycosuria):

Carbohydrate intake =   Insulin production

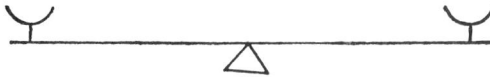

= Normal blood sugar level of 80–120mg/100ml

Carbohydrate intake   Insulin production inadequate

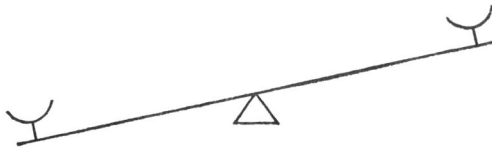

= Increase in blood sugar as in Diabetes Mellitus → Hyperglycaemia

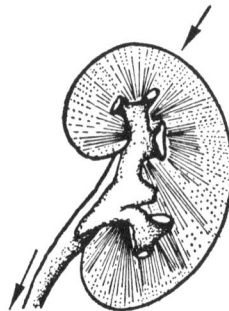

glycosuria

In the treatment of diabetes mellitus, the carbohydrate requirement for the day is estimated and divided between the various meals and snacks. Insulin required for the metabolism of the carbohydrate content of the diet is given in daily, or twice daily, doses. The urine is tested at regular, frequent intervals to give an indication of the blood sugar level.

As the fat content of the diet is sometimes restricted to prevent obesity which may predispose to complications later in life, it may be necessary to increase the protein content to suffice the energy needs of the child.

Foods of high carbohydrate concentration are restricted to prevent the development of a 'sweet tooth' and to avoid too rapid absorption of the food substances.

To stabilize a child on a suitable diet, with the required amount of insulin necessary to maintain the urine sugar-free for most of the twenty-four hours, a near normal life must be led while in hospital. Outdoor activities are encouraged so that the home situation may be simulated.

The twenty-four hour carbohydrate requirement is divided into 10g portions or lines, and these are distributed throughout the meals and snacks of the day. *Example:* A child of seven years of age requires approximately 160g of carbohydrate a day (TABLE 13). These may be divided as follows:

Breakfast	3 portions, i.e. 3 × 10g
Mid-morning	2 portions
Dinner	4 portions
High tea	3 portions
Bed-time	4 portions

The 10g portions are interchangeable with a wide range of foods. Tables of food exchanges, foods best avoided, and foods taken freely, together with recipes, are available from the British Diabetic Association (Appendix B).

If an ill child is unable to eat his diet, other 10g portions should be supplemented.

Each of the following contain 10g (1 portion) of carbohydrate:

> 2 rounded teaspoons glucose
> 2 level teaspoons sugar
> 60ml Lucozade
> 30ml orange or lemon squash
> 105ml fresh orange juice
> 2 large sugar lumps
> 5 small sugar cubes
> 210ml milk

GLUTEN-FREE DIET FOR COELIAC DISEASE

Coeliac disease is a condition where there is intolerance to gluten—the protein found in wheat and rye flour. As a result of this intolerance, the villi of the small intestine are flattened, preventing the absorption of essential nutrients. Wasting, failure to thrive and anaemia result, and the stools are bulky, greasy, offensive and frequent.

Dietary treatment of the condition is very satisfactory with a reversal of the clinical features. Foods containing wheat and rye and their products are substituted with foods containing wheat starch. Gluten-free wheat starch biscuits and bread can be made in the home, and are prepared by Welfare Foods (Stockport) Ltd. as Rite-Diet Gluten-free Products, available on prescription (E.C.10). With the exception of gluten-containing foods, the child may eat a normal diet. The fat content of the diet is often restricted in the early days of treatment to allow the more essential nutrients to be absorbed, skimmed milk being substituted for whole milk.

LOW FAT DIET
Indications for use
1 Where there is disturbance to the liver or biliary system, resulting in a lack of bile in the small intestine, e.g. hepatitis and congenital obliteration of the bile ducts.
2 In malabsorption syndrome, the presence of fat in the intestine may interfere with the absorption of other nutrients.
3 Following a large resection of gut, absorption of nutrients may be restricted. Reducing the fat content of the diet will allow greater absorption of the more essential nutrients.
4 In cystic fibrosis digestion and absorption of protein and carbohydrates may be inhibited if large quantities of fat are present in the intestine. Whole cow's milk may be given, but extra Pancrex will be needed.

The aim of this diet is to reduce the fat and to make up the energy requirement of the child by increasing the protein and carbohydrate content of the diet. The diet is monotonous, bulky and less palatable than the normal diet. The fat soluble vitamins A and D must be supplied as supplements in their water form. If bile is absent from the small intestine, vitamin K must also be given.

Snow Queen (Alfonal) and Cow and Gate Separated are two milks available with a fat content reduced to 0·1%.

MILK-FREE DIET
An infant who fails to thrive on cow's milk may have an intolerance or allergy to the protein caseinogen. This intolerance may also be due to lactose or galactose intolerance—see disaccharide intolerance. Velactin (Wander Ltd.) is a complete milk substitute where the protein is of soya bean origin, the fat is arachis oil and the carbohydrate content is supplied as starch, dextrose, sucrose and dextrins. Alternatively, Comminuted Chicken Meat (Trufood) may be prescribed. This may be diluted in water and given as a bottle feed. Each 100g contains 6·7g protein, 2g fat, thus producing 46kcal. Liquefied pressure-cooked

silverside beef may be added to a milk-free feed consisting of meat, Prosparol (providing fat) Caloreen or glucose, baby rice, etc.

Vitamin supplements are supplied in the form of Ketovite syrup and tablets.

MINIMAL LACTOSE DIET FOR GALACTOSAEMIA

Galactosaemia is a rare inborn error of metabolism, caused by deficiency of the enzyme essential for the conversion of galactose to glucose. Galactose accumulates in the liver, brain and lenses. Prognosis is poor unless early dietary treatment is given.

Galactose is a monosaccharide found in combination with glucose to form milk sugar—lactose. It is also found in some plant polysaccharides, e.g. soya and legumes—both of which are galactosides.

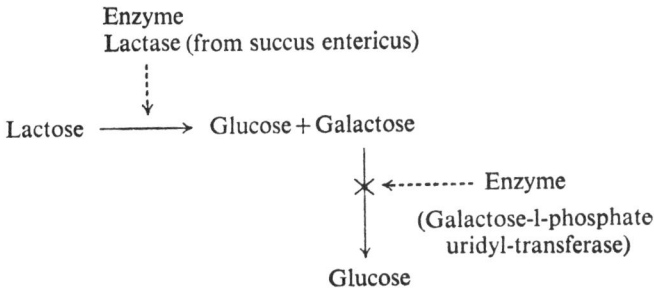

```
                Enzyme
                Lactase (from succus entericus)
                      ┊
                      ▼
    Lactose  ──────▶  Glucose + Galactose
                                    │
                             ╳ ◀------- Enzyme
                             │          (Galactose-l-phosphate
                             ▼              uridyl-transferase)
                        Glucose
```

Dietary treatment of the condition is exclusion of foods containing galactose. Milk substitutes available are:

Galactomin (Trufood)
Low Lactose Milk Food (Cow & Gate)
Nutramigen (Mead Johnson)
Velactin (Wander)—not used when there is galactoside intolerance.

Vitamin supplements, in the form of Ketovite syrup and tablets are essential.

DIET IN CARBOHYDRATE (DISACCHARIDE) INTOLERANCE

Increasing numbers of children suffering from persistent diarrhoea and failure to thrive have been found to have an intolerance to one or more sugars. The conditions may be due to an inborn error of metabolism or the result of a temporary disturbance of an enzyme system, due to gastro-enteritis, coeliac disease, or following resection of a large portion of gut.

When there is lactose intolerance, milk and milk products must be omitted. The lactose of cow's milk is replaced by one of the other sugars as in Cow & Gate Low Lactose feeds and Galactomin Formulae 17 and 19. A milk substitute such as Velactin may be given if intolerance to caseinogen is also suspected (page 184).

When it is found that a child suffers from sucrose or fructose intolerance, all foods containing these sugars are excluded from the diet. Household sugars, confectionery, root vegetables and fruits are excluded, and glucose is substituted for sweetening purposes.

The usual additional vitamin supplements are required.

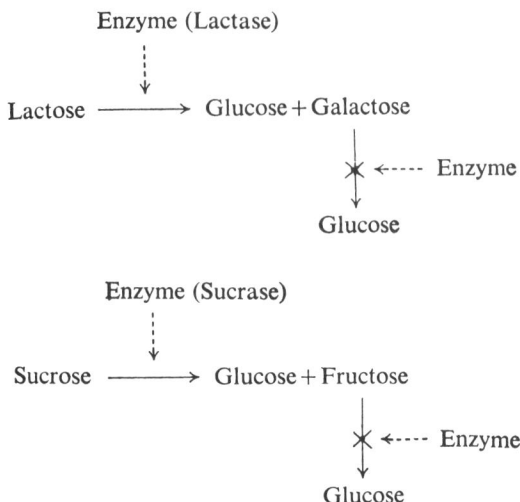

Enzyme (Lactase)

Lactose ──────→ Glucose + Galactose

⤬ ◄---- Enzyme

Glucose

Enzyme (Sucrase)

Sucrose ──────→ Glucose + Fructose

⤬ ◄---- Enzyme

Glucose

LOW PHENYLALANINE DIET IN PHENYLKETONURIA

Phenylketonuria is an inborn error of metabolism inherited as a recessive familial disorder, occurring in approximately 1–10,000 births. It is due to a deficiency of the enzyme phenylalanine hydroxylase, necessary in the metabolism of the essential amino acid phenylalanine to tyrosine.

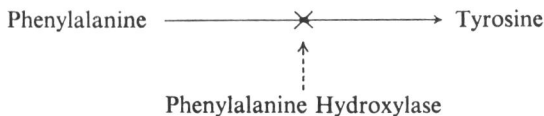

Phenylalanine ──────⤬──────→ Tyrosine

Phenylalanine Hydroxylase

In the absence of this enzyme, abnormal metabolites of phenylalanine accumulate in the body, resulting in irreversible brain damage causing convulsions and gross mental retardation. Tyrosine, necessary for the formation of melanin, is not formed so that the untreated European child with phenylketonuria usually has light-coloured hair and blue eyes.

The diagnosis is made by a raised plasma phenylalanine level measured by the Guthrie test (page 417), or by the presence of phenylpyruvic acid in a freshly-passed specimen of urine detected by a positive result to the Phenistix test (Ames). Diagnosis must be made and treatment instituted early if permanent brain damage is to be prevented. The treatment is dietary, and aims at giving a diet containing a small proportion of phenylalanine necessary to allow growth and development to take place.

The diet is expensive, restricted and monotonous. The protein intake of the child is given as a synthetic substitute low in phenylalanine content. Minafen (Trufood), Albumaid XP (Scientific Hospital Supplies) or Lofenalac (Mead Johnson) may be used for infants. In the first few months of life, the phenylalanine requirement is 50mg/kg/day to maintain a plasma level of around 2–3mg/100ml. This may be achieved by varying the supplement of fresh cow's milk which contains 171mg phenylalanine/100ml. For older children on mixed feeding who require comparatively less phenylalanine, a change to Cymogran or Aminogran (Allen and Hanbury) allows a more liberal diet to be given. An early change is advisable as difficulty may well be experienced introducing the child, at a later stage, to the unpleasant taste and smell of the food. Vitamin supplements must be given in the form of Ketovite tablets and syrup, daily.

The phenylalanine content of the diet is adjusted according to the plasma level of phenylalanine which is maintained at 1·0–5·0mg/ml. Frequent checks, using the Phenistix test, will give an indication as to whether the child is receiving too much phenylalanine in his diet. Regular Guthrie tests will give a more accurate estimation of the child's progress, and indicate any necessary adjustment in the diet.

The principles of dietary treatment of other inborn errors of metabolism such as histidinaemia, tyrosinosis and maple syrup urine disease are similar to those described above.

LOW CALCIUM DIET FOR HYPERCALCAEMIA

Hypercalcaemia results from:

i sensitivity to vitamin D in the early months of life;
ii overfeeding with vitamin D fortified foods in the first year of life.

Most of the proprietary artificial feeds and baby cereals are fortified with vitamin D and this must be taken into consideration when vitamin supplements are given to artificially-fed infants.

Locasol (Trufood) and Low Calcium Milk food (Cow & Gate) are two preparations low in calcium content used in hypercalcaemia.

LOW RESIDUE DIET

Roughage increases the amount of formed faecal matter excreted and is a necessary requirement in the prevention of constipation. A low residue diet is used:

i in the week prior to intestinal resection;
ii during the post-operative phase to allow healing to progress;
iii in ulcerative colitis;
iv in the control of diarrhoea.

Foods excluded from the diet are whole fruits and vegetables both raw and cooked, preserves, foods containing wholemeal cereals—bread, biscuits and crispbreads—fatty foods, and tinned or processed meats, fish and cereals.

The diet is deficient in vitamin C and should be supplemented with orange or blackcurrant juices.

For Further Reading

FRANCIS D. E. M. and DIXON D. J. W. (1969). *Diets for Sick Children*, 2nd edition. Blackwell Scientific Publications, Oxford.

CHAPTER ELEVEN

Fluid and Electrolyte Replacement

Water is essential for healthy functioning of the body. Dissolved in the fluids of the body are substances (solutes) called electrolytes which give the body fluids osmotic pressure.

Isotonic fluids contain the same proportion of solutes in solution as body fluids.

Hypotonic fluids have less solute in solution than body fluids.

Hypertonic fluids have a greater proportion of solutes in solution than the fluids of the body.

DISTRIBUTION OF BODY FLUIDS

Approximately 60% of the weight of an adult is water. Two-thirds of this volume are inside the cells (intracellular), the remaining one-third outside the cells (extracellular). The extracellular compartment can be divided into tissue fluid (interstitial fluid) and blood (intravascular).

Almost 75% of an infant's weight is water and a greater proportion of this fluid is extracellular.

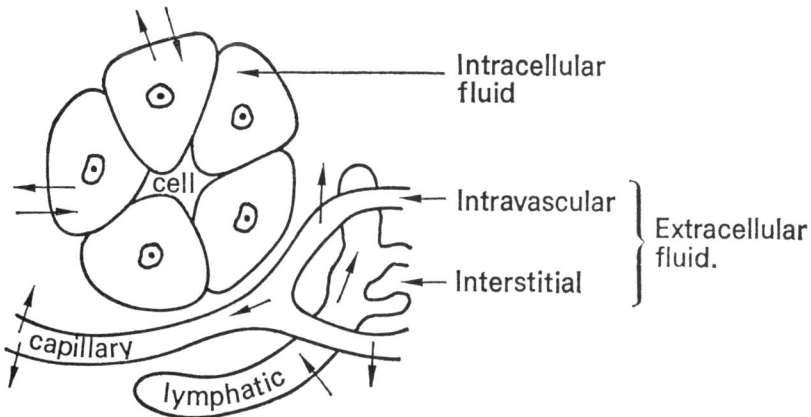

FIG. 30. Fluid compartments of the body.

189

TABLE 14. Distribution of Body Fluids in Adults and Infants

	Adult % weight	Infant % weight
Total body fluid =	60	60–70
Intracellular fluid =	40	40–45
Interstitial fluid =	15	25–30
Intravascular fluid =	5	8

To maintain fluid equilibrium within the body, the fluid requirement of an infant is far greater in proportion than that required by the adult. The fluid requirement for the average adult is approximately 50ml/kg; an infant requires 150ml/kg after the first five to seven days of life. This is due to the following reasons:

1 The metabolic rate of the infant is almost double that of the average adult, therefore, the loss of fluid through the skin, lungs and kidneys is relatively greater than in the adult.

2 Relatively large amounts of dilute urine are passed during the first few months of life as the immature kidneys are unable to concentrate urine.

Deprivation of fluid or excess fluid loss can rapidly give rise to serious fluid depletion in childhood and particularly in infancy.

FLUID EXCHANGE WITHIN THE COMPARTMENTS

The fluid compartments of the body are separated by semi-permeable membranes which maintain the definite chemical composition of the fluids on either side.

Osmosis is the process by which fluid is drawn through a semi-permeable membrane from an area of low concentration of solute to an area of high concentration until equilibrium is reached. The pressure exerted by this 'pull' is called the osmotic pressure.

Example 1. When there is excessive water loss from the body the volume of fluid in the extracellular compartment is reduced and the osmotic pressure increased. To restore the osmotic balance, fluid is withdrawn from the cells:

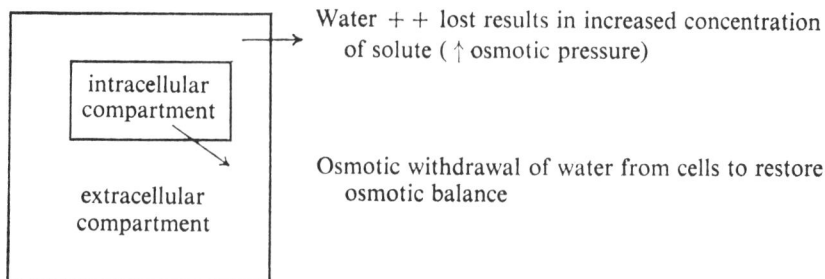

intracellular
compartment

extracellular
compartment

Water + + lost results in increased concentration of solute (↑ osmotic pressure)

Osmotic withdrawal of water from cells to restore osmotic balance

Example 2. When excess hypotonic solution is administered, as may occur with water absorption via the rectal route, the reverse situation occurs:

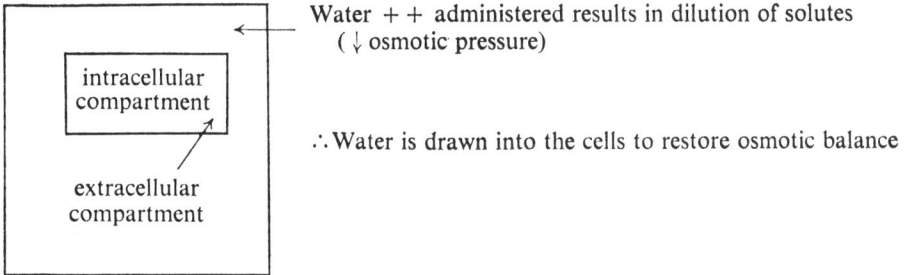

Water + + administered results in dilution of solutes (↓ osmotic pressure)

intracellular compartment

∴ Water is drawn into the cells to restore osmotic balance

extracellular compartment

Electrolytes

Inorganic acids, alkalies (bases) and salts, when in solution within the body, dissociate into charged atoms or ions. An electrolyte can be defined as a substance in solution which will conduct an electric current because it is dissociated into its charged molecules or atoms called ions. Positively (+ve) charged ions are called cations and negatively (−ve) charged ions, anions.

Electrolytes are estimated and expressed as the actual proportion of the solute present, i.e. milliequivalents per litre (mEq/1). Within the body fluids there are 300mEq of electrolytes per litre of solution, 150mEq cations and an equal number of anions.

The main extracellular cation is sodium (Na^+) and anion is chloride (Cl^-). The composition of the intracellular fluid consists mainly of potassium (K^+), phosphate (PO_4^-) and protein.

The normal range of serum electrolytes for healthy children is as follows:

Sodium	136–145	mEq/1
Potassium	4–5·5	mEq/1
Chloride	100–110	mEq/1

Acid-Base Balance

Acids are constantly being produced in the body as the result of metabolic processes. Acidity is conveniently expressed by the symbol pH, which stands for the negative logarithm of the hydrogen ion concentration. An increase in the hydrogen ion concentration lowers the pH. A decrease in the hydrogen ion concentration raises the pH (FIG. 31).

The body maintains the blood pH within the narrow range of 7·36–7·42 by means of powerful buffer systems which can accommodate acids and alkalies (bases) without the pH being greatly altered. Only when there is failure in the buffer systems does the pH fall outside the normal range. One of the best known buffer systems is the carbon dioxide, bicarbonate system. Its immediate readiness for action in the body is determined by the availability of bicarbonate and the

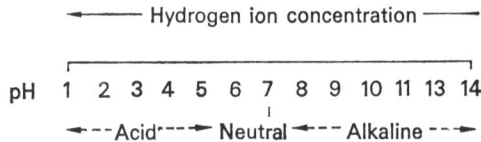

◄────── Hydrogen ion concentration ──────►

pH 1 2 3 4 5 6 7 8 9 10 11 13 14

◄‑‑Acid·‑‑‑► Neutral ◄‑‑‑ Alkaline ‑‑‑►

FIG. 31. pH notation. Water is neutral (pH7). Acids have a pH of less than 7. Bases or alkalies have a pH greater than 7.

rapid way in which the lungs can excrete carbon dioxide. Maintenance of the blood pH at 7·4 is dependent on the carbon dioxide in solution and bicarbonate remaining in the ratio of 1 : 20. Alterations which occur, due primarily to changes in the level of carbon dioxide in solution, are termed respiratory, whereas alterations which occur, due primarily to changes in the bicarbonate level, are termed metabolic or non-respiratory.

Acid-Base Disturbance

ACIDOSIS

Acidosis, due to a reduction in the bicarbonate level, is termed a metabolic acidosis, whereas that due to an excess of carbon dioxide in solution is termed a respiratory acidosis.

Metabolic acidosis occurs when there is retention of abnormal amounts of acid in body fluids. Diabetic ketosis and renal failure are conditions in which acid substances are increased. Initially there is a reduction in the bicarbonate level. Stimulation of the respiratory centre results in larger volumes of carbon dioxide being excreted from the lungs and a reduction in the carbon dioxide in the blood. A new equilibrium is established with the pH only slightly reduced from the normal value of 7·4, but with both the bicarbonate and carbon dioxide in solution reduced. This is referred to as compensated acidosis and is detected by a low standard bicarbonate value.

Inefficiency of the lungs to clear the blood of carbon dioxide causes *respiratory acidosis*. The kidneys excrete acid urine and retain bicarbonate in order to maintain the pH within the normal range.

ALKALOSIS

Alkalosis, due to an excess of bicarbonate, is termed metabolic alkalosis, whereas that due to a reduction in the carbon dioxide in solution is termed respiratory alkalosis.

Metabolic alkalosis arises when there is either excessive loss of acid products from the body or excessive intake of alkaline substances. Normally the hydrochloric acid of the gastric secretions is neutralized by the alkaline nature of the pancreatic juice. Should the acid gastric juice be lost by vomiting, the body will have a surplus of bicarbonate. Renal compensation increases the loss of base. Because of the rise in the pH of blood, the respiratory centre is depressed and as a result, carbon dioxide is retained in the blood. A new equilibrium is established with the pH only slightly increased from the normal value, but with both the bicarbonate and carbon dioxide in solution increased. This is referred to as compensated alkalosis and is detected by an increased standard bicarbonate value.

Respiratory alkalosis follows an excessive loss of carbon dioxide from the lungs during overbreathing (hyperventilation). Initial hyperventilation produces respiratory alkalosis following ingestion of excessive amounts of salicylates, i.e. aspirin, but this phase is usually short and is followed by metabolic acidosis. The kidneys excrete bicarbonate and retain acid in order to maintain the blood pH within the normal value.

SUMMARY

Acid-Base Disturbance	pH	P_{CO_2}	Standard Bicarbonate
Metabolic acidosis	↓	↓	↓
Respiratory acidosis	↓	↑	Normal or ↑
Metabolic alkalosis	↑	↑	↑
Respiratory alkalosis	↑	↓	Normal or ↓

The ability of the body to compensate for acid-base balance is limited. When the limit is reached, extra-corporeal compensating mechanisms have to be brought into use if the child is to survive, e.g. administration of intravenous sodium bicarbonate and the use of intermittent positive pressure ventilation in the treatment of profound respiratory acidosis.

BLOOD-GAS ANALYSIS

Capillary blood from a warm limb or arterial blood withdrawn under anaerobic conditions is necessary for the micro-Astrup analysis of acid-base balance. The pH, P_{CO_2} and standard bicarbonate are assessed. Base excess (which may be negative) is also frequently determined to assess the amount of base required to achieve correction of the balance. The normal range of base excess is -4 to $+2$ mEq/litre.

P_{CO_2} is the symbol used for the tension or partial pressure of carbon dioxide. (In a mixture of gases the pressure exerted by one gas is called its partial pressure.) The P_{CO_2} of plasma is controlled by respiratory mechanisms and is determined by the percentage of carbon dioxide in the alveolar air. The normal range is 32–46mmHg.

The bicarbonate level of plasma is a measurement of the non-respiratory component of acid-base balance and is controlled by the kidneys. The bicarbonate level is estimated under standardized conditions, i.e. on fully oxygenated whole blood ($P_{O_2} = 100$mmHg) when the P_{CO_2} is 40mmHg and the temperature 38°C, and is therefore referred to as the standard bicarbonate estimation. The normal range is 21·3–24·8mEq/litre.

Fluid and Electrolyte Imbalance

Dehydration is the state where the body is deprived of, or has lost water and salts.

In health, fluid and electrolyte equilibrium is maintained by a balance between fluid gain and fluid loss.

Fluid gain	=	*Fluid loss*
Fluid intake		Kidneys → urine
Food		Skin → sweating
Water of metabolism		Lungs → expired air
		Rectum → faeces

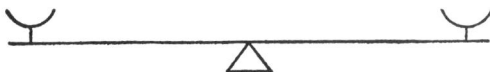

In illness, fluid and electrolyte imbalance may be due to:
1   a diminished intake;
2   an excessive output, e.g.
        diarrhoea,
        vomiting,
        sweating,
        polyuria,
        aspirate and drainage.

CLINICAL FEATURES OF DEHYDRATION
1   Dry tongue.
2   Scanty, concentrated urine.
3   Inelastic skin.
4   Sunken eyes and fontanelle.
5   Loss of weight.
6   Fever, particularly in severe dehydration.
7   Hypotonic muscles due to depleted potassium.

ROUTES AND METHODS OF REPLACEMENT
1   Fluid intake by mouth is increased (Chapter 10).

2   Intra-gastric feeding
    naso-gastric tube (Chapter 7).
    gastrostomy (Chapter 7).
3   Rectal infusion.
4   Subcutaneous infusion.
5   Intravenous infusion.
6   Intraperitoneal infusion.

The route and nature of fluid chosen for the replacement of body fluid depends on the severity of the dehydration and the type of fluid lost. With artificial means of fluid replacement, considerable care must be taken to prevent overloading the circulation.

Parenteral Administration

The intravenous route is the one giving the greatest control of fluid and electrolyte administration. The child is usually ill and dehydrated prior to the commencement of the infusion. The amount and nature of the fluid prescribed by the doctor will account for:

i   correction of initial dehydration;
ii   the child's usual daily requirement of fluid and electrolytes, according to weight;
iii replacement of abnormal losses such as occur in gastric aspirate, vomiting and diarrhoea.

An accurate record of the volume and nature of the fluid administered and of the child's output must be kept, and a urine collecting bag is applied if necessary.

Replacement Therapy

All solutions are prepared with special pyrogen-free water and sterilized in an autoclave.

1   ELECTROLYTE SOLUTIONS
    Normal (i.e. physiologically normal) *saline:* Sodium chloride 0·9%.
    Half-normal saline: Sodium chloride 0·45%.
    One-fifth normal saline: Sodium chloride 0·18%.

The weaker saline solutions may be used when water and a minimal amount of sodium are required by the body, as for example in the neonatal period, or they may be combined with dextrose 4·3% to produce an isotonic solution and some kilocalories.

Hartmann's solution and *Darrow's solution* contain sodium, calcium, potassium chlorides and lactate in varying proportions.

Sodium lactate and *sodium bicarbonate* are alkaline solutions used to correct or prevent acidosis.

Potassium chloride and *calcium gluconate* are available in ampoules for adding to bottles of parenteral fluid. Both potassium and calcium are necessary for co-ordination of neuromuscular activity, and therefore affect the rhythm of the heart beat if given in excessive amounts or if they are depleted in the body. They must be diluted in a quantity of electrolyte solution for administration.

2 DEXTROSE SOLUTIONS
Dextrose in water or *dextrose 4·3% in 0·18%* saline may be used as an isotonic maintenance fluid.

$$\text{Dextrose } 5\% \text{ in water} = 5\text{g dextrose}/100\text{ml}$$

Therefore each 100ml will produce 20kcal and each litre will produce 200kcal when oxidized in the body.

Dextrose 50% may be used in small quantities in the treatment of insulin overdosage.

3 FAT EMULSION COMPOUND, e.g. *Intralipid* (Vitrum, Stockholm).
This emulsion provides a large number of kilocalories in a small volume of fluid for intravenous nutrition, and is of value during prolonged intravenous therapy. No electrolyte solutions, vitamin supplements, or drugs are added to the solution as these will cause the fine emulsion to form large fat particles.

Intralipid is prepared as:
   10% solution, i.e. 10g/100ml = 90kcal/100ml or 900kcal/litre.
   20% solution, i.e. 20g/100ml = 180kcal/100ml or 1800kcal/litre.

The recipient set must be renewed before and following the administration of Intralipid.

4 PROTEIN REPLACEMENT, e.g. *Aminosol* (Vitrum, Stockholm).
This preparation contains a mixture of the essential amino acids necessary for the synthesis of body protein.

Aminosol is prepared as:
   Aminosol 10% i.e. 10g/100ml = 40kcal/100ml or 400kcal/litre.

To ensure that the protein is 'spared' for repair of tissues, the child must receive sufficient kilocalories. Aminosol and Intralipid may be administered simultaneously through a Y-shaped connection, or a solution containing amino acids and glucose or amino acids, fructose and ethanol is given.

Aminosol-Glucose solution produces 307kcal/litre
   3·3%   5%

Aminosol-Fructose-Ethanol produces 875kcal/litre
   3·3%   15%   2·5%

5 PLASMA SUBSTITUTES

Dextran 6% in normal saline or in dextrose is used to expand the vascular compartment. This may be desirable when shock, resulting from a diminished blood volume, has led to a fall in the blood pressure. Proprietary preparations of dextran such as Dextraven, Intradex or Macrodex may be used to maintain the arterial blood pressure while awaiting arrival of compatible blood. Blood for grouping and cross-matching must be taken before dextran is administered as it causes rouleaux formation of the red blood cells.

Intravenous Infusion

There are four methods used in childhood for administering fluid by the intravenous route:

  i   Venepuncture or 'stab' method;
 ii   Vein dissection or 'cut-down' method;
iii   Umbilical cannulation;
 iv   Scalp vein method.

The requirements for the various methods differ, but the maintenance of the infusion and the nursing care of the child are the same.

Venepuncture ('stab' method)

This is the method of choice but, as the veins of infants and small children are small, fragile and difficult to enter by percutaneous puncture, the method is of limited use in paediatrics.

REQUIREMENTS

The basic trolley is prepared as described on page 258 with the addition of the following equipment:

BOTTOM SHELF

Mask and gown for the doctor.
Covered splint and bandage to immobilize the limb.
Bottle of prescribed intravenous fluid.
Bottle clip.
Recipient set.
Suitable needle, e.g.
    No. 1 hypodermic needle.
    Guest's cannula.

Batemann needle.

or

Small vein set.

Mediswab.

Receiver for excess fluid.

Narrow adhesive tape.

Sphygmomanometer.

Fluid balance chart.

Waterproof protection for the bed.

At the bedside:

Anglepoise lamp.

Infusion stand.

PREPARATION OF THE CHILD

A simple explanation is given to an older child. Sedation may be necessary if the child is restless or apprehensive. The child is placed in a comfortable position in bed with the clothing removed from the selected limb. A vein in the arm or dorsum of the hand is usually preferred. A padded splint of suitable size is applied to the arm, care being taken not to restrict the circulation. It may be necessary to restrain the other arm of a small child to avoid interference with the infusion.

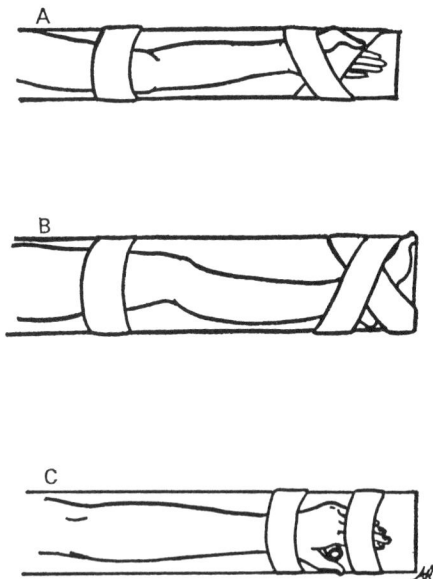

Fig. 32. Splinting of a limb for intravenous therapy into:
    A. a vein in the antecubital fossa;
    B. the long saphenous vein;
    C. a vein in the dorsum of the hand.

METHOD

The fluid to be administered is checked by the doctor and nurse. The bottle seal is broken and the rubber cap cleansed prior to the needle of the recipient set being introduced into the inverted bottle. The flow regulator is opened to allow the fluid to run through the whole apparatus to expel the air. The flow of fluid is interrupted by closing the flow regulator, and the sterile end for insertion into the needle or cannula is covered with its protective sheath.

While the doctor washes and dries his hands, the nurse ensures that everything required for the procedure is on the top of the trolley. The bedclothes are protected with the waterproof sheet.

In order that the veins may be made more prominent, the nurse may be asked to apply manual pressure around the upper arm, or a sphygmomanometer cuff may be placed in position and the pressure raised to 50mmHg.

The needle is inserted after cleansing the skin. Pressure is withdrawn from the upper arm. The primed recipient set is attached to the needle and the fluid flow regulated. A piece of gauze is placed over the needle and lengths of adhesive tape are used to secure the needle and tubing in position. The limb is bandaged to the splint, leaving the extremity exposed for inspection.

The child is made comfortable, ensuring that the locker of an older child is placed in a suitable position; if the infusion is in the left arm, the locker is placed on the patient's right hand side.

Vein Dissection ('cut-down' method)

This method is used when intravenous fluids are needed urgently by a collapsed, dehydrated infant, and when difficulty is encountered inserting the needle by the venepuncture method. A small incision is made over the site of a vein which is exposed for cannulation. The long saphenous vein, exposed just above the internal malleolus of the ankle, is the site most often chosen. The cephalic vein in the antecubital fossa may also be used.

REQUIREMENTS

The basic trolley is prepared as described on page 258 and as for venepuncture, with the addition of the following equipment (all sterile; these will be included in a composite pack):

2 towel clips.
1 Bard Parker handle and blade.
3 pairs mosquito forceps.
1 pair curved mosquito forceps.
1 pair toothed dissecting forceps (heavy).
1 pair non-toothed dissecting forceps (fine).
1 aneurysm needle.
1 pair dressing scissors.

1 pair fine pointed scissors.
1 needle holder.
Bottom shelf
Sterile gloves for the doctor.
Mersuture.
3/0 plain catgut.
Intravenous cannula or catheter.
2ml syringe ⎫
Lignocaine 1% ⎬ for local anaesthetic.
Nos. 17 and 12 hypodermic needles ⎭
5ml syringe ⎫
No. 1 hypodermic needle ⎪
Ampoule of normal saline ⎬ for displacing air in intravenous catheter.
File ⎭
Requirements for restraint, if necessary.

PREPARATION OF THE CHILD
The patient is prepared as for venepuncture. A padded splint of suitable size is applied to the limb, using lengths of adhesive tape. If the long saphenous vein is to be cannulated, the splinted limb is tied to the foot of the cot and the other leg is securely restrained.

METHOD
The procedure is essentially as for venepuncture. No manual pressure is required above the site of the vein. Following local cleansing and insertion of local anaesthetic, a small incision is made in the skin over the site of the vein to be exposed. The flow of blood through the vein is interrupted by a distal catgut ligature and the cannula is gently inserted through a small opening in the vein. It is threaded several centimetres into the lumen of the vein and secured in position, the primed recipient set is attached to the cannula and the flow rate regulated. The incised skin edges are brought together by sutures and the wound is covered with gauze, secured in position with lengths of adhesive tape. The limb is bandaged to the splint.

Scalp Vein Infusion

This is the method of choice during infancy when the scalp veins are prominent, permitting easy entry of a fine needle, thus avoiding the use of the veins of the arms and legs.

REQUIREMENTS
The basic trolley is prepared as described on page 258, with the addition of the following equipment: 1 pair of sterile Spencer Wells artery forceps.

Bottom shelf

Tray of equipment for shaving the area:
  Gauze swabs.
  Razor and blade.
  Soap solution.
Mask and gown for the doctor.
Requirements for arm restraint.
Bottle of prescribed intravenous fluid.
Bottle clip.
Infant's recipient set.
Scalp vein needle (small vein set).
Mediswab.
Receiver for excess fluid.
5 ml syringe ⎫
Ampoule of normal saline ⎬ for displacing air in scalp vein needle.
No. 1 hypodermic needle ⎪
File ⎭
Collodion *or* ⎫
Plaster of Paris, bowl of warm water ⎪
and waterproof protection and ⎬ for securing needle.
Narrow adhesive tape ⎭
Fluid balance chart.
At the bedside:
Anglepoise lamp.
Infusion stand.

PREPARATION OF THE INFANT:

The infant is dressed in an open-back gown. The elbows are splinted and the infant secured in a treatment blanket. If he is active, a sedative should be given half-an-hour prior to commencement of the procedure.

When the infusion site has been chosen by the doctor, the appropriate anterior lateral aspect of the scalp is shaved.

METHOD

The top shelf of the trolley is prepared with the sterile equipment from the lower shelf. Lengths of narrow adhesive tape are prepared.

The recipient set is primed as described on page 199. Normal saline is used to displace the air from the fine tubing attached to the scalp vein needle.

The nurse positions the infant across his cot and places her hands on either side of his head with her forearms alongside his body. She may be asked to apply pressure with her thumb over the selected vein. Pressure is released when blood is seen to flow into the scalp vein set. A small quantity of normal saline is injected through the tubing and the syringe is replaced by the primed recipient set. The rate of flow is regulated.

Plaster of Paris or cotton wool strips soaked in collodion and lengths of adhesive tape are used to secure the needle in position.

The infant is nursed with the infusion site uppermost. Sandbags may be used to maintain the head in position. Adequate sedation is required if the child is at all restless.

Umbilical Cannulation

Cannulation of the umbilical vein is possible during the first week of life.

The requirements for this procedure are as for vein dissection (page 199) with the addition of the following sterile equipment:

Sterile silver probe.

Ruler.

Selection of umbilical catheters.

Adequate restraint of the limbs is essential. Observing a meticulous aseptic technique, the doctor shortens the umbilical cord to within 1cm of the abdominal wall and threads an umbilical catheter 8–12cm or 3–4 inches into the inferior vena cava via the umbilical vein. The primed recipient set is inserted into the cannula and the fluid flow regulated. The umbilicus is covered with gauze, secured in position with lengths of adhesive tape.

Maintenance of Intravenous Therapy

Frequent observation of both the patient and the infusion are essential to ensure that everything possible is done to keep the infusion running as ordered by the doctor.

Care of the Child Receiving Intravenous Therapy

As the child is going to be confined to bed, all basic nursing care is required to fulfil his needs. Frequent change of position will prevent the occurrence of redness over areas of pressure and hypostatic pneumonia. As with all children receiving fluids by an artificial means, the mouth needs four-hourly care to keep it clean and moist.

Restlessness in the smaller child and infant is controlled by the use of sedatives and by allowing an infant to suck an occluded teat. Increased pressure in the scalp vein of a restless infant will slow down the rate of infusion. Frequent checks are made to ensure that any restraint is not causing pressure or restriction to the blood flow. An older child, with the limb adequately splinted, should be encouraged to move about his bed and be given suitable occupation.

A careful record should be maintained of the child's pulse and respiration rates so that early signs of overloading of the circulation may be detected. Any abnormal behaviour of the infant or child, e.g. twitching, should be reported.

Care of the Infusion

RATE OF FLOW

Nurses working with adults think in terms of litres and drip rates of anything up to sixty drops a minute. In paediatric work, thinking is in terms of millilitres and drip rates of anything down to two or three drops a minute.

A continuous slow administration of parenteral fluid can be achieved with the use of a Palmer Constant Rate Infusion pump and may be preferred by those caring for low birth weight infants requiring minimal quantities of fluid to maintain adequate hydration (PLATE 9).

With the use of a conventional recipient set, it is important that the intravenous fluid drips at a steady rate, as requested by the doctor (TABLE 15).

TABLE 15.

Drip Chart (when 15 drops = approximately 1ml)

ml/hour	Drops/minute (approximate)
5	1
10	2–3
15	4
20	5
25	6
30	7–8
35	9
40	10
45	11
50	12–13
75	19
100	25

The figures in TABLE 15 have been obtained by using the following formula: Where 15 drops equals approximately 1ml, as in most standard recipient sets:

$$ml/hour \times 15 = \text{number of drops/hour}$$

$$\text{Therefore } ml/hour \times \frac{15}{60} = \text{number of drops/minute}$$

thus formula for estimation of rate of flow =

$$\frac{ml/hour}{4} = \text{drops/minute}$$

If the rate of flow is prescribed as X number of drops per minute, multiply by 4 to obtain the ml/hour, i.e.

$$\text{drops/minute} \times 4 = ml/hour$$

If the doctor has prescribed X ml to be absorbed in H hours, divide the volume of fluid by the number of hours to give ml/hour and divide this by 4 to obtain the drops/minute, i.e.

$$\frac{X\text{ml}}{H \times 4} = \text{drops/minute}$$

When 60 drops equals approximately 1ml, as in micro-drips from a Metroset (McGaw Laboratories), the number of millilitres per hour is equal to the number of drops per minute.

IF THE INFUSION SLOWS OR STOPS

i   The fine lumen of the needle or cannula will limit the rate of fluid flow, but if the infusion is not running as quickly as it should, raising the infusion bottle will increase the head of pressure;

ii   A kink in the tubing of the recipient set will result in slowing of the infusion and is readily rectified;

iii   The needle may have become lodged against the wall of the vein and adjustment to the position of the limb may result in more rapid infusion. At no time should the needle be advanced or withdrawn;

iv   When bandaging the limb to a splint, it is advisable to leave the site of infusion easily accessible for regular inspection. Unnecessary disturbance to the site will be caused if this step is not taken. If the needle slips out of the vein, fluid will run into the surrounding tissues and will cause pain and swelling. At the same time, the infusion will slow down and eventually stop. A further site is chosen for continuation of the infusion;

v   Veins of small children are liable to go into spasm, particularly when the limb is cold or when cold blood is being administered. The limb should be kept warm and a loop of recipient set tubing should be strapped parallel to the limb to allow warming of the advancing fluid. Gentle massage along the vein may help to relieve the spasm;

vi   Thrombophlebitis may occur if the infusion has been running into the same vein for some days, and particularly if quantities of dextrose have been given or if any infection has entered the site. The route taken by the vein is seen to be inflamed and the doctor will decide whether to discontinue the infusion into that site;

vii   The needle may have become blocked with blood clot. While awaiting the arrival of the doctor, a tray for aspirating the blood clot should be prepared with sterile equipment:

5 or 10ml syringe.

No. 1 needle.

Ampoule normal saline.

File.

CHANGING THE INTRAVENOUS BOTTLE

Second and subsequent bottles of intravenous fluid should be prepared ready for changing shortly before they are due to be commenced. The bottle label is checked with the patient's prescription sheet, and any additions prepared under strict aseptic conditions and added by inserting a needle through the cleansed rubber cap.

The flow regulator on the recipient set is closed while the neck of the spent bottle contains a small quantity of fluid. The infusion bottle must not be allowed to run dry. If ever this happens, the entire recipient set must be renewed to prevent air being driven into the vein. To prevent the cotton wool air filter becoming wet, the air inlet is occluded with a pair of artery forceps. The bottle seal is broken and the rubber cap cleansed with spirit lotion and allowed to dry.

The spent bottle is removed from the intravenous stand and the needle(s) removed. These are inserted into the indentation in the cap of the new bottle. At no time should the needle(s) touch anything except the cleansed rubber cap. If the infusion fluid is contained in a polythene envelope, the air inlet is omitted or occluded with a pair of Spencer Wells artery forceps. The bottle clip is attached and the new bottle hung on the intravenous stand. The prescribed rate of flow is again adjusted by opening the flow regulator and a record is made on the fluid balance chart.

CHANGING THE INTRAVENOUS RECIPIENT SET

To prevent reactions in the vein and blockage of the needle or cannula, the recipient set should be changed at the following times:
  i   Every twenty-four hours during prolonged intravenous therapy;
 ii   Following a blood transfusion;
 iii If blood is to follow a dextrose infusion;
 iv   If a saline solution is to be given before or after administration of Intralipid.

RECORDING OF INTRAVENOUS FLUIDS

As comparatively small quantities of fluids are required by children, it is essential to have some accurate method of estimating the amount of fluid administered. With older children requiring larger quantities of fluid, the markings on the bottle or a paper strip attached to the bottle give a fairly accurate guide, and allow for the quantity of absorbed fluid to be recorded at hourly intervals.

When small quantities of intravenous fluids are to be administered, an infant's recipient set, incorporating a graduated burette, gives an accurate guide to the amount of fluid being absorbed. The burette may be used as either a reservoir or a dispensing chamber. The amount of fluid in the bottle or burette must be read at eye-level for accuracy and recorded on the fluid balance chart every hour or half-hour.

Below are two examples of methods for recording intravenous therapy using a 30ml graduated burette as incorporated in the infant's recipient set produced by Avon Medical Supplies Ltd. (FIG. 33).

Example 1.

Using the burette as a reservoir, the graduated burette is filled to 0ml at the commencement of the infusion and on every hour if the infant is to have 30ml/hour or less.

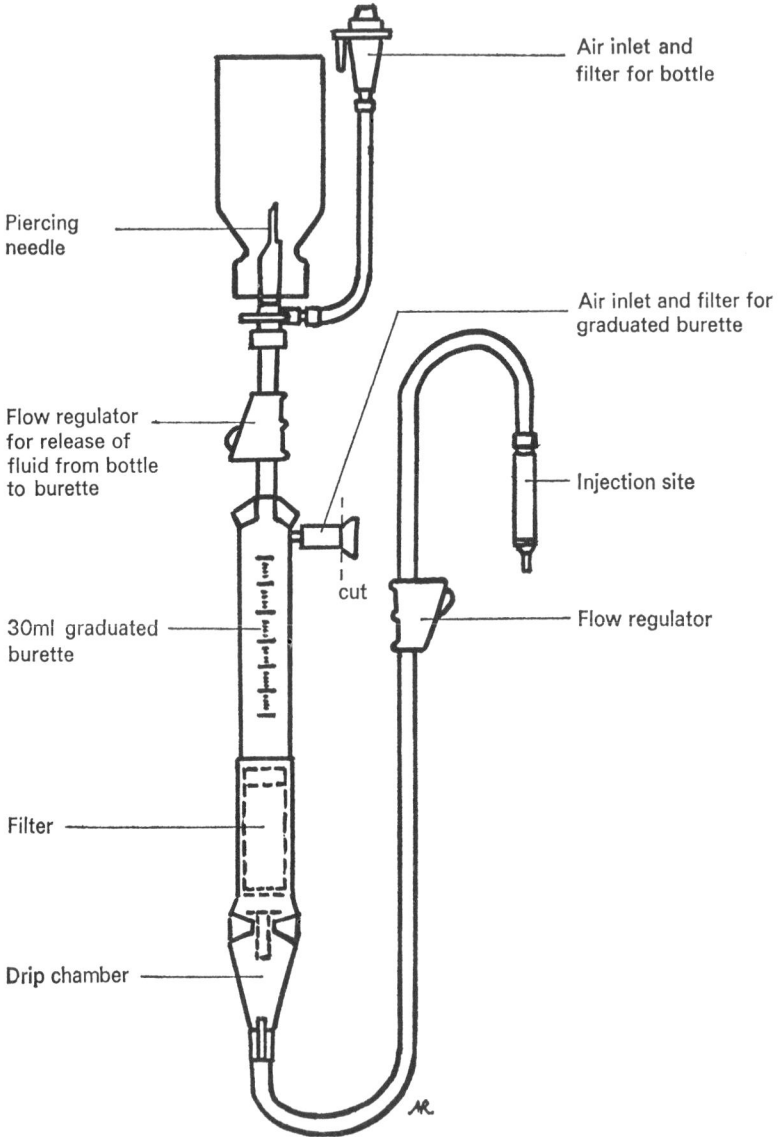

FIG. 33. Infant's recipient set (as produced by Avon Medical Supplies Ltd.)

The burette reading at the end of each hour (should be the volume required per hour) is recorded over 0—the level to which the burette is filled.

If the infant is to receive more than 30ml/hour the burette is filled every half-hour.

For an infant commencing intravenous therapy at 01.00 hours, to run at 20ml/hour or 5 drops/minute, the chart would read as follows:

Time hours	Nature of fluid	Rate per hour ml	Reading on burette ml	Amount absorbed ml	Cumulative total ml
01·00	4·3% dextrose in 0·18% saline	20	/0	—	—
02·00			20/0	20	20
03·00			20/0	20	40
04·00			15/0	15	55
05·00			25/0	25	80
06·00			20/0	20	100

Example 2.

Using the burette as a dispensing chamber, the graduated burette is filled at the commencement of the infusion, and on every subsequent hour, with the quantity of fluid to be absorbed in one hour. Drugs to be administered by the intravenous route may then be inserted into the graduated burette and will reach the vein without too great dilution or delay.

The volume of fluid in the burette at the end of each hour—which should be nil—is recorded over the volume of fluid to be absorbed in the following hour (the volume to be absorbed per hour + any residue from the previous hour).

For the same infant commencing intravenous therapy at 01.00 hours, to run at 20ml/hour or 5 drops/minute, the chart would read as follows:

Time	Nature of fluid	Rate per hour ml	Volume of fluid in burette ml	Amount absorbed ml	Cumulative total ml
01·00	4·3% dextrose in 0·18% saline	20	/20	—	—
02·00			0/20	20	20
03·00			0/20	20	40
04·00			5/25	15	55
05·00			0/20	25	80
06·00			0/20	20	100

Removal of Intravenous Needle and Cannula

i   Venepuncture;

ii Scalp vein infusion.

When the infusion is no longer required, the flow regulator is closed and the needle removed, using an aseptic technique.

REQUIREMENTS

A tray containing sterile equipment.
Gallipot for skin lotion.
Cotton wool balls.
Gauze swabs.
2 pairs dressing forceps.
Additional equipment:
Narrow adhesive tape.
Receptacle for disposable items.

METHOD

The surrounding area is cleansed with spirit lotion and the needle withdrawn. Pressure is applied over the site until bleeding has ceased. The area is covered with a piece of gauze maintained in position with lengths of adhesive tape. The splint is removed and the limb inspected.

iii   Vein dissection.

The requirements for removing the cannula are the same as listed above with the addition of one pair of sterile stitch scissors. If a ligature has been used to secure the cannula in position, this will need to be cut prior to withdrawal of the cannula.

The surrounding area is cleansed and the cannula slowly withdrawn. Slight pressure may be required over the site of insertion for a short time. The cannula is inspected to see that it is intact. The sutures which are then covered with an Airstrip dressing or a piece of gauze secured with lengths of adhesive tape are removed on the fifth day. The splint is removed and the limb inspected.

If the needle has been removed because of thrombophlebitis, glycerin ichthammol or a kaolin poultice may be applied to relieve local discomfort.

Intraperitoneal Infusion

The large area of highly absorptive healthy peritoneum supplies an effective route for administering fluid and blood. This route has lost popularity in Britain.

The requirements for this procedure are as for venepuncture (page 197). A No. 1 hypodermic needle is used.

The infant is nursed in the supine position. Sedation and adequate restraint of all limbs is essential. A urinary catheter is passed if requested by the doctor, but as the infant is frequently dehydrated, this preliminary is not usually necessary.

The procedure is essentially as for venepuncture. Observing a meticulous aseptic technique, the doctor inserts the needle at a point to one side of the mid-line just below the umbilicus. The primed recipient set is attached to the needle and the rate of flow regulated. The needle is secured, or preferably held, in position during rapid infusion of fluid. With the careful use of this route, there is rapid absorption of fluid with little danger of overloading the circulation. Temporary distension of the abdomen is the usual cause for dyspnoea.

Subcutaneous Infusion

Isotonic solutions of saline or Hartmann's solution may be injected into the subcutaneous tissues as a means of replacing water and electrolytes. Glucose fluids are best avoided as they can cause tissue necrosis.

This is a useful method for a nurse to administer small quantities of fluid to a child who is not receiving his full fluid requirement by other routes. With improvement in intravenous equipment and techniques and better facilities for biochemical analysis, this route has proved less popular than in the last decade. However, it still has a useful place in paediatrics and every paediatric nurse should be familiar with the procedure.

The middle-third of the upper and lateral aspect of the thighs are practical sites for administering fluids into the subcutaneous tissues. Alternative sites are the axillae and the area of tissue between the two scapulae, but immobilization of the child is difficult. Two sites—both thighs or both axillae—may be used simultaneously using a Y-shaped connection and additional lengths of tubing, or two separate recipient sets may be used.

Absorption of fluid from the tissues is enhanced by the use of the enzyme hyaluronidase (Hyalase). It is dispensed in powdered form in single dose vials of 1500 units, and is reconstituted with 1 ml of sterile distilled water, and injected either directly through the needle into the tissues or into the lumen of the lower end of the recipient set. Its maximum effect lasts about half-an-hour.

METHODS USED
1   When small quantities of fluid are to be administered, the fluid may be injected by using a syringe and needle.
2   When larger amounts are necessary, the drip method is the procedure of choice, using two sites simultaneously or consecutively.

REQUIREMENTS
The basic trolley is prepared as described on page 258 with the addition of the following equipment:
Bottle of prescribed intravenous fluid.
Bottle clip.
Infant's recipient set (with graduated burette).
No. 1 hypodermic needle(s).
Ampoule of hyaluronidase.
Ampoule of sterile distilled water.
2 ml syringe.
Mediswab.

Narrow adhesive tape.
Requirements for leg restraint.
Receiver for collection of excess fluid.
Fluid balance chart.
At the bedside:
Intravenous stand.

PREPARATION OF THE CHILD

As the procedure is more frequently carried out in infancy, that given below is pertaining to infancy. If the infant is at all restless, a sedative is given prior to commencement of the procedure. Two nurses work together. Assuming that the thighs are the chosen site for infusion, the infant is placed on a clean napkin folded in such a way that it can be readily applied once the infusion is in progress. It is most essential that the infant's legs are adequately restrained for this procedure. The chest and abdomen are protected with a folded treatment blanket.

METHOD

Both nurses wash their hands. The fluid to be administered is carefully checked with the prescription sheet, the bottle seal broken and the rubber cap cleansed. The needle of the recipient set is introduced into the inverted bottle and the fluid run through the whole apparatus to expel the air. The flow regulator is closed to occlude the flow of fluid and the sterile end for insertion into the needle is covered with its protective sheath.

Working together, the two nurses check and prepare the hyaluronidase.

Three lengths of adhesive tape, each 10cm (4 inches) long, are cut.

The nurse who is going to insert the needle then washes and dries her hands and, using an aseptic technique, cleanses the site for insertion of the needle. A sterile towel is placed around the area. The needle is passed through a fold of gauze and inserted at an angle of 45° or less into the subcutaneous tissues (as for hypodermic injection). $\frac{1}{2}$ or 1ml of hyaluronidase is injected, the amount depending on whether one or two sites are to be used to administer the amount of fluid prescribed by the doctor. The primed recipient set is attached to the needle and the flow of fluid regulated by adjustment to the flow regulator. The gauze swab is strapped firmly into position and a further length of adhesive tape is used to fasten the tubing to the leg.

The rate of flow should not exceed the rate of absorption of the fluid from the tissues. The rate of infusion should be slowed or temporarily stopped if there is blanching, redness or induration of the site. One site will absorb only 50–75ml at any one time and a second site is prepared in the same way if a larger volume of fluid is to be administered.

When the infusion is running satisfactorily, the napkin is fastened into position and the infant made comfortable. The nurse should remain with the infant for the short time the infusion is in progress (half-an-hour, or so).

When the infusion is completed, the needle is withdrawn and the puncture wound covered with sterile gauze. The infant is then restored to a comfortable position in bed. The quantity of fluid given is recorded on the fluid balance chart.

When the axillae are used, the child's wrists are restrained. When the subscapular region is used, the infant is similarly restrained in the prone position.

Rectal Infusion

This route may be used to administer small quantities of normal saline to supplement a poor oral fluid intake. For example, following repair of a cleft palate, the toddler may not be able to maintain a satisfactory oral fluid intake in the first twenty-four to forty-eight hours post-operatively, and this may be supplemented by giving 90–150ml (3–5oz) of rectal saline at six hourly intervals.

No diarrhoea should be present and the rectum must be prepared by the use of a suppository.

The normal saline is made up by mixing one 5ml spoonful of salt in 540ml (1 teaspoon to 1 pint) of tap water. Isotonic solutions are administered to avoid water intoxication which may occur if large quantities of hypotonic solution are given (page 191).

METHODS USED
1 90–150ml may be given over a period of twenty minutes or so and repeated six-hourly (intermittent rectal infusion).
2 Larger quantities of fluid may be dripped slowly into the rectum over a longer period (continuous rectal infusion).

REQUIREMENTS
Tray.

For Intermittent Rectal Infusion.
Measuring jug containing solution.
Lotion thermometer.
Funnel, length of tubing and graduated connection.
Catheter size 12 F.G., 6 E.G.
Lubricant.
Waterproof protection for the bed.
Additional requirements:
Bed blocks.

For Continuous Rectal Infusion.
Bottle of prepared saline.
2 lengths of tubing, each of 50cm or 18 inches.
Drip chamber.
Graduated connection.
Catheter size 12–15 F.G., 6–8 E.G.
Flow regulator.
Lubricant.
Waterproof protection for the bed.
Safety-pin.
Narrow adhesive tape.
Scissors.
Additional requirements:
Infusion stand and bottle clip.
Bed blocks.

PREPARATION OF THE CHILD

The child is offered facilities for emptying his bladder. Low bed blocks are placed at the foot of the bed and the child is made comfortable in the left lateral position. The bedclothes are arranged so that only the buttocks are exposed. Waterproof protection is placed under the buttocks.

METHOD

The temperature of the saline is checked to ensure that it is 38°C (100°F). The apparatus is assembled and the air expelled by displacement with warm saline.

The fine catheter is lubricated and inserted 8–12cm (3–5 inches) through the anus into the rectum and the fluid flow is released. The fluid is allowed to run in slowly over the next twenty minutes or so, the height of the funnel being raised or lowered to increase or decrease the rate of flow. The funnel is at no time allowed to become empty.

On completion of the procedure, the catheter is gently withdrawn and the child left comfortable. The foot of the bed is lowered and the waterproof protection removed half-an-hour after completion of the procedure. The volume of fluid administered is recorded on the child's fluid balance record.

If a continuous rectal infusion is to be given, the catheter is secured in position with a length of adhesive tape and the flow of fluid regulated by adjustment to the flow regulator. To prevent undue strain on the catheter, the tubing is secured to the drawsheet with a safety-pin. The child is placed in a comfortable position in bed and the bedclothes are replaced.

For Further Reading

BLACK D. A. K. (1968). *Essentials of Fluid Balance*, 4th edition. Blackwell Scientific Publications, Oxford.
DICKENS M. L. (1970). *Fluid Electrolyte Balance: A Programmed Test*, 2nd edition. Blackwell Scientific Publications, Oxford.
HARRIS F. (1971). *Paediatric Fluid Therapy*, 1st edition. Blackwell Scientific Publications, Oxford.
TAYLOR W. H. *Fluid Therapy and Disorders of Electrolyte Balance*, 2nd edition. Blackwell Scientific Publications, Oxford.

CHAPTER TWELVE

Administration of Drugs

In its broadest meaning, a drug may be defined as any substance—solid, liquid or vapour—which may be applied to the body either externally or internally for the prevention, diagnosis or treatment of disease. In actual practice, the term 'drug' is usually used to refer to a substance which can only be obtained on prescription. In this chapter, however, the term is used in its broadest sense.

The storage and administration of some drugs is regulated by statute, and the registered nurse is under a legal obligation to see that the rules are carried out. In addition, every hospital has its own regulations concerning the administration of drugs controlled under these acts and these must be carefully followed.

Legislation Controlling the Storage and Administration of Drugs

The Dangerous Drugs Act

This act controls the use of certain powerful drugs of dependence and includes:
Opium and its derivatives, containing 0·2% Morphine and over, e.g. Papaveretum ('Omnopon'*).
Cocaine and preparations containing 0·1% and over.
Pethidine.
Methadone ('Physeptone').
Drugs controlled by this act are commonly referred to as D.D.A.'s or D.D.'s. The ward stock of these drugs is the responsibility of the ward sister. The ward sister or her deputy may order further supplies from the hospital pharmacist using a special D.D.A. order book which in many hospitals is also signed when the drugs are received.

The drugs are stored in a separate locked cupboard which is clearly labelled D.D.A. and is often found inside another locked cupboard which contains the drugs controlled by Schedules 1 and 4 of the Pharmacy and Poisons Act. The

* See page 219.

key to the cupboard is kept on the person of the ward sister, and entrusted to the senior nurse on the ward in her absence.

When drugs controlled by this act are prescribed for a patient, the order must be clearly written and signed by a qualified medical practitioner. The drug may not be repeated unless clearly indicated on the patient's prescription sheet.

When administering these drugs, an accurate record must be made in the D.D.A. ward register. This register may be inspected by the hospital pharmacist at any time and must be retained on the ward for two years after the date of the last entry.

Although not required by law, in hospital practice it is usual for two nurses, one of whom is a state registered nurse, to check and administer any drug governed by the Dangerous Drugs Act.

The Pharmacy and Poisons Act

Certain drugs which are dangerous if taken in excess are controlled by Schedules 1 and 4 of this Act. They include the majority of drugs which act on the central nervous system, for example tranquillizers and barbiturates, the sulphonamides, and digitalis and its preparations. These drugs must be prescribed in the same way as the drugs controlled by the Dangerous Drugs Act and stored in a locked but separate cupboard from the drugs of addiction. The bottle labels are marked 'Schedule Poison' or 'Poison' to indicate that their contents are controlled by this act.

Individual hospitals have their own routine for checking and recording the administration of these drugs. It is usual for two people to check the drug and the recording is made in the appropriate column on the patient's prescription sheet (FIG. 34).

Therapeutic Substances Act

Many new drugs are listed in this more recent act and are only available to the public on prescription. Included in this list are the antibiotics and many hormones, e.g. cortisone and its derivatives and insulin.

General Care of Drugs in the Ward

1 All drugs should be stored in the correct cupboards, all of which should be inaccessible to children.

    i *The Dangerous Drugs Cupboard* must only contain the drugs controlled by the Dangerous Drugs Act.

    ii *The Poisons Cupboard* contains the drugs controlled by Schedules 1 and 4 of the Pharmacy and Poisons Act.

iii   *The Medicine Cupboard.* Medicines not listed in either the Dangerous Drugs Act or the Pharmacy and Poisons Act are stored in separate cupboards. Mixtures and pills are stored in a separate cupboard from those drugs intended for external use

The ward medicine cupboard should be kept locked. Stock preparations for internal use and prescriptions dispensed for individual patients are stored in this cupboard. Some drugs need to be stored in a cool, light cupboard, while others require storage away from light.

iv   *The Lotion Cupboard.* Preparations for external use such as antiseptics, creams, ointments and drops, unless controlled by the Pharmacy and Poisons Act, should be stored away from preparations which may be taken by mouth. In addition, lotions are dispensed in ridged bottles as a further indication that they are intended for external use only.

Great care must be taken in any hospital ward, and particularly in a children's ward, to ensure that lotion bottles are not left around in the ward or annexes, and that the door of the lotion cupboard is kept locked. The same stringent control should be applied to the cupboard containing the urine testing equipment.

v   *Refrigerator.* Some medicines and other drugs have to be stored in a refrigerator in order that their potency is maintained, e.g. some antibiotics and antitoxins.

2   Adequate stores of stock preparations should be maintained to avoid borrowing from other wards and departments. It is wasteful to hold large stocks of drugs which are rarely used as these may be very expensive and have a short 'shelf' life, i.e. the period in which they may safely be used.

3   Drugs should be used in rotation to avoid old stock becoming out of date. Certain drugs such as antibiotics and insulin are clearly marked with an expiry date after which they should be returned to the pharmacy.

4   The labels on the containers should be clear and firmly attached to the body of the container and not the lid. If the label becomes illegible or detached, the container should be returned to the pharmacy.

5   At no time should ward staff alter the label on a container; such alterations should be made by the pharmacy staff.

6   Drugs dispensed for an individual patient but no longer required should be returned to the pharmacy to prevent over-congestion of the drug cupboards.

7   It should not be permitted at any time to transfer the contents of one bottle to another bearing the same label, or for a drug to be returned to its container if it is not required.

8   Once a drug container is removed from its locked cupboard it should not be left unattended.

Prescribing Drugs for Children

Tolerance to drugs in childhood varies considerably, some being very well tolerated whilst others, like morphia, are best avoided.

Many formulae are used to determine the size of a dose of a drug to be given to a child. Some rely on the weight of the child, others on age and, more recently, surface area has been taken as a guide to paediatric drug dosage. To assist the medical staff in estimating a suitable drug dosage, the child is weighed accurately on admission and as required during his stay in hospital.

Children of the same age group vary considerably in size, so age alone may prove a poor guide to dosage calculation, particularly where very sick children are concerned.

The three formulae given below will give the nurse some idea of methods used as a guide to estimate the dose of a drug for a child, when the adult dose is known.

1 Young's Rule

Calculating the child's dose of a drug according to age.

$$\frac{\text{Age of child}}{\text{Age} + 12} \times \text{Adult dose} = \text{Child's dose}$$

Example: A child aged 8 years, suffering from tuberculosis, requires Intramuscular Streptomycin

Adult dose = 1g daily, divided into two doses.

$$\frac{8}{8 + 12} \times 1000\text{mg (1g)} = \text{Child's dose}$$

$$= \frac{8}{20} \times 1000\text{mg}$$

$$= \frac{800}{2}\text{mg}$$

$$= 400\text{mg daily, i.e. 200mg twice daily.}$$

2 Clark's Rule

Calculating the child's dose of a drug according to body weight

$$\frac{\text{Weight of child in lb}}{150} \times \text{adult dose} = \text{child's dose.}$$

Example: A child weighing 20lbs requires Intramuscular Streptomycin

Adult dose = 1g daily, divided into two doses.

$$\frac{20}{150} \times 1000mg\ (1g) = \text{child's dose}$$

$$= 133mg\ \text{daily, i.e. } 66\cdot5mg\ \text{twice daily.}$$

In this instance the doctor would prescribe a dose that is readily and accurately calculated, i.e. 62·5mg or 75mg, as the drug is prepared as a 1 gramme in 4ml solution.

3 Percentage Method of Estimating Paediatric Drug Dosage

As a child has a relatively greater surface area than an adult, he requires relatively larger doses of a drug than his weight alone would suggest; most paediatricians therefore use this method.

Using surface area, a child's dose may be estimated by the following formula:

$$\text{Child's dose} = \frac{\text{Surface area of child}}{\text{Surface area of adult}} \times \text{adult dose}$$

Example: A seven-year-old child of 'normal' height and weight has a surface area of 0·85 square metres.

Using the formula, his drug dosage can be calculated as:

$$\frac{0\cdot85}{1\cdot70} = \frac{1}{2} \text{ or } 50\% \text{ of the adult dose.}$$

TABLE 16 gives the values at other age levels.

TABLE 16. The Percentage Method for Estimation of Paediatric Dosage
after Catzel

Approximate Age	Weight kg	lb	Surface area m²	% of Adult dose
20 years	65	145	1·70	100
16 years	54	120	1·53	90
14 years	45	100	1·36	80
12 years	40	88	1·28	75
11 years	36	80	1·20	70
10 years	30	66	1·00	60
7 years	23	50	0·85	50
5 years	18	40	0·68	40
3 years	15	33	0·56	33·3
18 months	11	25	0·50	30
1 year	10	22	0·42	25

(Catzel, Pincus (1966) *Paediatric Prescriber*, third edition. By kind permission of Blackwell Scientific Publications, Oxford.)

For the infant under one-year-of-age, the drug dose is usually calculated on a weight basis, the dose/kg body weight being estimated from the required dose for a one-year-old child, i.e. 25% of the adult dose. Since the child of one year weighs about 10kg, calculation is easy.

Example: If the adult dose of a drug is 60mg the dose for a child of 1 year = 15 mg.

Therefore for an infant weighing 6kg, the dose

$$= \frac{6}{10} \times 15\text{mg}$$

$$= \frac{3}{5} \times 15\text{mg}$$

$$= 9\text{mg}$$

General Principles for Administration of Drugs

Only drugs prescribed by the doctor on the patient's prescription sheet may be given to a patient in hospital. This sheet must state clearly:

1   The name and age or date of birth of the patient.
2   The date of the prescription.
3   The time(s) the drug is to be given.
4   The approved name of the drug.
5   The dose of the drug.
6   The route by which the drug is to be administered.

Each prescription must be signed by a medical practitioner.

It is advisable for two people to check together the preparation of any drug to be administered to a child. When small doses are prescribed a fraction of the stock mixture must often be administered. There is much truth in the old proverb 'two heads are better than one'.

1   The date of the prescription is checked to confirm it is current treatment. A check should also be made to see that the drug has not already been given.
2   Timing of administration of some drugs is of importance. Some drugs are prescribed to be given before meals or feeds, for example atropine methonitrate is necessary to relax the pyloric sphincter to allow a feed to pass through. It is, therefore, futile to give this drug either with or following a feed. Other drugs may be prescribed to be given following a meal or a feed. To maintain a constant blood level, antibiotics must be given punctually and at regular intervals. When caring for infants with regular feed-times, the doctor should be asked to prescribe the drugs to be given orally at times which are convenient to the infant's routine—six-hourly medicines for an infant fed three-hourly, and four or eight-hourly medicines for an infant fed four-hourly.

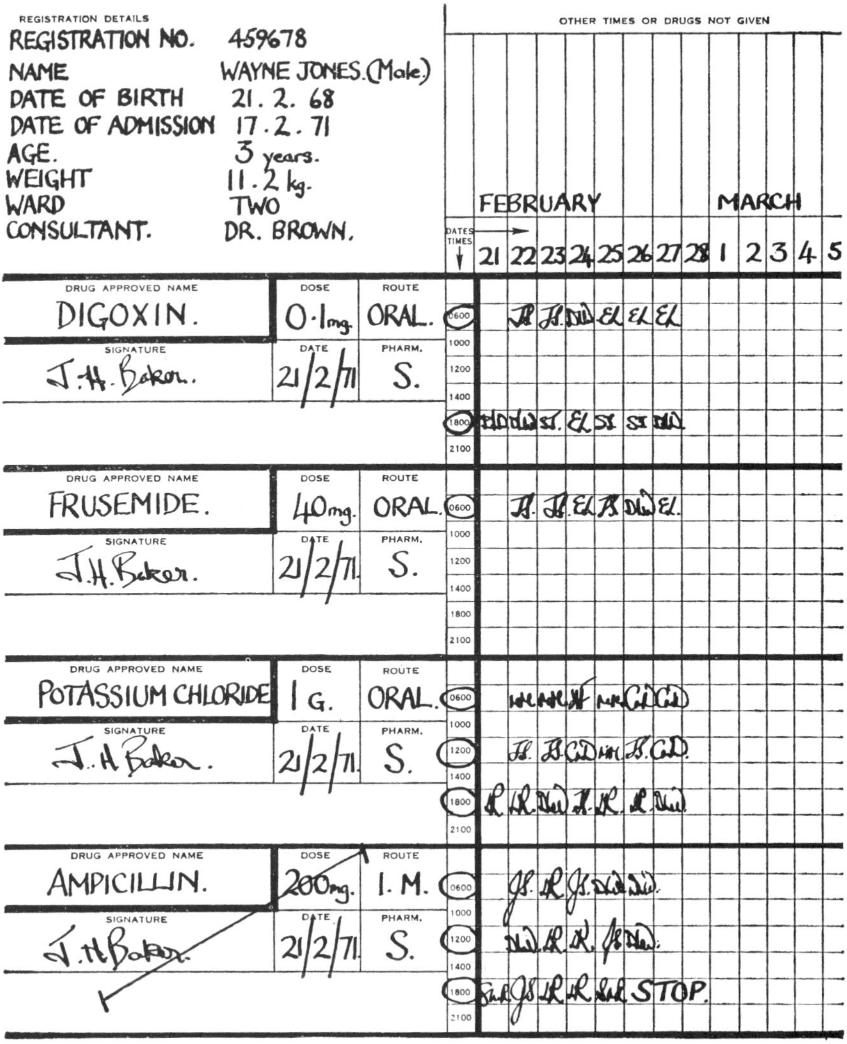

FIG. 34. Prescription sheet.

3 Some drugs are called by their proprietary or trade names particularly when their official names in the British Pharmacopoeia are long and difficult to pronounce. The practice is not recommended, and the approved name must be given in writing by the pharmacist or doctor on the prescription sheet and bottle label, so that nurses preparing the drug for administration are left in no doubt regarding its true identity. When in doubt, do not assume, always ask.

4 A nurse must be able to calculate the dose of a medicine or injection as prescribed by the medical staff. If she is unable to calculate the amount of drug to be given then she must ask for help.

Calculation of Drugs

Formula: Divide the strength required by the strength available. The resulting fraction gives the amount of stock solution of a drug required.

$$\frac{\text{Strength required}}{\text{Strength available}} = \text{fractional amount of stock solution required}$$

Example 1. Stock bottle of Streptomycin for intramuscular use contains: 1g or 1000mg/4ml

$$\text{Dose prescribed is 100mg}$$

$$\frac{\text{Strength required}}{\text{Strength available}} = \frac{100}{1000 \text{ in 4ml}}$$

$$\text{Therefore amount required} = \frac{1}{10} \text{ of 4ml}$$

$$= \frac{4}{10} \text{ ml}$$

$$= 0\cdot4\text{ml}$$

Example 2. Stock bottle of Elixir of Digoxin is prepared as 0·05mg or 50 microgrammes in 1ml.

$$\text{Dose prescribed is 0·125mg or 125mcg.}$$

$$\frac{\text{Strength required}}{\text{Strength available}} = \frac{0\cdot125}{0\cdot05} \text{ in 1ml or } \frac{125}{50} \text{ in 1ml}$$

$$\text{Therefore amount required} = \frac{125}{50} \text{ of 1ml}$$

$$= \frac{25}{10} \text{ of 1ml}$$

$$= \frac{5}{2} \text{ of 1ml}$$

$$= 2\cdot5 \text{ or } 2\tfrac{1}{2}\text{ml.}$$

Example 3. Intramuscular Cloxacillin is prepared as 250mg in 2ml.

$$\text{Dose prescribed is 62·5mg.}$$

$$\frac{\text{Strength required}}{\text{Strength available}} = \frac{62\cdot5}{250} \text{ in 2ml}$$

$$\text{Therefore amount required} = \frac{625}{2500} \text{ of 2ml}$$

$$= \frac{1}{4} \text{ of 2ml}$$

$$= 0\cdot5 \text{ or } \tfrac{1}{2}\text{ml.}$$

Some drugs are expressed as percentage solutions. Per cent, or the international symbol % means 'for every hundred'. A 10% solution means that in every 100 parts there are 10 parts of concentrate. This may be a mixture of two fluids or a solute (solid) in a solvent (liquid).

When the percentage solution is referring to a solid in solution, the percentage indicates the number of grammes of solute in 100ml of solution.

For example a 1% solution contains:

1g in 100ml or 1000mg in 100ml or *10mg in 1ml.*

Example: Calcium Gluconate is prepared as a 10% solution.
Dose prescribed is 100mg (0·1g).
A 10% solution contains 10g in 100ml.
Therefore 100ml contains 10g
          10ml contains 1g
          1ml contains 0·1g
Therefore 1ml of 10% solution would contain 100mg (0·1g) of Calcium Gluconate.

5 The route by which the drug is to be administered must be clearly indicated on the prescription as the dosage varies with the route of administration.

6 Before a drug is administered, the nurses should check that the name on the child's bracelet, or other means of identification in use, is the same as that on the prescription sheet.

7 Both nurses take the checked drug together with the prescription sheet to the child's bedside and administer it by the prescribed route.

8 When the drug has been administered, a record should be made in the appropriate place, e.g. D.D.A. register and/or the patient's prescription sheet, depending on the nature of the drug. If the drug is prescribed as a single dose the prescription is cancelled.

9 The child should be observed for side-effects of the drug.

Routes for Administration of Drugs

1 By mouth—oral.
2 Rectal.
3 By injection
    i Intradermal (page 418).
    ii Hypodermic (Subcutaneous).
    iii Intramuscular.
    iv Intravenous.
    v Intrathecal.
4 Inhalation.

5 Topical.
    i Inunction (page 330).
    ii Eye.
    iii Nose.
    iv Ear.

The obvious route for the administration of drugs is by way of the alimentary tract. When drugs are given by injection, the term parenteral administration is used. The route chosen by the doctor depends on several factors:

1 *The nature of the drug.* Some drugs cannot be given by mouth as they are destroyed in the stomach, e.g. insulin is destroyed by the proteolytic action of pepsin. Streptomycin is not absorbed from the alimentary tract so is of no value in the treatment of tuberculosis, but is used as a means of destroying the normal intestinal flora (commensals) prior to major intestinal surgery.

2 *The desired speed of action.* Drugs administered by injection, especially by the intravenous route, have a much more rapid action than those administered orally.

3 *The physical disabilities of the patient.* If the child is unable to tolerate oral fluids then an alternative route must be chosen for administration of essential drugs.

4 *The age of the child.* When possible, drugs are given to a child by mouth unless his serious condition makes it necessary for the drug to be given by intramuscular injection. Injections are painful and traumatic to the child, but nevertheless have to be given in the interests of recovery. If an intravenous infusion is in progress, the intravenous route is often used for parenteral administration of drugs.

Oral Administration of Drugs

Paediatric medications are prepared as tablets (which can be crushed), powders, granules, mixtures, emulsions, elixirs and syrups. Older children may be persuaded to swallow capsules which are considerably less expensive than their equivalents dispensed as an elixir or syrup. Bitter medicines are made acceptable to children by the addition of fruit flavouring in the syrup or alcohol. Capsules should not be opened as the contained powder is unpalatable.

Sweets are of basic necessity on a medicine trolley. Even the most bitter medicine will be taken by a small child if he is assured of a reward in the form of a chocolate drop or Smartie.

REQUIREMENTS
Prescription sheets.
Oral medications—tablets, syrups, etc.
Medicine measures.
Millilitre measures.

1ml syringe.
5ml spoons.
Small trays or plates.
Jug containing fruit juice or water.
Sweets.

METHOD
Each child's prescription sheet is read carefully by two nurses and the general principles for administration of drugs, as given on page 218, are carefully followed.

POURING MEDICINES
Having confirmed that the medicine contained in a bottle is that prescribed for the child, one finger is placed on the bottle stopper while the bottle is shaken to mix its contents. The bottle stopper is removed and held in the crook of the little finger. The measure is held so that the markings are at eye-level and the thumb-nail is placed at the appropriate graduation. With the bottle label uppermost, the medicine is poured to the appropriate level in the measure (FIG. 35).

The bottle stopper is replaced and the measure containing the medicine placed on a small tray and taken to the child's bedside, with the prescription sheet. If a small quantity of medicine has been measured in a conical measure, this is tipped into a spoon and the measure rinsed with some water to remove the residue. A 1ml syringe provides a safe, accurate method of measuring minute doses of a drug, e.g. elixir of digoxin.

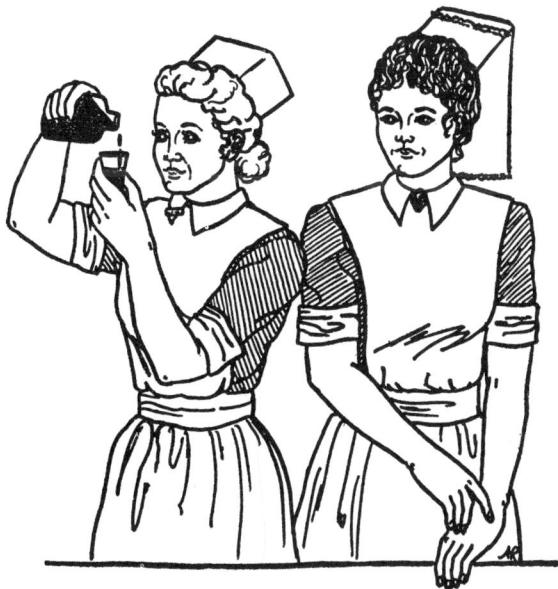

FIG. 35. Pouring a medicine. The measure is held so that the markings are at eye-level.

DISPENSING TABLETS

The prescribed number of tablets is tipped from the container into either the bottle lid or a spoon. A tablet can then be crushed to a powder between two spoons before mixing with milk, fruit juice or jam.

ADMINISTERING ORAL MEDICAMENTS TO SMALL CHILDREN

Drugs should never be put into an infant's feeding bottle as they cling to the bottle and are retained. A crushed tablet is mixed with boiled water or a little feed so that the spoon is not more than half-full. Medicines are best offered before a feed unless contra-indicated. The half-full spoon is placed at the infant's lips while he sucks the medicine from it. Rejected medicine can thus be carefully collected and re-administered. The medicines are followed by a feed or boiled water to rinse the mouth of the strange taste.

Much ingenuity is necessary to encourage a doubting toddler to take his medicine. A calm, matter-of-fact approach is preferable. A preliminary chat while fastening his bib is time well spent. Having watched his fellow patients taking their medicines, most toddlers will co-operate. On the occasions when co-operation is not forthcoming it may be better to return again later when his mood may have changed. It is sometimes best to take the child from his cot and sit him on the nurse's knees. To achieve control, the child may be restrained in a blanket or sat with his right arm tucked under the nurse's left arm. The nurse can then control his left arm as she administers the medicine. Great care must be taken to ensure that a struggling child does not inhale the medicine. A fruit juice drink or sweet will take the unpleasant taste away and may help to improve relationships for another time. It is important that a child swallows the medicaments he has been prescribed and that he understands that the drug will be given despite his protests. It should always be borne in mind that alternative methods cause physical as well as psychological trauma.

On completion of drug round. The bottles are wiped clean and returned to their appropriate cupboards. Empty, or almost empty, containers are returned to the pharmacy. The used measures, spoons and trays are thoroughly washed, rinsed and dried before being returned to the cupboard.

Administration of Drugs by the Rectal Route

A drug may be administered by the rectal route in the form of a suppository or enema for either its systemic or local effect. Details of reasons for rectal administration of drugs, requirements for, and techniques are to be found under rectal procedures on pages 124–129.

Administration of Drugs by Injection

An injection is an unpleasant experience for a person at any age and is particularly traumatic to the small child who often lives in fear of the next 'needle'.

Children should be told the truth at all times or their trust in human nature is lost. An injection hurts and this the child must be told, but in addition he should be told that the pain will soon be over and that the 'prick' is to help him to get better so that he can soon go home.

To allay anxiety, the drug should be prepared away from the bedside so that the procedure is over before the small child is fully aware of the situation. Two nurses are essential for this procedure, one to restrain and comfort the child, the other to administer the drug. Most small children cry during the injection and need immediate reassuring love and comfort.

SYRINGES
Disposable plastic syringes have almost replaced the non-disposable glass and metal, and all glass, syringes. They are individually packed, with or without

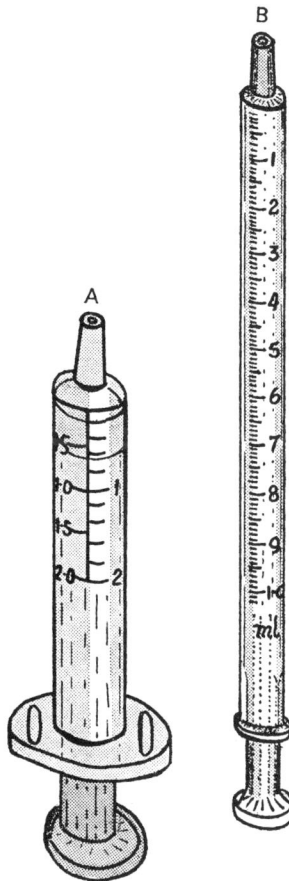

Fig. 36. A. A 2ml syringe
B. A 1ml Mantoux syringe bearing 0·01 ml graduations.

B.S. 1619 Syringe
1-millilitre model

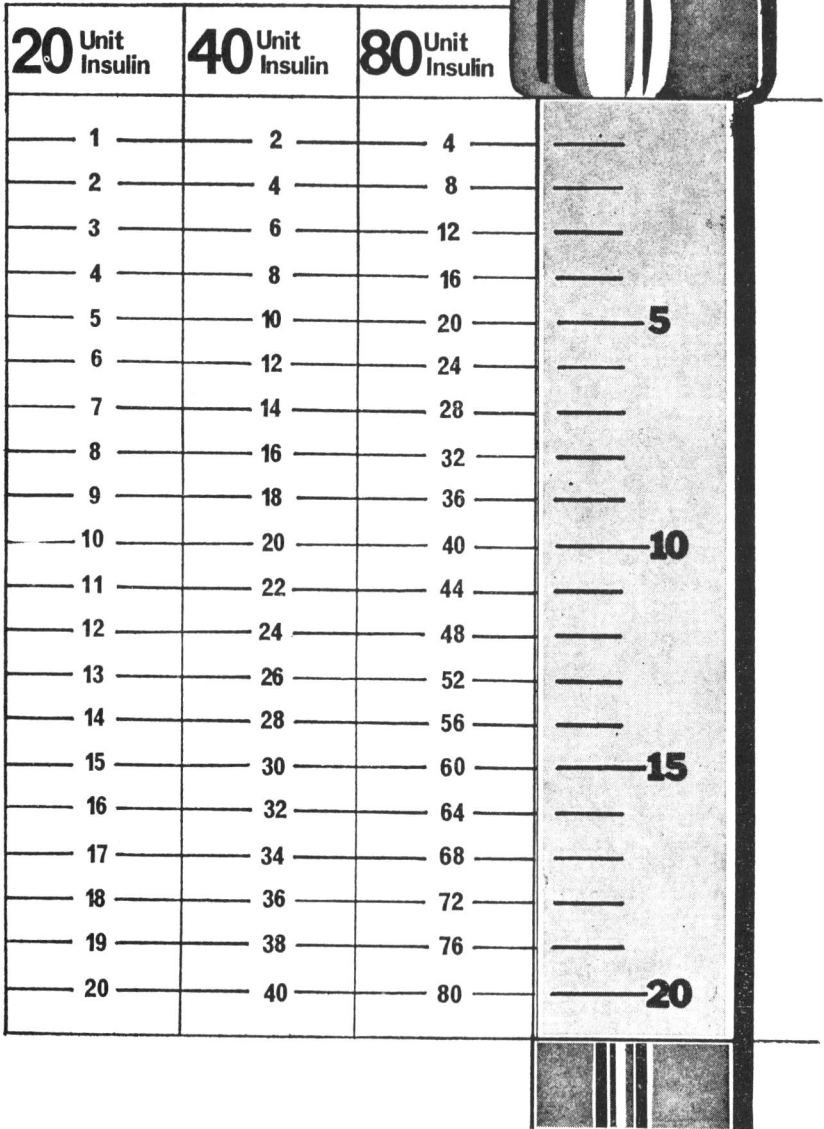

20 Unit Insulin	40 Unit Insulin	80 Unit Insulin	
1	2	4	
2	4	8	
3	6	12	
4	8	16	
5	10	20	5
6	12	24	
7	14	28	
8	16	32	
9	18	36	
10	20	40	10
11	22	44	
12	24	48	
13	26	52	
14	28	56	
15	30	60	15
16	32	64	
17	34	68	
18	36	72	
19	38	76	
20	40	80	20

FIG. 37. Insulin syringe. Levels to which to fill the B.S. 1619 Syringe using 20-unit, 40-unit and 80-unit insulins.

needles, sterilized by gamma irradiation and are suitable for the administration of nearly all drugs, with the common exception of paraldehyde. 2ml, 5ml, 10ml 20ml and 50ml pre-packed syringes are available, the 2ml syringe being the one most frequently used by the nurse. Rarely is a drug for administration to a child contained in more than 2ml.

Standard 2ml syringes are graduated in 0·1ml (1/10ml) divisions so that drug dosage requiring multiples of 0·1ml can be accurately administered (FIG. 36A).

For administration of a drug contained in less than 0·1ml, a 1ml Mantoux syringe bearing 0·01ml (1/100ml) graduations is essential (FIG. 36B).

Special syringes for administration of insulin are graduated in 20 units/ml divisions (FIG. 37).

Syringes with an eccentric nozzle may be requested by a doctor for administering a drug by the intravenous route.

Disposable syringes should be disposed of immediately following use to avoid the transmission of serum hepatitis. Syringes make excellent water pistols, but a nurse must realize that a used syringe is a potentially dangerous toy.

NEEDLES

Disposable needles are used almost exclusively, a sharp, straight needle for each injection being guaranteed. Needles vary in length and diameter of the lumen; the higher the gauge number (standard wire gauge—S.W.G.) the smaller the diameter of the lumen. Manufacturers adopt a colour code system which is peculiar to their own brand of needles.

No. 1⎫
No. 2⎭ for intramuscular and intravenous injections.

No. 12   for intramuscular injections for infants.

No. 15⎫
No. 17⎭ for hypodermic (subcutaneous) injections.

No. 20   for intradermal injections and for hypodermic injections for the diabetic child.

Disposal of hypodermic needles demands care on the part of the nursing staff. Needles readily penetrate paper sacks and are of danger to the ward refuse collector. To avoid unnecessary accidents, used needles, blades and ampoules may be collected into a waxed or plastic container, e.g. a disposable sputum carton, the lid being firmly secured and the full carton disposed of in the refuse collecting bag.

Preparation of a Drug for Injection

REQUIREMENTS

Tray.

Sterile equipment:

    Syringe.

Needle.
Spirit lotion in container and swabs *or*
Mediswab.

Additional requirements:
  Prescription sheet.
  Drug to be administered
    Multidose vial.
    Single dose ampoule.
  Ampoule of sterile distilled water if required.
  File, if required.
  Record book if required (e.g. D.D.A.).

METHOD

The administration of drugs by injection demands a strict aseptic technique. The protective skin is punctured and micro-organisms could gain entry. The equipment used must, therefore, be sterile and the hands thoroughly washed and dried before handling the syringe. At no time should the sterile needle be touched.

The patient's prescription sheet is read carefully by two nurses and the appropriate drug taken from the cupboard and checked with further reference to the prescription sheet.

The syringe and needle containers are opened and the syringe held at the piston end. The sheathed needle is attached to the syringe and left protected until required.

Using a Multidose vial. If necessary, the drug is reconstituted with the manufacturer's recommended quantity of diluent—usually water for injection or normal saline. The quantity of diluent added is of considerable importance, particularly as a single dose container intended for one dose for an adult may well be used for fractional doses for children. For example, Ampicillin 250mg is diluted with 1·8ml (not 2ml) of water for injection to give a resulting strength of 125mg in 1ml. The administration of a drug of too high a concentration could cause the child more discomfort than necessary.

The rubber diaphragm of the multidose container is cleansed with a medicated swab and allowed to dry. The swab is discarded. To prevent the formation of a vacuum in the bottle, a small quantity of air is injected; 1ml is inserted if 1ml of solution is to be withdrawn.

The needle is inserted at a right angle through the rubber diaphragm of the inverted vial and the air is injected. Negative pressure is applied to the syringe by withdrawing the piston to the appropriate level. The charged syringe is read at eye-level and adjusted with the point of the needle still in the bottle. Sensitization to a drug, particularly an antibiotic, can be prevented by avoiding ejection of excess drug into the air. For the same reason, except when iron or paraldehyde is to be administered, the one needle is used both for charging the syringe and administration of the drug.

The needle is re-inserted into its sheath until ready for use.

Using a single dose ampoule. When the drug is contained in a single dose glass ampoule, the drug is collected into the body of the ampoule and the top (filed if necessary) is snapped off at the neck, care being taken to ensure that the fingers are clear of the neck. The syringe is charged to the required level and the excess solution ejected into the ampoule which is held at right angles to the needle. The needle is re-inserted into its sheath until ready for use.

Hypodermic (Subcutaneous) Injection

Drugs administered into the subcutaneous tissues are eventually absorbed into the blood stream by way of the lymphatic drainage. Their absorption is slower than when given intramuscularly, and only small quantities of a drug can be administered by this route, e.g. 0·5–2ml.

A fleshy area is chosen for the administration of a drug into the subcutaneous tissues, the outer aspect of the upper arm and the anterior or lateral aspects of the thigh being common sites.

The area is cleansed with a medicated swab and allowed to dry. The skin is pinched between the thumb and first or second finger of the left hand and the needle is inserted at an angle of 45° to within 2mm of the hilt. The left hand then supports the needle on the syringe while the right hand injects the fluid smoothly and slowly into the subcutaneous tissues. When the contents of the syringe have been ejected, the needle is withdrawn and the medicated swab held over the site. Massage in an upward direction will help to disperse the fluid.

For the diabetic patient requiring daily, or twice daily, hypodermic injections of insulin for a lifetime, the sites of injection must be rotated, the abdominal wall often being used. The insulin is given via a short, fine No. 20 needle which is inserted at an angle of 90° to reduce the formation of fibrous tissue.

Intramuscular Injection

A drug is administered by intramuscular, as opposed to subcutaneous injection when:

i   a more rapid action is required;

ii when the drug would prove irritating to the subcutaneous tissues.

The sites used for intramuscular injection must be areas where there is a reasonable amount of muscle with no underlying nerves and blood vessels that could be damaged. The following sites are normally used:

1   The gluteal muscle in the upper and outer quadrant of the buttock (FIG. 38).

2   The vastus lateralis muscle in the outer aspect of the thigh mid-way between the hip and the knee (FIG. 39).

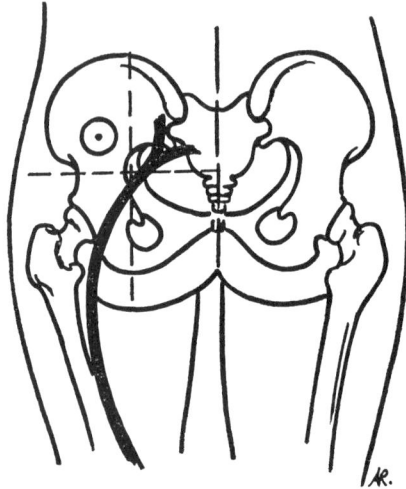

FIG. 38. Site for administration of an intramuscular injection into the buttock. The upper and outer quadrant of the buttock is used. The sciatic nerve passes through the other three quadrants.

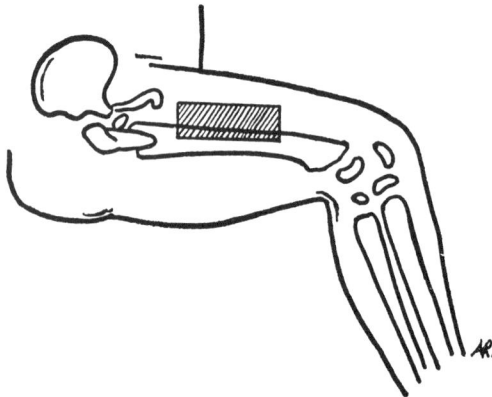

FIG. 39. Site for administration of an intramuscular injection into the lateral aspect of the thigh.

3   The deltoid muscle in the upper outer aspect of the arm just below the shoulder joint.

When injections have to be administered at frequent intervals, a definite rotation of sites must be used to obtain maximum absorption with minimum fibrosis. The deltoid muscle is best avoided in childhood, and definitely in infancy, as it is poorly developed.

The area is cleansed with a medicated swab and allowed to dry. The skin is then stretched between the thumb and forefinger of the left hand to prevent the drug exuding back on withdrawal of the needle (FIG. 40). The needle is inserted quickly at an angle of 90° to within 2mm of the hilt, depending on the size of the muscle. The full length of the needle is not inserted, thus avoiding difficult withdrawal should the needle break off at the hilt.

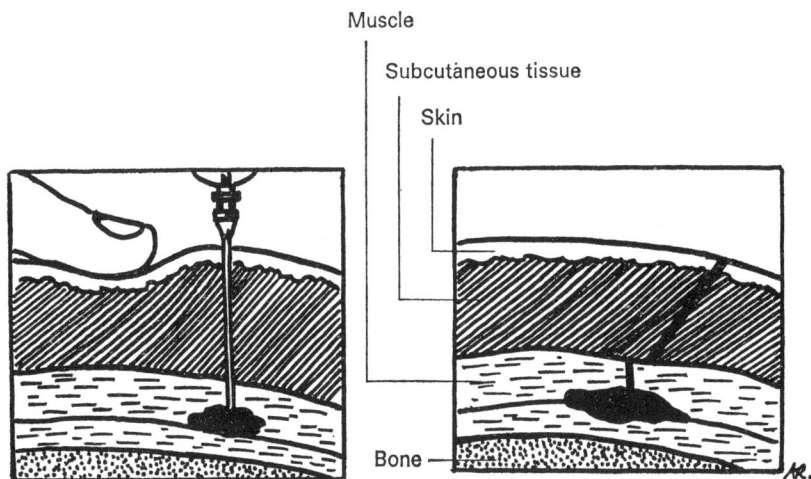

FIG. 40. Intramuscular injection technique. The skin is stretched between the thumb and forefinger to convert the needle track into a zig-zag which prevents leakage of the drug into the subcutaneous tissues.

Negative pressure is created in the syringe by slight withdrawal of the piston. If blood is revealed, the needle must be withdrawn and re-inserted.

The content of the syringe is injected slowly and smoothly by exerting even pressure on the piston to avoid sudden tension within the tissues, resulting in unnecessary discomfort. The needle is withdrawn quickly, a medicated swab being placed over the puncture. Movement of the limb allows more rapid dispersal and absorption of the drug from the site.

To avoid staining of the tissues following injection of iron (Imferon or Jectofer) the needle is withdrawn ten seconds after injection of the drug to allow time for the muscle to accommodate the drug.

Multiple injections. When a child has been prescribed more than one drug to be given by the intramuscular route at the same time, it is considered less traumatic to the child to give all the drugs through one needle. However, no more than 2–3ml should be administered into one site at any one time and there are many drugs in common use that should be given through individual needles—the barbiturates, cortisone acetate, digoxin, chloramphenicol, tetracyclines, erythromycin, procaine penicillin, parentrovite and phenytoin, to mention a few. The advice of the pharmacist or doctor should be sought before mixing the drugs.

GENERAL ADVICE

An injection can be made less painful if a good technique is adopted, and the following points are remembered:

1   A relaxed child experiences less discomfort than one who is tense and agitated.

2   Firm but gentle restraint is necessary to prevent movement of the limb as the needle is inserted. The needle should never be inserted to the hilt as this is the weakest point.

3   When a long course of injections has to be given, the sites should be used in strict rotation.

4   A strict aseptic technique is essential to avoid subsequent abscess formation.

5   Spirit irritates and is painful, therefore, just sufficient lotion is used to cleanse the area which is allowed to dry before the skin is pierced.

6   Choice of needle size depends on the type of injection to be given, i.e. No. 15 or 17 for hypodermic injections, and No. 12 or 1 for intramuscular injections. Fluid injected under pressure through a fine bore needle causes more discomfort than one administered through a wide bore needle.

7   The needle is swiftly inserted and withdrawn, but the fluid is injected slowly and evenly to avoid rapid painful distension of the tissues.

8   The manufacturer's recommended concentration of solution should not be exceeded—too great a concentration of solution can cause painful irritation of the tissues, leading to aseptic necrosis.

9   Excessive distension of the tissues is painful. One intramuscular injection should not exceed 2–3ml in volume. 0·5ml–2ml may be given by hypodermic injection.

10   A small child needs immediate love and comfort, and an older child should be thanked for his co-operation.

Intravenous Injection

This route is used by the doctor when rapid action of a drug is necessary, as in the administration of glucose to terminate hypoglycaemia, insulin in diabetic coma and thiopentone to induce anaesthesia.

A syringe with an eccentric nozzle is often preferred.

A vein in the antecubital fossa, i.e. the cephalic or median basilic is usually selected and the elbow extended. The vein is made prominent by constriction of the arm above the site with the hand of the assisting nurse. A pocket tourniquet or length of rubber tubing may be applied over an older child's sleeve to achieve the same result. Similarly, the veins on the dorsum of the hand may be chosen when digital constriction is applied around the wrist. At no time should the constriction be tight enough to occlude the radial pulse.

The skin is cleansed and allowed to dry. Once the vein has been entered, the pressure is released and the injection made. On withdrawal of the needle, firm pressure is applied over the injection site and the limb is elevated for about one minute.

When an intravenous infusion is in progress, the freshly reconstituted drug may be given through a two-way tap connecting the cannula with the recipient set, into the tubing near to the cannula, into the burette of an infant's recipient set or into the reservoir. The method used depends on the nature of the drug and the policy adopted by the hospital authority. Drugs should not be given with blood or Intralipid. Alternatively, continuous slow parenteral administration of a drug is achieved with the use of a Palmer Constant Rate Infusion Pump (PLATE 9) or a Chronometric Infusion Pump (PLATE 10). A Watkins (U.S.C.1) 'Chronofusor' Chronometric Infusion Pump is a portable infusor for continuous around-the-clock administration of drugs. Originally designed as a method of administering prolonged cancer chemotherapy to ambulatory patients, it is of particular value in maintaining morale and activity in children suffering from leukaemia. The self-contained portable apparatus carried in a harness or bodice ejects a constant flow of heparanized drug solution into a cannulated blood vessel at the rate of 0·2ml/hour. With care, the infusion can be continued over a period of several weeks.

Intrathecal Injection

Some chemotherapeutic agents do not readily pass from the blood into the cerebrospinal fluid (the blood-brain barrier) so may be injected directly into the cerebrospinal fluid following a lumbar puncture or ventricular tap, or inserted into a ventriculostomy reservoir. Small dilute doses of freshly prepared drugs are injected, using a strict aseptic technique. Penicillin may be injected in purulent meningitis, streptomycin in tuberculous meningitis and methotrexate to control leukaemic infiltration of the meninges. Contrast medium is injected for radiological detection of spinal lesions.

Details of requirements and technique are to be found under methods of obtaining a specimen of cerebrospinal fluid on pages 378–383.

Administration of Drugs by Inhalation

1 Oxygen therapy.
2 Humidification
    cool mist therapy
    steam therapy.
3 Administering local medicaments.

Oxygen Therapy

Oxygen therapy is necessary to control anoxaemia which may be due to:
  i A lack of O_2 in the inspired air.

ii Depression of the respiratory centre, due to a raised intracranial pressure or administration of excessive doses of morphine derivatives or barbiturates.

iii Obstruction within the lumen, in the wall or from outside the respiratory passages.

iv Inadequate gaseous exchange at lung level due to:
   a. pulmonary inefficiency
      collapse
      oedema
   b. cardiac inefficiency
      cardiac failure
      shock
   c. a reduction in the oxygen carrying power of the blood
      severe anaemia
      carbon monoxide poisoning.

Children with pulmonary and cardiac inefficiency account for all but a few of those requiring administration of oxygen.

The clinical features of decrease in the oxygen concentration of circulating blood include:

i   anxious restlessness;
ii tachypnoea—rapid difficult inspiratory effort;
iii tachycardia;
iv cyanosis (except in severe anaemia).

Estimation of the blood Po_2 and gas levels using the Astrup technique confirms the diagnosis.

Oxygen is a colourless, odourless, tasteless gas which readily supports combustion. It is supplied to hospitals in metal cylinders (black with a white top) of various capacities and by bulk transfer from a transporter tank to the hospital's liquid oxygen store. A system of pipes carries a constant flow of oxygen from a central oxygen supply to the wards and departments. Where this service is not available, oxygen is supplied from a cylinder at the child's bedside. Non-kink pressure tubing is used to carry oxygen from its source to tent or mask, the rate of flow being controlled by adjustment to a dry-bobbin flow-meter. As dry oxygen is an irritant to the delicate epithelial lining of the respiratory passages, humidification is necessary.

Oxygen may be administered as follows, the choice of method depending on the child's age and the reason for administration:

i   into an incubator (page 75);
ii into a tent;
iii by disposable polythene mask.

1 Oxygen Tent

The pattern of oxygen tents is constantly being improved, but the basic principles involved remain essentially unchanged.

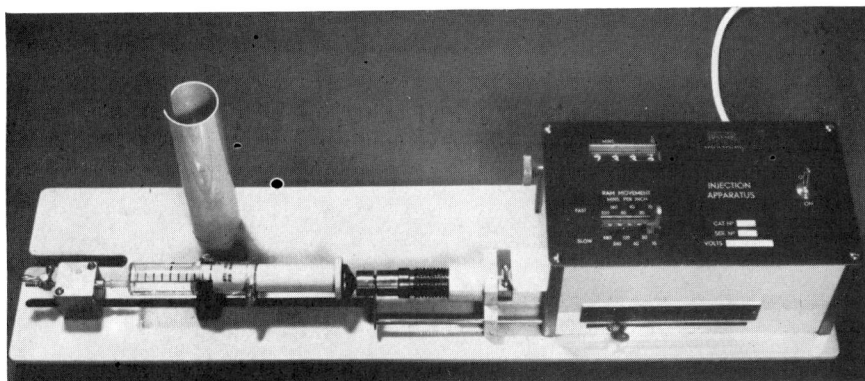

PLATE 9. Palmer Constant Rate Infusion Pump.

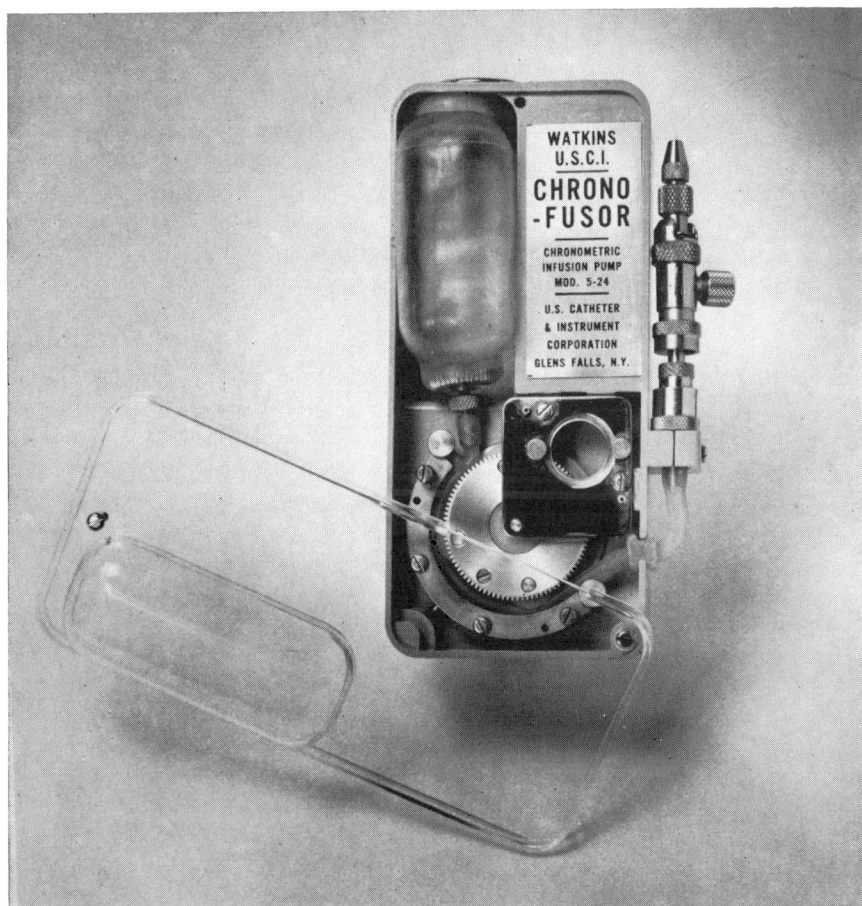

PLATE 10. Watkins (U.S.C.I.) 'Chronofusor' Chronometric Infusion Pump.
(The front has been removed to reveal the working principle.)
(Reproduced by kind permission of Chas. F. Thackray Ltd.)

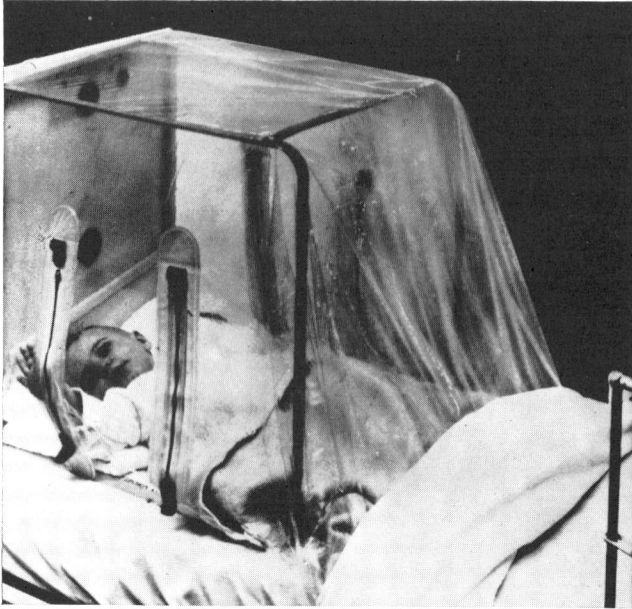

(a)

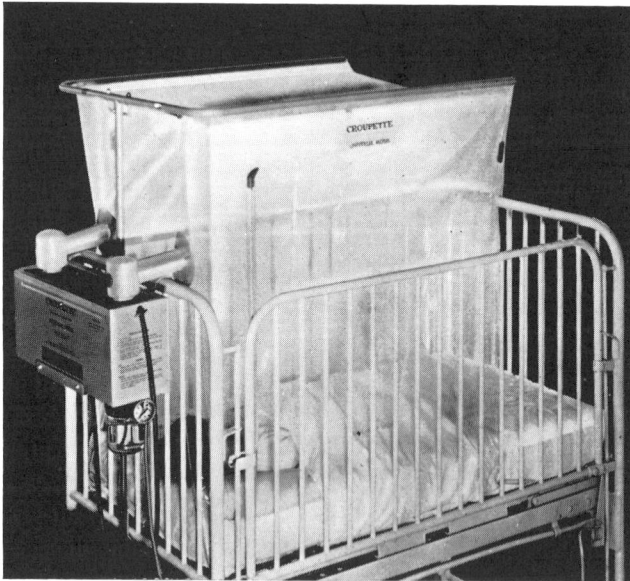

(b)

Plate 11. Cool Mist and Oxygen Tents.
(Reproduced by kind permission of Air-Shields (U.K.) Ltd.).
(a) Croupette—Model D. (b) Universal Croupette in use with a cot.

An oxygen tent consists of a metal frame from which is suspended a transparent air-tight plastic canopy which completely envelops the bedding. Access to the child is through horizontal and/or vertical openings closed by zip fasteners. Adequate humidification and cooling is achieved by diverting the oxygen supply through an electrically controlled refrigeration unit or container of ice (PLATE 11). The relative percentage humidity can be increased, if necessary, by the use of a humidifier, atomizer or nebulizer, as described below.

METHOD

The child will be supported in an upright position as required by his degree of dyspnoea. Care must be taken to ensure that his pillows do not obstruct the oxygen inlet. His favourite toy can share the experience, provided it is not a mechanical sparking toy.

The claustrophobic effect of confinement within a tent can prove most frightening to a small child, and every effort should be made to allay apprehension and anxiety. A nurse should remain within sight in an endeavour to overcome feelings of loneliness. When the need for oxygen therapy is anticipated, the child may be introduced to his little house in a playful way, thus making acceptance more tolerable.

The manufacturer's instructions regarding preparation and use of the tent should be carefully followed. The oxygen supply is turned on before the skirt of the canopy is tucked well under and all around the mattress to prevent escape of oxygen. Flushing of the tent with up to 10 litres of oxygen/minute is necessary for twenty minutes at the commencement of the therapy and each time the child has received attention through the openings. The rate of flow is then adjusted to that prescribed by the doctor.

POINTS TO CHECK WHILE IN USE

i Oxygen supply. A cylinder requires replacement when the dial indicates three-quarters empty.

ii Temperature. The temperature within the tent should be maintained at about 18–21°C or 65–70°F. Ice is replenished as necessary and the controls of a refrigeration tent are adjusted accordingly.

iii The ice water tray requires emptying at intervals.

iv Humidifiers, atomizers or nebulizers are replenished to maintain the required level of humidity.

v If the child is nursed in an oxygen tent for a prolonged period of time, the tent air is analysed as described on page 75. Because of the child's need for frequent attention, high concentrations of O_2 are rarely achieved.

vi The child's general condition is assessed at frequent intervals—colour, respiration and pulse rates and general behaviour.

Precautions. No electrical apparatus should be used inside the tent and the child is discouraged from playing with toys which may produce a spark. Oil and grease are not used on the oxygen supply apparatus because of the increased risk of fire.

On discontinuation of treatment, the oxygen supply and control knobs are turned off and the tent is removed from the bedside. The canopy is thoroughly washed with soap and water, rinsed and dried. Solvents such as ether and methylated spirit should not be used. When dry, the canopy is inspected for tears, and stored for re-use or returned to the suppliers.

2 DISPOSABLE POLYTHENE MASKS

Face masks are not well tolerated by small children but, with adequate explanation and reassurance, the co-operation of an older child may well be obtained.

A disposable polythene mask of suitable size is attached to the oxygen supply and the oxygen turned on. The mask is made to fit snugly over the child's nose, mouth and chin and the elastic ear-pieces are shortened if necessary. The oxygen flow is then adjusted to the prescribed rate. Additional humidification is not necessary as the inflowing oxygen mixes freely with the water-saturated expired air within the mask.

Tension on the non-kink delivery tubing is prevented by securing the tubing to the pillow, using a safety-pin.

Humidification

Steam or cool mist are used with or without the addition of drugs. Their local soothing effect on the respiratory passages relieves congestion and loosens viscid secretions, thus facilitating expectoration or aspiration.

The choice of method depends on the child's age and the reason for increasing humidity.

Increased atmospheric humidity is beneficial:

i   to infants of low birth weight;
ii to children with inflammatory conditions of the respiratory passages—due to infection or chemical irritation;
iii following tracheostomy when inspired air has by-passed the warm, moist mucous membrane of the nose;
iv to sufferers of cystic fibrosis when mucolytic drugs are administered in an aerosol;
v   for the local relief of nasal congestion and sinusitis.

Cool Mist Therapy

The passage of oxygen or compressed air through water, Alevaire and other drug containing solutions contained in a humidifier, atomizer or nebulizer produce a fine spray of minute water droplets. These may be administered:

i   into an incubator (page 70);

ii   into the confines of a tent;
iii into the atmosphere of a room;
iv   by mouth-piece or tracheostomy collar.

1   CROUPETTE AND HUMIDAIRE TENTS

Both tents are designed to achieve cool super-saturation of the contained air with minimal wetting. Both can be used with or without oxygen and the addition of aerosol drugs.

The Croupette is one of a large range of humidifiers manufactured by Air-Shields (U.K.) Ltd. (PLATE 11(a)). Both the infant and universal models can also be used as oxygen tents—50–60% oxygen concentration being achieved. A Dia-Pump, produced by the same firm, may be used to supply the tent with compressed air, or provide an efficient suction apparatus at the child's bedside. Explicit instructions are inscribed on the ice box. The Humidaire tent (Oxygen-aire) achieves both a high humidity and a high oxygen concentration as required. An Oxygenaire Air Compressor may be used to supply gas to the tent. Alternatively, gas is supplied from a cylinder or piped from a central dispenser.

REQUIREMENTS

Croupette or Humidaire tent.
Dia-Pump or Air Compressor   *or*   Piped air/oxygen or appropriate cylinder.
Pressure tubing.
Distilled water.
Ice.
Wall thermometer.

METHOD

The method of preparing and erection of the tent is described on page 235. The manufacturer's instructions regarding preparation and use of the tent should be followed carefully.

The water jar is filled to the appropriate level with distilled water and the atomizer is attached. Ice is put into the ice container if necessary and tubing is attached to nipples draining the ice box and the inside wall of the tent. The wall thermometer is placed to one side of the tent.

POINTS TO CHECK WHILST IN USE

i   Each time the infant requires attention, the following should be checked:
    a. the pressure dial;
    b. the water jar, which is refilled with distilled water as required;
    c. the temperature of the tent—which should not exceed 21°C or 70°F;
    d. the ice box, which is replenished as necessary;
    e. the ice water tray, which is emptied as necessary;
    f. the child's general condition.

ii The water jar is emptied and cleaned at least daily;

iii The inside of the canopy is wiped as necessary to ensure an unobstructed view of the child.

Hydration of the respiratory passages with super-saturated air demands frequent attention to the air-passages. Oro-pharyngeal suction should be carried out if the child is too young to expectorate excessive secretions. Clothing should be minimal for comfort, and changed as necessary; overheating is thus avoided.

On completion of treatment, the control knobs are turned off and the tent removed from the bedside. The canopy is cleaned as described on page 236. The atomizer is dismembered, washed under running water, checked for efficiency and replaced for re-use.

2 DIRECTIONAL MIST THERAPY (WITHOUT TENT)

The Croupaire and Hydrojette I and II manufactured by Air-Shields (U.K.) Ltd. are designed to direct cool mist within close proximity of the child's face. No restricting mask or tent is necessary. Both are simple to use and are safe and effective for both hospital and home use.

3 DIRECTIONAL MIST THERAPY (USING TRACHEOSTOMY COLLAR)

An Ultrasonic Nebulizer (Air Shields (U.K.) Ltd.) provides larger volumes of mist containing more uniform particle sizes. It is of particular value for use with a tracheostomy collar, mouth-piece or intermittent positive pressure ventilator, but can also be used to increase the humidity of a tent. The Hydrojette can also be used with a fitted collar for a child with a tracheostomy.

NEBULIZATION OF DRUGS

Drugs may be administered as aerosols, produced by nebulization of the pre-scribed medicament for their local effect on the respiratory passages. This method of administration is of particular value in reducing the viscosity of the thick tenacious respiratory secretions in cystic fibrosis by the use of mucolytic agents, e.g. 0·9% sodium chloride. The aerosol may be administered into a tent or through a face mask, tracheostomy collar or mouth-piece, or included in the circuit of an intermittent positive pressure ventilator. The most penetrating mist can be obtained from an Ultrasonic Nebulizer (Air-Shields) for either direct inhalation therapy or to increase the humidity of a tent.

The manufacturer's instructions should be carefully read before attempting to use a nebulizer. Basically, its use is simple, air or oxygen being used to break up the prescribed solution contained in the nebulizing chamber into a very fine mist.

INSUFFLATION OF DRUGS

With the individual use of a simple Spinhaler (Fisons Pharmaceuticals Ltd.) drugs may be inhaled orally in ultrafine powder form. Only drugs specially supplied in a sealed gelatin capsule 'Spincap' (Fisons) can be used with this tube-like inhaler. Following perforation of the capsule, deep inspiration allows its content to be evenly distributed in the inspired air by the action of a tiny propeller. Patient acceptance of this treatment is excellent, and care must be taken to ensure that the inhaler is not used by other children or once the capsule is emptied. An increase in respiratory effort over a period of time could result in giddiness and fainting. At present, use of the inhaler is confined to administration of 'Intal' in the control of asthma.

Steam Therapy

Warm moist air may be administered:
i into a steam tent;
ii by Nelson's inhaler;
iii from a large jug.

The administration of warm moist (medicated) steam has been virtually superseded by more efficient, less dangerous methods of increasing the water vapour content of the air. Warm, moist air, rather than cool mist is, however, beneficial to toddlers suffering from stridor, croup and acute laryngo-tracheo-bronchitis, and may still be preferred.

1 Steam Tent

A tent or canopy erected over the top third of a cot or bed can be used to confine the circulation of warm moist steam produced by a kettle to the immediate vicinity of the child. This is the only practical way of administering warm, moist air to a small child unless he is nursed in a small single cubicle in which steam from a boiling kettle is allowed to circulate freely.

REQUIREMENTS
Four-sectioned screen or special frame.
2 sheets ⎫
          ⎬ or special cover.
1 drawsheet ⎭
Safety-pins.
Wall thermometer.

Large Tray:
Electric steam kettle with long spout.
Tincture of benzoin compound, if prescribed.
5ml spoon.
Stool or low table.

METHOD
The screen covers are removed from a four-sectioned screen which is then ar-

ranged around the head of the bed or cot. The frame is draped with sheets and drawsheet in the following manner:

As the ceiling of the tent requires frequent changing, this is applied last. The length of the drawsheet is pinned to cover the height of one section of the screen frame. One large sheet is draped around the remaining three sections and secured with safety-pins. The opening between the sheet and drawsheet thus allows the passage of the steam kettle spout.

The second sheet is draped over the top of the screen so that a 30–45cm (12–18 inches) fall at the front allows adequate observation of the child. The excess sheet is folded at the corners and neatly secured with safety-pins (FIG. 41).

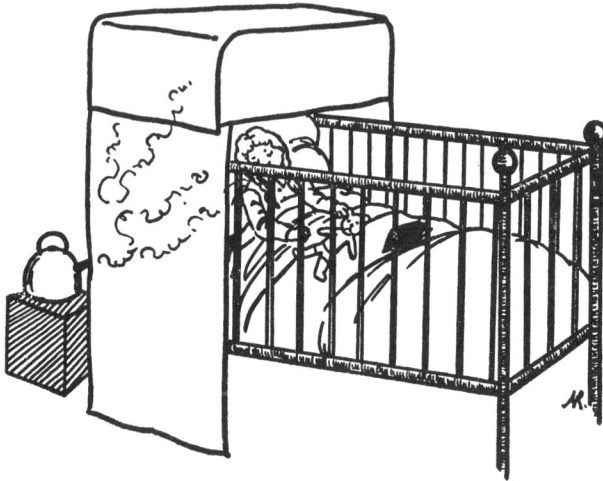

FIG. 41. A steam tent confining the warm moist air produced by a kettle to the immediate vicinity of the child, while allowing for adequate observation.

The electric kettle, filled with the required amount of water and two 5ml spoonfuls of tincture of benzoin compound, if prescribed, is brought to the boil. The kettle is placed on the tray on a stable stool or low table with the long spout directed through the opening into the tent. The spout is directed in a space between the head of the bed and the cotton tent, well out of the reach of the child. The wall thermometer is pinned to the inside of the tent on the opposite side to the kettle.

As the child is usually suffering from dyspnoea, he is nursed sitting up, supported by waterproof-protected pillows and restrained in such a way that he cannot reach the kettle. Constant vigil is desirable, both for the safety of the child receiving steam therapy and the other children in the ward. Often the child's ill state demands constant observation. Once the child is convalescent, a story told by his mother or just her presence will distract his attention from the surrounding apparatus.

Bed, tent and personal linen require frequent changing as they become damp. The child should be safeguarded against overheating by ensuring that there is adequate ventilation in the tent, that his temperature is recorded at four-hourly intervals and more frequently if necessary, and that the temperature in the steam tent does not exceed 24°C (75°F). The temperature recorded by the wall thermometer should be charted hourly when the kettle is replenished with 500–1000ml of boiling water, as required. Maintenance of a written record helps to ensure that the kettle does not boil dry.

2   Nelson's Inhaler and Open Jug Methods

The following procedures are dangerous in the hands of children and are used infrequently for this reason. They may serve a useful purpose, however, in the relief of nasal congestion and sinusitis for an older, co-operative child while under constant supervision.

REQUIREMENTS

Nelson's Inhaler   *or*   Graduated litre jug.

Cover   Towel.

Gauze   Face towel.

Measure.

Flat bowl or tray.

Drug as prescribed, e.g. tincture of benzoin compound and 5ml spoon   *or*   1–2 menthol crystals.

Paper handkerchiefs.

Sputum carton.

METHOD, USING A NELSON'S INHALER

The measure is filled with 540ml (1 pint) of boiling water. 300ml of this water is poured into the Nelson's inhaler, followed by one 5ml spoonful of tincture of benzoin compound, if prescribed, and the remainder of the boiling water. The water should not be above the level of the air inlet. The gauze protected glass mouth-piece is replaced so that it points in the opposite direction to the air inlet. The cover is secured around the inhaler which is placed in the flat-bottomed bowl or on the tray.

The child is supported with pillows at a table or bed-table on which the tray is placed. He is instructed to place the gauze-protected mouth-piece between his lips and to breathe in through his mouth and out through his nose, while the nurse remains constantly at his side. With subsequent loosening of secretions, the child should be encouraged to expectorate into the sputum carton and to blow his nose.

METHOD, USING AN OPEN JUG

When a Nelson's inhaler is not available, a large jug may be similarly used. Boiling water is mixed with cold water in a 5:1 ratio, with the jug not more than half-filled. The towel is folded around the jug to form a funnel and the jug is placed on the flat tray. The prescribed drug is added just prior to administration of the inhalation.

While under constant supervision, the child is instructed to breathe in through his nose with his face over the jug, and to raise his head to expire. His face should be dried as necessary.

Both procedures should be continued for seven to ten minutes and may be repeated every four to six hours.

Methylated spirit may be used to remove residual stains of tincture of benzoin compound from the apparatus.

Administration of Topical Drugs

Instillation of Eye Drops and Ointment

Soothing topical eye medicaments may be prescribed as:
1   Eye drops (guttae) dispensed in a dropper bottle or single dose container.
2   Ophthalmic ointments dispensed in collapsible tubes with long slender nozzles. Eye ointments are preferable in childhood as their oily base is less readily diluted with tears.

Eye medications are instilled for many purposes, the drug being absorbed by the conjunctiva or cornea:
1   To dilate the pupils in order to facilitate local examination. Mydriatic drugs inhibit the action of acetylcholine released by the parasympathetic nerve fibres, thus leaving the sympathetic nervous system to influence the size of the pupils. Atropine 1% has a lasting effect and homatropine 1 or 2% is usually preferred for its quick action for a shorter period.

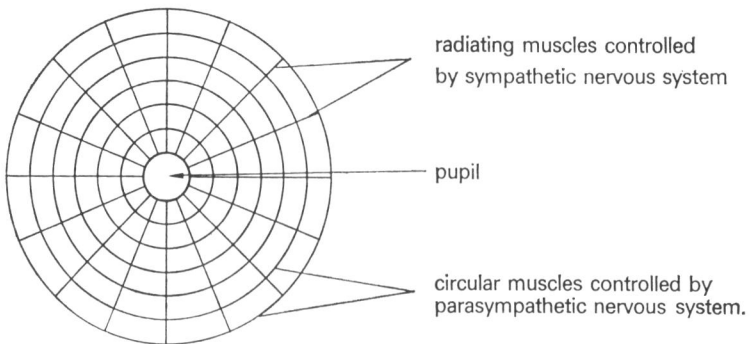

radiating muscles controlled by sympathetic nervous system

pupil

circular muscles controlled by parasympathetic nervous system.

2   To constrict the pupil. Miotic drugs enhance the action of the acetylcholine released at the neuromuscular junction of the parasympathetic fibres, causing greater constriction of the pupil. Apart from counteracting the action of mydriatic drugs, their use in paediatric work is limited. Pilocarpine 0·5% and Physostigmine 0·25% give miotic action.

3   To prevent or control infection. Prophylactic chemotherapeutic agents, such as sulphacetamide (Albucid) and antibiotic preparations, may be prescribed for children undergoing ophthalmic surgery. Conjunctivitis, which may be unilateral or bilateral, is treated topically (locally).

4   To lubricate the eye ball. When reflex blinking is inhibited, bland oily drops of castor oil or liquid paraffin are used to prevent drying and irritation of a cornea exposed to air or anaesthetic vapours. They may also be used for their soothing effect in the treatment of burns and abrasions.

5   Prior to examination of the cornea, a fluorescein 2% eye drop is instilled. Abrasions or ulceration are then seen as vivid green concentrations.

6   To induce local anaesthesia prior to removal of a foreign body from the cornea as, for example, cocaine hydrochloride 1 or 2%.

7   To reduce inflammatory response, prednisolone eye ointment may be used.

REQUIREMENTS

Eye drops⎫
Pipette   ⎬ *or* tube containing ophthalmic ointment.
            ⎭
Small sterile lint squares or wool swabs.
Prescription sheet.
Receptacle for soiled swabs.

METHOD

The eyes' normal response to overt stimulation is protective reflex closure of the lids. This procedure is frightening to the small child and little co-operation can be achieved. It is best carried out quickly and efficiently by an experienced nurse.

Prior to instillation of drops or ointment, the eye-lids are bathed, or the eyes irrigated with sterile sodium chloride (see below).

Two nurses are essential for this procedure unless the child is co-operative. A small child is restrained in a blanket and placed supine. The prescription is checked. After washing and drying her hands, the nurse fills the dispensing pipette, stands behind her patient and rests her right hand on the child's forehead. With the index finger of her left hand placed near the margin of the lower lid, the lower fornix of the conjunctival sac is exposed by applying gentle, downward and backward digital pressure. The child's attention is attracted so that his gaze is upward. The pipette is lowered to within a few millimetres of the exposed conjunctival sac and one or two drops are released. Excess medicament is mopped from the cheek and the child comforted in a face upward position for two to three minutes to discourage dilution with tears and drainage into the lacrimal passages.

If ophthalmic ointment is used, the tip of the nozzle is wiped with a cotton wool swab and a thin strip of ointment is applied to the exposed lower fornix of the conjunctiva and lid traction is released.

Eye Bathing

REQUIREMENTS

Tray.

Sterile Equipment	*Composite pack*
Gallipot.	Gallipot.
Bowl containing cotton wool balls or lint squares.	6 small lint squares or cotton wool swabs.

Additional requirements:

Bottle of sterile 0·9% sodium chloride, i.e. normal saline, standing in a jug of warm water.

Receptacle for soiled swabs.

METHOD

The child is positioned as for instillation of eye drops. Sterile saline is poured into the gallipot and the nurse washes and dries her hands. Two or three swabs are soaked in warmed saline and the excess solution is squeezed out before the unaffected eye is bathed.

The closed eye-lids are bathed from the inner canthus outwards, using the swabs once only, care being taken not to exert any pressure on the eye ball. The lids are then gently dried and the procedure is repeated for the other eye.

Irrigation of the Eye

REQUIREMENTS

Tray.

Sterile Equipment:

Small jug of warmed sterile saline (38°C or 100°F).

Lotion thermometer.

Undine standing in a small bowl.

Small lint squares or cotton wool swabs.

Additional Equipment:

Receiver.

Receptacle for soiled swabs.

Waterproof protection for the bed.

METHOD

The child is placed, restrained if necessary, in a supine position with the head slightly towards the affected side. The receiver is supported on the waterproof protection, just below the eye which is to be irrigated. The temperature of the lotion is checked.

The nurse washes and dries her hands and on return to the child's side fills the undine with the prepared solution and stands behind her patient, resting her right hand on the child's forehead. The lotion is first allowed to run on to the child's cheek to accustom him to the sensation, and then directed from the inner canthus to the outer while the eyelids are gently separated with the thumb and finger of the left hand. The rate of flow can be controlled by adjusting the tilt of the undine or by a finger placed over the air inlet. The outlet should be held at a sufficient distance to prevent injury should the child suddenly move. To achieve thorough cleansing, the child is encouraged to move his eyes up and down, right and left.

On completion of the procedure, the eye-lids are gently dried, using each cotton wool ball once only.

Instillation of Nasal Drops

Nasal decongestants in the form of ephedrine hydrochloride $\frac{1}{2}$ or 1% drops are effective in shrinking the nasal mucosa, permitting greater air entry and adequate drainage of the middle ear through the Eustachian tube. They are frequently prescribed prior to feeding a 'snuffly' infant and for the relief of upper respiratory tract and middle ear infections.

REQUIREMENTS

Nasal drops in dropper bottle.
Cotton wool balls.
Receptacle for soiled swabs.
Prescription sheet.

METHOD

An infant is placed on the nurse's knees with his body parallel to and supported by her thighs and his head hyperextended over the nurse's left hand. A bigger child is asked to blow his nose before being placed supine with his head hyperextended over the side of the bed or over a pillow placed under his shoulders (FIG. 42). For the decongestant to reach the naso-pharynx the position is important. The tip of the primed pipette is directed to just inside each nostril and the prescribed solution is instilled. The position is maintained for five minutes to permit gravitational drainage into the naso-pharynx.

Nasal sprays are rarely used during childhood.

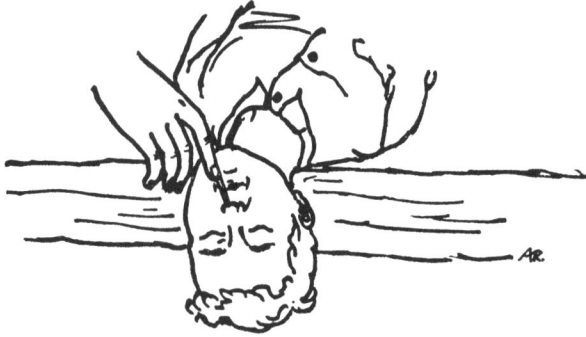

FIG. 42. Position of a child for insertion of nasal drops.

Instillation of Aural Drops

Ear drops may be instilled:
  i to soften wax, e.g. 4% sodium bicarbonate, olive oil and wax solvents such as Cerumol or spirit ear drops B.N.F.;
 ii to relieve the pain of otitis media, e.g. phenol ear drops B.N.F.;
iii for the treatment of infection of the external auditory meatus (otitis externa), e.g. chloramphenicol or neomycin ear drops;
 iv to float out small insects, e.g. olive oil;

REQUIREMENTS
Ear drops.
Pipette.
Prescription sheet.

METHOD
The ear drum is examined to exclude perforation.

The child is placed in the lateral position on his unaffected side or in a sitting position with his head tilted towards the unaffected side. The warmed ear drops are instilled and the child's position is retained for two to three minutes to assist deep penetration by gravitational flow. A small piece of well-loosened cotton wool is placed in the outer meatus to absorb excess solution.

Aural Insufflation

Following cleansing of the external auditory meatus, drugs may be administered in powder form in the local treatment of otitis externa. The primed insufflator is directed into the canal and the bulb is gently but deliberately squeezed.

Cleansing of the External Auditory Meatus

Prior to aural examination, insertion of drops and insufflation, the auditory canal requires thorough cleansing. Mopping is the method of choice, although the doctor may ask for the ear to be irrigated. Clear vision is essential or the tympanic membrane could be damaged. The S-shaped auditory canal is increased in size and straightened by pulling the pinna backwards and upwards (backwards only during infancy). An aural speculum is held just inside the canal while the beam from a reflected light on a head mirror or head lamp is focussed on to the tympanic membrane. Alternatively, an auroscope is used.

Dry Mopping an Ear

REQUIREMENTS
Tray.
Sterile Equipment:
Wool carrier and cotton wool.
Aural speculum.

Additional Equipment:
Head mirror ⎱
Lamp   ⎰ *or* Auroscope.
Receptacle for soiled swabs.

METHOD
The child is sat on a chair or restrained on a nurse's knee with his affected side facing the operator. A wisp of cotton wool is securely attached to the wool carrier ensuring that the end is safely protected. The canal is thoroughly cleansed while under direct vision, as described above. To prevent an unpredictable move causing injury, the aural speculum is held in position with the left hand resting on the child's head.

Syringing an ear

This procedure is only carried out in experienced hands on the instructions of a doctor. It is used exclusively for removal of wax and non-vegetative foreign bodies and only when the tympanic membrane is intact. Ear drops may be prescribed to soften hard wax prior to syringing.

REQUIREMENTS
As for dry mopping, with the addition of the following equipment:
    Aural syringe and nozzle, or Higginson's syringe.
    Jugs of lotion, e.g. normal saline or tap water.
    Aural angled forceps.
    Lotion thermometer.
    Receiver.
    Waterproof protection.

METHOD

This procedure may prove distasteful to a child, and his co-operation should be sought by explanation and reasoning. He is sat on a chair or on a nurse's knees with his affected ear towards the operator. The lotion is prepared at 38°C (100°F) so that it enters the external canal at body temperature. Much discomfort, nausea and giddiness may be experienced if the semi-circular canals are affected by the introduction of fluid of a higher or lower temperature.

The waterproof protection is placed around the child's shoulders and the receiver supported immediately below the affected ear. After ensuring that the lotion is of the correct temperature, the syringe is primed, the nozzle firmly secured in position and the air expelled. To prevent an unpredictable move causing injury, the hand straightening the canal also supports the syringe nozzle placed at the canal entrance, and the lotion is directed in a gentle stream on to the roof of the canal. The lotion thus directed flows over the tympanic membrane and floor of the canal before being collected in the awaiting receiver.

When it is thought that the meatus is clear, it is mopped dry and the tympanic membrane is inspected.

For Further Reading

BOYLES KORKIS F. (1965). *Ear Nose and Throat Nursing*, 2nd edition. J. & A. Churchill, London 1965.
GARLAND P. (1966). *Ophthalmic Nursing*, 5th edition. Faber and Faber, London.

CHAPTER THIRTEEN

Wounds and Wound Care

Wounds may be incised, punctured, lacerated or contused. The majority of wounds seen on a surgical ward are incised wounds healing by 'first intention'.

Healing by 'First Intention'

An incision made to perform an operation has been intentionally inflicted under strict aseptic conditions. The two cut edges of skin are held in close apposition by sutures, clips or adhesive strips until new connective tissue has formed in the clot. The wound may be covered with a plastic skin such as Nobecutane or a dressing.

Unless otherwise indicated for the reasons listed below, the dressing covering a 'clean stitched' wound should be left undisturbed:

1 A rise in body temperature.
2 Reluctance of an infant to feed.
3 Obvious discharge from the wound.
4 Local discomfort.
5 Contamination with excreta.

Unnecessary removal of the dressing and wound toilet increase the risk of introducing micro-organisms and disturbing the formation of connective tissue and delicate new epithelium.

Healing by 'Second Intention'

Abscess cavities and burst sutured wounds heal by 'second intention' Daily insertion of a diminishing quantity of moistened sterile ribbon gauze maintains separation of the skin edges until the cavity has healed from the bottom. Excessive granulation tissue is controlled with a single cauterizing application of silver nitrate.

Factors Essential for Wound Healing

The relatively rapid healing power of children is influenced by many factors:
1   A good nourishing diet is important. Protein for growth and repair of damaged tissues, vitamin C for the formation of connective tissue and iron to prevent or treat anaemia, should all be well represented. The doctor may prescribe vitamin C and iron supplements.
2   Sleep and local rest are important. The affected part of the body requires rest to allow healing to take place; for example, the two cut edges of an incised wound are held together with sutures or clips, a fracture is reduced and splinted, an anastomosis of the alimentary tract is given opportunity to heal by temporary discontinuation of oral feeding.
3   Infection interferes with the natural healing process. Interference with dressings should therefore be reduced to a minimum and a non-touch technique used at all times.

Factors Delaying the Healing Process

1   The presence of infection, foreign body or haematoma in the wound.
2   A wound sutured under tension.
3   General debility.
4   Lack of vitamin C.
5   Ischaemia (a reduced blood volume affecting the oxygen supply to the part).
6   Corticosteroids interfering with the normal inflammatory reaction delaying the healing process.

Burst Abdomen

Evisceration is an uncommon, but nevertheless alarming complication of abdominal surgery, occurring usually seven to fourteen days post-operatively. It is often precipitated by local infection in a debilitated child and should be suspected if a hitherto dry wound discharges blood-stained watery fluid.

The 'burst' may be merely separation of the superficial skin layers (dehiscence) or complete breakdown of the wound with expulsion of the distended loops of bowel (evisceration).

A dressing trolley containing additional large sterile towels should be prepared for inspection of the area. The child will naturally be very frightened, and the nurse must do everything possible to reassure her patient. If the 'burst' involves an area of superficial skin and muscle, the nurse may use long strips of non-stretch adhesive tape to approximate the two edges. The doctor will then decide on the necessity for a secondary suturing.

In total evisceration, the doctor should be informed immediately and the exposed loops of bowel covered with a large, sterile towel. On no account should the nurse try to replace the abdominal contents or use gauze swabs and cotton wool on the area.

Shock is inevitable and the child should be placed flat in bed and oral fluids withheld. A naso-gastric tube is passed and the doctor will prescribe a sedative and erect an intravenous infusion prior to the child's prompt return to theatre for a secondary repair of the abdominal wall.

The parents should be informed of the nature of this complication and their child's impending surgery, and should be encouraged to visit in the immediate post-operative period.

Dressing Materials

Gauze. Made of cotton threads or polyester fibres woven into a wide mesh, gauze is soft, pliable, porous and absorptive for use next to wounds. Gauze swabs are made commercially, but may be made from gauze rolls supplied to hospitals in varying widths. Short lengths are cut and folded in such a way that the swab is of four to eight thicknesses and the frayed edges are turned in.

Ribbon gauze. Rolls of close woven gauze of various widths may be sterilized for light packing of abscess cavities or to provide a wick type of drainage.

Lint. This is an expensive material and should not be mis-used where cheaper alternatives are available. (Old linen is quite satisfactory for poultices and for use as a temporary flannel.)

Non-adherent dressings. Petroleum jelly impregnated cotton net material (tulle gras) provides a non-adherent surface application to raw areas. Supplied commercially, it can be re-sterilized by dry heat. Melolin XA (Smith and Nephew Ltd.) is made of soft extra absorbent cotton and polyester fibres faced with a non-adherent microporous plastic film. The advantage of non-adherent dressings is that their removal does not disturb the underlying healing process. The ease with which they can be removed is more acceptable to the small child.

Cotton wool. Prepared as balls or pads, cotton wool is widely used for its absorptive property and for padding. As supplied by the manufacturers, cotton wool is firmly compressed into a roll. To increase its effectiveness, the roll of wool is unwound, split into thicknesses and warmed before being made into balls and pads.

Gamgee. This consists of a layer of wool enclosed in gauze. Its effective absorptive property is increased by warmth.

Cellulose tissue. Comparatively cheap and very absorptive cellulose tissue provides a suitably effective outer packing when large quantities of fluid have to be absorbed, as for example, in colostomy care. Unlike the other dressing materials mentioned above, it can be safely disposed of in the lavatory.

Means of Securing Dressings

Instead of an unnecessarily cumbersome and often inadequate dressing, many surgeons prefer to spray a 'clean stitched' wound with Nobecutane. Subsequent care is minimal. Following removal of the sutures, Nobecutane solvent is used to clean the surrounding area.

When dressings are used to protect the wound from friction or contamination and to absorb discharge, these must be comfortably and adequately retained in position using one of the following methods:

1 Bandages

Roller bandages may be of cotton mesh, Kling, crêpe, elastic (Robert Jones) or of plaster of Paris. Bandages are best secured with adhesive tape.

Special bandages include:

i A many-tailed bandage used to retain an abdominal dressing in position. Many-tailed bandages are tedious to make, difficult to retain in position, and may interfere with respiratory function. Their use has been virtually superseded by more efficient methods.

ii A T-bandage used to retain a perineal dressing in position.

Tubegauz (Scholl), a seamless tubular gauze bandage available in five sizes, is quick to apply with the use of applicators, and provides an efficient, comfortable covering for dressings applied to most parts of the body. It is of particular value in skin disorders and as a means of restraining a small infant.

Netelast (Roussel), a cotton and elastic wide mesh tubular net, is available in seven sizes. It is quick to apply, comfortable to the wearer and self-securing, thus avoiding the use of safety-pins. No applicators are necessary and it can be re-used.

2 Adhesive (not used when there is a history of sensitivity).

Short lengths of *zinc oxide plaster* (Johnson & Johnson) are used to secure a piece of gauze over a wound.

Non-allergic adhesive tape such as *Micropore* (Minnesota Mining & Mfg. Ltd.) is less difficult to remove and leaves no residual mark and is therefore of particular value in paediatrics.

Elastic, porous *Elastoplast* (Smith & Nephew Ltd.) gives support as well as adequate coverage to the wound of an ambulant child. It is also of value to use as a corset dressing (FIG. 43) when there is tension on an abdominal suture-line or when the wound requires frequent attention.

CORSET DRESSING (suitable for an infant)

1 Four lengths of 7·5cm Elastoplast are cut (two for each side). These should

be of sufficient length to extend laterally over the iliac bones to just beyond the umbilicus, medially.

2   Each pair is prepared by joining length-ways with a 1–5cm overlap (depending on the size of the infant).

3   One end is turned under 3–5cm and eyelets are cut 1 cm from the resulting fold.

4   The corset is applied to the skin leaving a 2–4cm gap between the two sides to allow for tightening.

5   Narrow tape laced through the eyelets secures the corset over the dressing and is unlaced for each change of dressing.

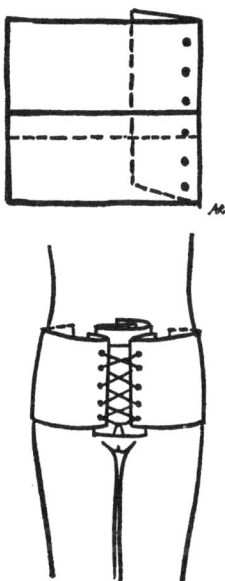

FIG. 43. Corset dressing.

Sleek (Smith & Nephew Ltd.) provides complete occlusion of the wound with a waterproof dressing. Perforations in the plaster allow air to reach the skin and moisture to escape, thus avoiding softening of the skin (maceration) and delay in the healing process.

Individual plasters incorporating a strip of gauze or lint, Band-Aid (Johnson & Johnson) or Melolin, Airstrip (Smith & Nephew Ltd.) are of particular value when there is a 'clean stitched' wound adjoining a discharging colostomy or drainage area, and for small children. Supplied in individual sterile packs, they are easy to apply, comfortable to the wearer and cause little discomfort when removed.

REMOVAL OF ADHESIVE

To a small child, removal of the old dressing is the most fearful part of the dressing procedure. Adhesive should never be pulled away from the skin. A corner is lifted and the skin eased down away from the adhesive. Swabs soaked in solvent, such as methylated ether or carbon tetrachloride, may be used to assist removal and also to clear the skin of adhesive marks.

Aseptic Technique

This technique is adopted for procedures when it is imperative that micro-organisms are not introduced.
1   Where the continuity of the skin surface is broken, e.g.
    dressing of wounds—intentional
                          accidental.
    all percutaneous injections.
2   Where a cavity of the body is to be entered, e.g.
    the bladder.

Principles of an Aseptic Technique

1   All the equipment and dressings used must be sterilized.
2   The participating staff must wash and dry their hands before the procedure.
3   All dressings and other sterile equipment are handled with forceps (non-touch technique) except when sterile gloves are worn.
4   All soiled dressings and disposable equipment are placed in a suitable closed container and incinerated as soon as possible.
5   The trolley must be cleared, cleaned and re-set with further sterile equipment before another procedure is carried out.

Sterilization of Equipment

Sterilization means rendering an article free from living micro-organisms. An article is therefore either sterile or unsterile and never 'almost sterile'. The effect of the killing agent on both the micro-organisms and the object to be sterilized have to be considered.

Methods of Sterilization

PHYSICAL
This method is used in preference to chemical sterilization which is more difficult to control.

1 *Dry heat*

Hot air oven at a temperature of 160°C for one hour.

Infra-red oven at a temperature of 200°C for half-an-hour.

This method is suitable for stainless steel and all glass equipment, particularly syringes which can be sterilized assembled ready for use. The method is not suitable for rubber, cloth, plastic or paper.

2 *Moist heat*

i Boiling is quick and simple but, unfortunately, resistant spores are not killed by a temperature of 100°C (212°F) even if boiling is prolonged. This traditional method of sterilizing ward equipment is on the decline.

ii The autoclave is a method of sterilization using pressurized steam. Both micro-organisms and spores are killed. Dressings lightly packed in metal drums, cardboard boxes, paper or nylon, metal and polypropylene containers and instruments, rubber gloves and fluids for parenteral administration may all be sterilized in an autoclave. A temperature of 134°C (274°F) and a pressure of 32lb per square inch is maintained for $3\frac{1}{2}$ minutes.

Various methods are used to test the efficiency of the autoclave as a sterilizer, and to indicate sterility. Impregnated paper strips which change colour if the correct temperature is maintained for the correct length of time are incorporated on the outside of a pack. Likewise, a Browne's tube put in the centre of a lightly packed dressing drum changes colour.

iii Ionizing radiation is being used extensively in the pharmaceutical industry to sterilize much of the pre-sterilized disposable equipment now in use. This is clearly labelled 'sterilized by gamma radiation'.

CHEMICAL

Chemical sterilization of articles required for aseptic techniques is not common and ranks as a poor second best. Chemicals are, however, used extensively to sterilize feeding equipment and to disinfect contaminated articles. Additional factors have to be considered:

Physical sterilization.

1 Time.

2 Temperature.

3 Moisture content.

Chemical sterilization.

1 Time, which varies with strength and nature of disinfectant.

2 Article must be free from organic matter—pus, blood and faeces.

3 Concentration of the chemical.

4 Complete immersion is essential.

5 Nature of the micro-organisms.

Central Sterile Supply Department (C.S.S.D.)

Pre-packed sterile, often disposable, equipment prepared in a local C.S.S.D. or supplied from a pharmaceutical company is quickly replacing the traditional method of sterilization and preparation of equipment for procedures demanding an aseptic technique.

During the last decade, paper has been substituted for cloth, tinfoil for stainless steel, plastics for rubber and glass, so that much of the equipment in use today is used once and then destroyed. Although expensive to initiate, dressing packs and composite packs for special procedures supplied from a central depot have many advantages both to patients and staff. What should be sterile is sterile because steam under pressure using an autoclave is an efficient means of destroying all micro-organisms, including spores.

Individual dressing packs reduce the risk of contamination that exists when a dressing drum containing the requirements for more than one dressing is opened repeatedly. The use of pre-sterilized composite packs is quick and easy compared with traditional methods—a point often not appreciated by the young

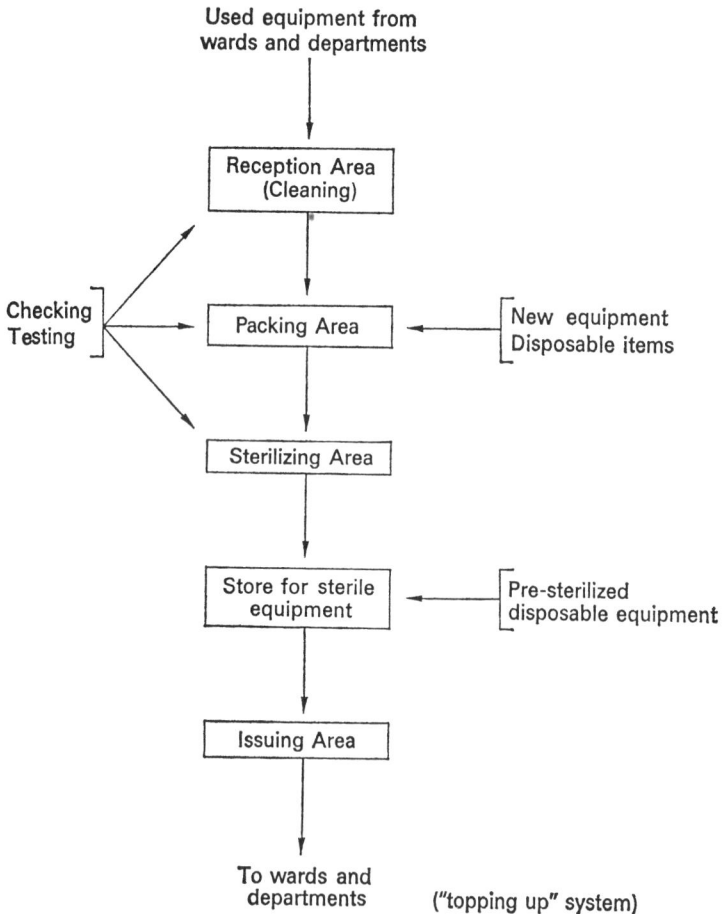

Used equipment from wards and departments

↓

Reception Area (Cleaning)

Checking Testing ← Packing Area ← New equipment Disposable items

↓

Sterilizing Area

↓

Store for sterile equipment ← Pre-sterilized disposable equipment

↓

Issuing Area

↓

To wards and departments   ("topping up" system)

FIG. 44. The service supplied by a Central Sterile Supply Department (C.S.S.D.).

student who may never have practised any other method. Wastage should be avoided by choosing a pack of minimal content for each purpose.

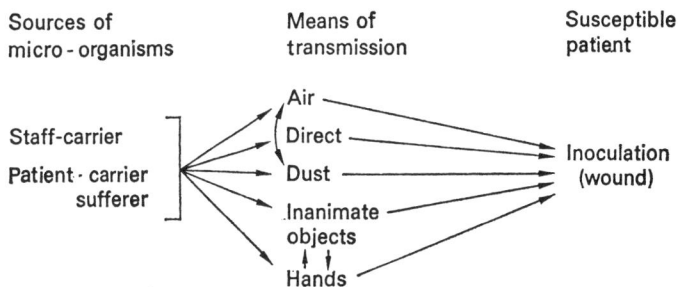

FIG. 45. Transmission of wound infection.

Surgical Dressing Technique

The Environment

An air conditioned room is the ideal area in which to perform procedures demanding an aseptic technique. This is not possible in the majority of older hospitals, but is a goal to be achieved in future planning.

From the psychological aspect, it is an advantage for a child to be taken into a separate room for dressing of wounds and for painful procedures to be performed, so that other children are not upset by his distress. Unless the room is air conditioned, the concentration of micro-organisms in the confined area may prove an additional hazard. Where there is no special room or when the child is nursed in isolation, the prepared trolley is taken to the child's bedside.

To reduce the dust in the immediate vicinity of the patient, activities such as cleaning and bed-making should be completed at least half-an-hour before the wound is exposed.

Nurses' Preparation

Prior to preparing for any aseptic technique, the hands must be washed with soap and water before drying on a clean towel. A mask may or may not be worn. A paper mask is efficient while it remains dry, and should be disposed of at the end of each dressing or procedure. It is invariably necessary to talk to a small child while carrying out an aseptic technique. A mask may be worn to prevent droplets reaching the broken skin surface.

A child may be very frightened when he sees a nurse wearing a mask. So that he is assured of her familiar face, the nurse should put on her mask in his presence. If the child is still frightened, it is better that the mask is removed than for the nurse to attempt to perform the procedure on a distressed, unco-operative patient.

Preparation of Equipment

The dressing trolley is washed with soap and water daily, and sprayed with spirit lotion and dried with a clean paper towel before each procedure.

Two or three receptacles are clipped to the sides of the trolley:
1   for disposable equipment and soiled dressings;
2   for instruments and other non-disposable equipment;
3   for bandages, cotton dressing towel, etc. (if required).

USING C.S.S.D. EQUIPMENT

The sterile composite or dressing pack is checked to ensure:
1   that the outer cover is intact;
2   that the seal is not broken;
3   that the pack is dry;
4   that the autoclaving process has converted the colour coding;
5   that the expiry date has not been exceeded.

BASIC DRESSING TROLLEY

Top shelf:
Initially empty but for dressing pack containing:
Gauze swabs.*
Cotton wool balls.*
1 paper towel.*
1 gallipot.*
4 pairs dressing forceps, Dissecting or Bryant's (may be in a separate pack).*

Bottom shelf:
Dressing pack.
Additional packs as required.

USING TRADITIONAL METHOD

The equipment required is completely immersed in boiling water for five minutes. Using Cheatle's forceps stored in a cylindrical jar of disinfectant, the equipment is lifted from the sterilizer and placed on the top shelf of the trolley. Care is taken to ensure that the Cheatle's forceps touch only sterile objects and always point in a downward direction. Cheatle's forceps are also used to transfer the necessary cotton wool and gauze dressings and towels from the sterile dressing drums (with closed perforations) to the sterile bowls.
Large bowl for towel(s).
Small bowl for wool and gauze swabs.
2 gallipots for lotions.
Instrument tray containing 4 pairs of dressing forceps.
All the receptacles are covered with lids.

Lotions for wound and skin toilet:
   Spirit for skin preparation and 'clean stitched' wounds.
   Aqueous antiseptics for open and drained wounds.
Solvent for removing adhesive plaster marks.

* Wrapped in disposable trolley cover and sealed in a paper bag.

Adhesive tape, bandages, etc. as required.
Trolley scissors.

METHOD
Two nurses are necessary to carry out a dressing, however simple. One assists her colleague with preparing the requirements on the top shelf of the trolley; her responsibility then lies entirely with ensuring the comfort and safety of the child.

The second nurse remains 'clean', touching only the sterile objects necessary to carry out a strict aseptic technique.

Both nurses wash their hands and dry them on clean towels.

USING C.S.S.D. EQUIPMENT	USING TRADITIONAL METHOD
First Nurse. Using the trolley scissors, the bag containing the composite dressing pack is opened to allow the sterile pack with corners uppermost to slide on to the trolley top. (The emptied bag may then be attached to the side of the trolley to receive the soiled dressings.)	Removes the lids from the stainless steel equipment.
Second Nurse Opens the pack by handling only the outside of the wrap so that the trolley surface is completely covered.	
First Nurse. Opens the instrument pack (if separate) and additional packs as required to allow their contents to slide on to the sterile trolley cover.	

Suitable lengths of adhesive tape are cut and attached to the side of the trolley.

Second Nurse.
Using one pair of forceps, the sterile content of the trolley top is re-organized. The gallipot is held away from the trolley while the first nurse pours the lotion.

First Nurse.
Pours the lotion into the gallipot. Her full attention is then given to her patient. She reassures her charge, exposes the area and loosens the strapping securing the dressing.

USING C.S.S.D. EQUIPMENT   USING TRADITIONAL METHOD

Second Nurse

Using the initial pair of forceps | Taking one pair of forceps
the soiled dressing is carefully removed and inspected before discarding into the receptacle for soiled dressings. These forceps are then discarded into the receptacle for non-disposable equipment (unless disposable).

Using two further pairs of dressing forceps, the dressing towel is placed in the best position to avoid contamination of the bedclothes. Retaining the forceps in her hands, the nurse inspects the wound to assess the necessary toilet.

A discharging wound is cleansed first with a mild aqueous antiseptic solution, the swab being used once only. Fresh swabs are then used for each side and the surrounding area. One pair of forceps is used for transferring the lightly moistened swab from the trolley to the second pair of forceps which is reserved for the actual wound toilet. The second pair of forceps is discarded after use and the remaining sterile pair of forceps from the trolley top is used to apply sterile gauze and cotton wool dressings to the wound.

Both pairs of forceps are then discarded into the instrument container.

First Nurse.

Maintains the dressing in position.

Second Nurse.

Pours solvent into the gallipot and removes the resistant adhesive marks. The noxious smell and chill of the solvent is unacceptable to small children and should only be used following prior warning and in areas away from the face.

The dressing is then secured.

Both nurses ensure that the child is comfortable and suitably rewarded.

Care of equipment following use.

The disposable contents of the trolley top shelf are discarded into the bag for soiled dressings. Excess lotion may be absorbed by the paper towel. The top of the bag is screwed before being placed in a receptacle for burnable rubbish. The non-disposable equipment is retained for return to C.S.S.D. in the recognized manner. | The top of the bag containing soiled dressings is screwed before being placed in a receptacle for burnable rubbish. The stainless steel equipment is washed in hot, soapy water, rinsed, boiled for five minutes, removed from the sterilizer and stored dry for re-use.

Both nurses wash and dry their hands.

Sterile disposable gloves may be used when an aseptic technique using instruments is not practical, as for example, following an operation for hypospadias and care of the umbilical cord.

Removal of Sutures

The length of time sutures remain in position depends on:

1 *The rate of healing.* Healthy tissues heal well, but when the child is generally debilitated or the local tissues are devitalized, healing is slow.

2 *The site.* To lessen the possibility of an unsightly scar, some sutures are removed as early as possible. This is particularly so of wounds of the face and neck where there is a rich blood supply and the suture-line is not usually under tension. Facial sutures may be removed as early as the fourth and sixth post-operative days for this reason. Clips used to close transverse incisions in the loose skin folds of the neck are removed on the second and fourth post-operative days. When the sutures are under tension, they are not removed until much later—usually six to ten days after insertion, or they may be left as long as fourteen days if healing has been delayed.

In all instances, it is the surgeon who decides when his patient's sutures should be removed.

Principles Involved

1 The stitch is cut in one place only to ensure that no part of it is left under the skin.

2 Suture material which has been above the skin must not be drawn through the underlying tissues.

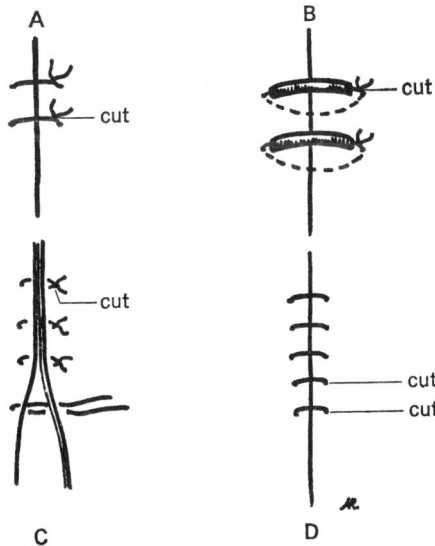

Fig. 46. Varieties of suture. A = Interrupted. B = 'Deep tension'. C = Mattress. D = Continuous.

Types of Suture

1 *Interrupted.* Each stitch is tied separately and the ends cut short. This suture is most commonly used.

2 *Deep tension sutures* are designed to withstand strain. A short length of narrow rubber tubing prevents the suture cutting into the skin.

3 *Continuous.* Used infrequently. One length of suture material is used to oversew the skin edges together.

4 *Continuous subcuticular suture.* One length of suture material is inserted in a zig-zag fashion through the subcuticular tissues. The suture is drawn tight, the free ends tied across a piece of gauze and covered with Elastoplast. Dressing and suture are removed in one simple action (FIG. 47).

REQUIREMENTS

In addition to a basic dressing trolley, a pair of fine sterile stitch scissors or a disposable stitch cutter is required.

METHOD

The procedure is as for surgical dressing technique.

The exposed wound is inspected to confirm adequate union of the skin edges. Cleansing is not necessary and adds to the risk of introducing micro-organisms.

A gauze swab is placed on the dressing towel to receive the cut sutures. With plain dissecting forceps in one hand and stitch scissors or cutter in the other, the nurse proceeds to remove alternate sutures.

The knot securing the stitch always lies against the skin on one or other side of the suture-line. This is gently lifted in the forceps so that 1–2mm of stitch from below the skin surface is drawn above it. The stitch scissors are opened just sufficiently to allow the point of one blade to pass between the knot and the skin and the stitch is cut. Gentle traction on the forceps directed towards the suture-line allows the stitch to slide easily out without dragging the skin edges apart. The procedure is repeated until alternate or all of the sutures have been removed, as necessary. A dressing may be applied for twenty-four hours, after which the wound is cleansed and left exposed. The adhesive marks are removed.

A small child is often very proud of his stitches and is pleased to take them home for his school friends to admire.

To remove a continuous suture, the stitch is cut at each point where it enters the skin along one side of the suture-line. Gentle traction on the forceps allows each portion to be removed.

Removal of Clips

Metal clips are rarely used in childhood. They are retained in position by sharp points which penetrate the skin on either side of an incision. Michel clips require a special remover to straighten the clip to disengage first one sharp point and then the other. Kifa clips are removed by approximating the centre wings with a pair of dissecting forceps. The straightened clip can thus be similarly disengaged.

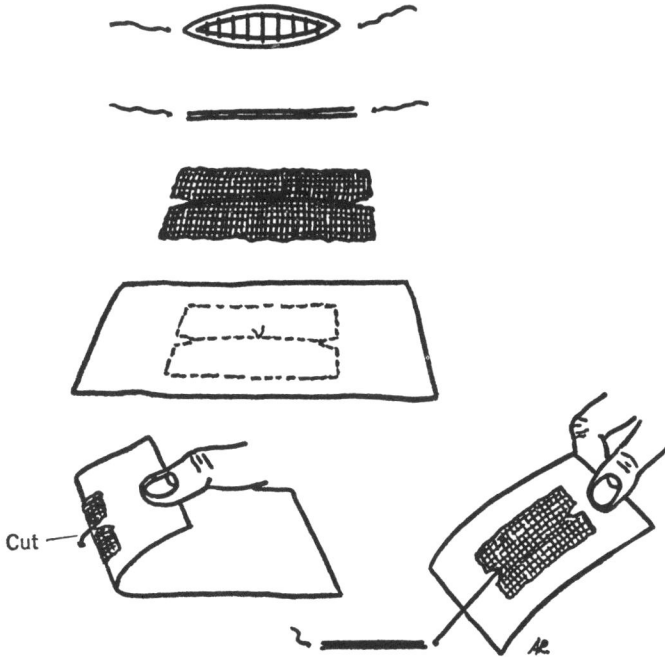

FIG. 47. Continuous subcuticular suture. The skin edges are brought together and the suture is tied across a piece of gauze. The dressing is covered with a length of Elastoplast adhesive strapping until the suture is removed.

Removal of Adhesive Strips

Incisions closed with adhesive strips are left undisturbed for at least twelve days before the strips are carefully removed (FIG. 48).

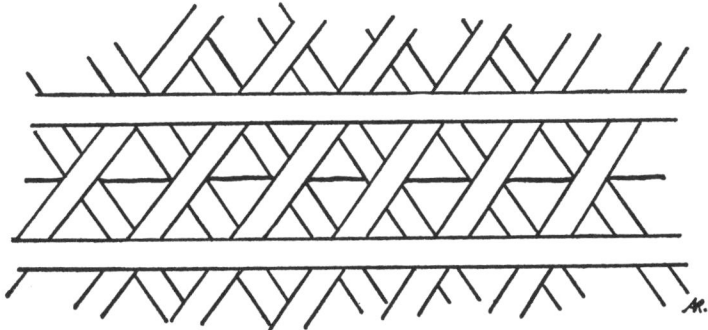

FIG. 48. Closure of an incised wound with the use of adhesive strips.

Care of Infected Wounds

Infected wounds heal by 'second intention', that is from the bottom upwards, over a period of several days or possibly weeks. The cavity may be lightly packed with diminishing quantities of gauze or a drainage tube may be inserted to ensure that the skin edges do not unite before the underlying structures are adequately drained and healed.

Dressing

Although infected, such wounds must be dressed with the same meticulous aseptic technique as is used for incised wounds. The daily dressing is often painful and distressing to a fractious small child and sedation is advisable.

REQUIREMENTS
In addition to a basic dressing trolley:
1 pair sinus forceps ⎫
1 pair dressing scissors ⎬ all sterile.
1 roll ribbon gauze ⎭
Proflavine ⎫
EUSOL and paraffin ⎬ as requested.
Lotio rubra (red lotion) ⎭

METHOD
The basic procedure is as for surgical dressing technique.
   The pack is gently removed, and the forceps and pack are discarded.
   A shorter length of ribbon gauze is cut and soaked in a soothing lotion. The gallipot containing the lotion and wick is placed on the sterile towel surrounding the immediate area. One end of the wick is taken in the tips of the sinus forceps and gently passed to the bottom of the open cavity, care being taken to ensure that the wick does not touch the surrounding skin. The procedure is repeated until the cavity is lightly packed. The ribbon gauze is trimmed to within 4cm of the skin, and a gauze dressing and cotton wool pad are secured in position.

Wound Irrigation

Discharging sinuses and granulating cavities may be irrigated with sterile lotion administered at body temperature with a sterile disposable balloon-type syringe and fine catheter. Sterile forceps are used to insert the fine catheter and the out-flow is collected into a large receiver suitably placed on the waterproof protected bed. The irrigating fluid may be a weak solution of aqueous solution of chlorhexidine, EUSOL or normal saline.

Baths

Saline baths may be prescribed when there is a large area of granulating tissue. The bath must be thoroughly cleaned both before and following such a procedure.

Drainage of Wounds

Wound drainage is used:

1 To prevent accumulation of blood and serous fluid in the depths of a wound. Tubes inserted for this purpose are usually removed within forty-eight hours of insertion.

2 To prevent collection of pus, blood, urine, bile or other fluid deep down in the wound—usually the abdominal cavity. The tube is removed by repeated shortening over a period of several days, as directed by the surgeon.

Two methods are employed:
1 Open wound drainage using a length of:
     i   corrugated drain;
     ii simple tubing;
     iii latex strip.
2 Closed wound drainage using a closed suction Redi-vac system (Zimmer Orthopaedics Ltd.).

Open Wound Drainage

The drainage tube is usually inserted at one end of the main suture-line or preferably through a separate stab wound nearby. The main suture-line can then be sealed off.

At the time of operation, the drain is anchored with a skin stitch and a sterile safety-pin inserted through the projecting end to avoid the risk of its slipping into the peritoneal cavity. To move the drain, the stitch has to be cut and a further sterile safety-pin is inserted each time the tube is shortened. All tubes should be moved every forty-eight hours to prevent their becoming adherent in the depths of a wound.

Shortening Drainage Tubes

REQUIREMENTS
In addition to the basic dressing trolley (all sterile):
2 additional pairs of dressing forceps.
1 pair stitch scissors.
1 safety-pin.
1–2 pads of cotton wool.

METHOD

The basic procedure is as for surgical dressing technique.

The anchoring skin stitch is removed by cutting between its knot and the drain (FIG. 49). Gentle traction on the dressing forceps grasping the drain allows 1–2cm of tubing to be withdrawn. Using forceps, a sterile safety-pin is inserted just above the skin level, and closed. The protruding length of drain is cut off and discarded. With wound toilet completed, the drain is surrounded

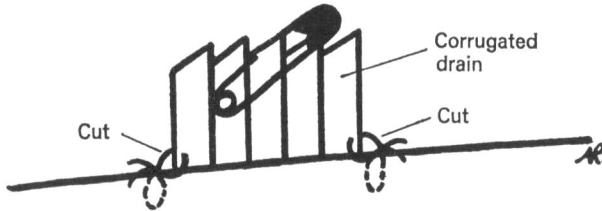

FIG. 49. Open wound drainage.

with gauze, covered with adequate absorptive cotton wool packing and secured in position.

The top dressing may be changed as frequently as is necessary, so avoiding unnecessary exposure of the wound.

Closed Wound Drainage

Accumulations of serous fluid in the depths of a wound, with associated risk of bacterial invasion, are prevented by gentle negative pressure created by a Redivac closed suction drainage (FIG. 50). Dressings and pressure bandages are not required as all accumulations of fluid are drained into the evacuator bottle and the underlying tissues become adherent.

The perforated suction tube is inserted at the time of operation and attached to an evacuator bottle. On return from theatre, the antennae on the rubber stopper are 100° apart, indicating maximum vacuum of 600mmHg. As the evacuator bottle fills, this angle is decreased until the antennae are parallel. This means that the suction is no longer effective because the vacuum has fallen to 40–50mmHg and a second evacuator bottle is necessary.

PREPARATION OF A REDI-VAC BOTTLE

The sterile bottle is prepared by securing the manometric rubber stopper in position with the screw-cap and placing the shut-off clamp over the stopper tube. A high vacuum capacity aspirator is attached to the stopper tube until the antennae are 100° apart. The stopper tube is then closed with the shut-off clamp and the connecting tube is attached. The evacuator is then ready for use.

Replacing a Redi-vac bottle. The catheter system is occluded at the rubber coupling to prevent back-flow, and the exhausted bottle is replaced. The shut-off clamp on the manometric stopper is released first, then the clamp on the rubber coupling.

Removal of the perforated tube. When suction is no longer necessary, the tube is removed by disconnecting the evacuator bottle to release the vacuum and withdrawing the tube slowly from the tissues.

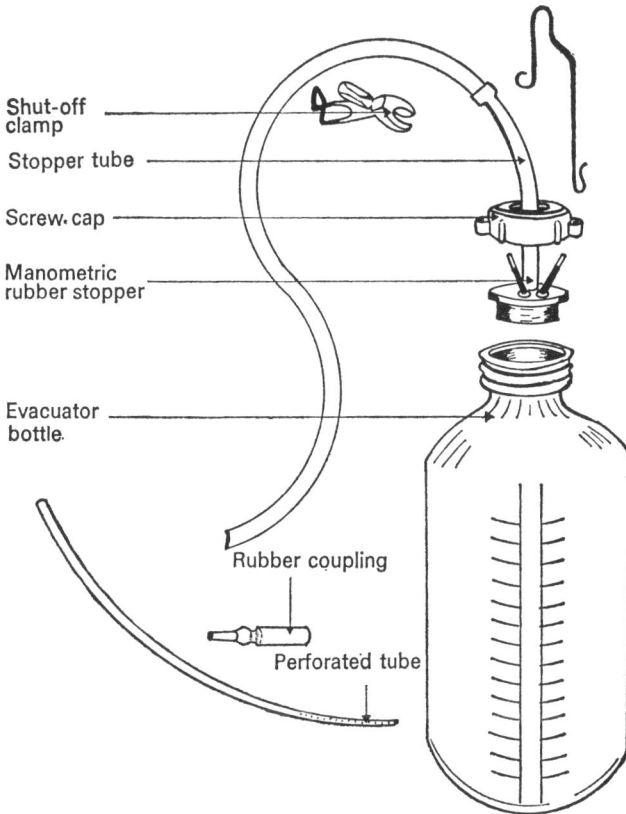

FIG. 50. Closed wound drainage. Redi-vac wound suction apparatus (Zimmer Orthopaedic Ltd.).

Burns and Scalds

Skin destruction due to hot fluid or steam (scalds), dry heat, electricity and strong acids and alkalies (burns), cause partial or complete skin loss. Skin destroyed by any agent is repaired by regeneration of epidermal cells and resurfaced by proliferation of surface epithelium. A burn frequently involves a large area of skin, thus reducing the number of epithelial cells available to restore a covering to the skin. Healing is therefore slow, with the exposed devitalized tissues highly susceptible to infection. If free from infection, partial thickness or superficial burns regenerate into normal skin by spontaneous epithelization from hair follicle and sweat gland remnants. This healing process takes two to three weeks and leaves no scar. When the burn has destroyed all the epithelial elements, i.e. it is deeper than the sweat glands, regeneration is from the edge of the burn. Healing is slow and is superseded by formation of granulation tissue with subsequent scarring, contracture and deformity. Skin grafting reduces disfigurement and promotes healing and, if carried out early, protects the child from toxaemia and hypoproteinaemia from toxic absorption and excessive serum exudation, respectively.

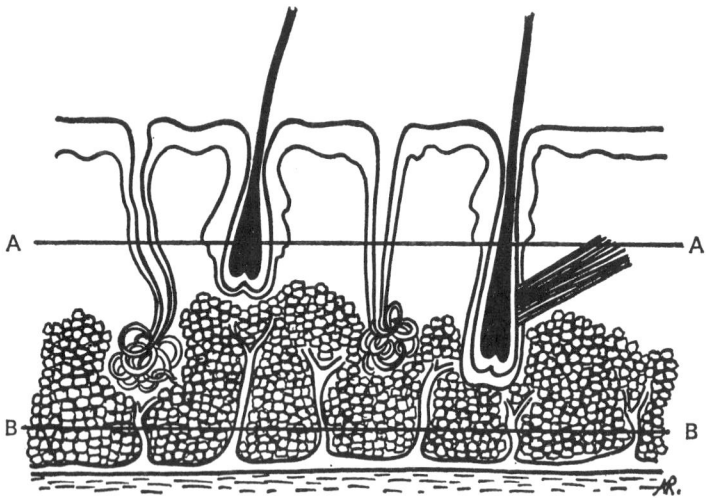

FIG. 51. Cross section through the skin.
A——A Depth of skin lost in a superficial burn (partial skin loss). Split skin grafts cut at this level.
B——B Depth of skin lost in a deep (full thickness) burn. Full-thickness skin grafts (Wolfe grafts) cut at this level.

As the result of burning, there is increased vascularity and permeability of the capillaries of the affected area. The contained plasma leaks into the surrounding tissues to cause oedema, and between the layers of skin to form blisters. If the burned area exceeds more than 10% of a child's body surface, the circulating blood volume is considerably reduced and the child may die from oligaemia unless plasma replacement is sufficient to compensate for protein loss. Superficial skin destruction exposes the sensitive nerve endings and the inevitable pain will increase the degree of shock unless adequately controlled. Deep burns are painless as the nerve endings have been destroyed.

The extent and not the depth of the burn determines plasma replacement necessary to prevent shock. The percentage of body surface area burned can be estimated using the 'Rules of Nine'; the body surface area being divided into areas of 9% of the total:

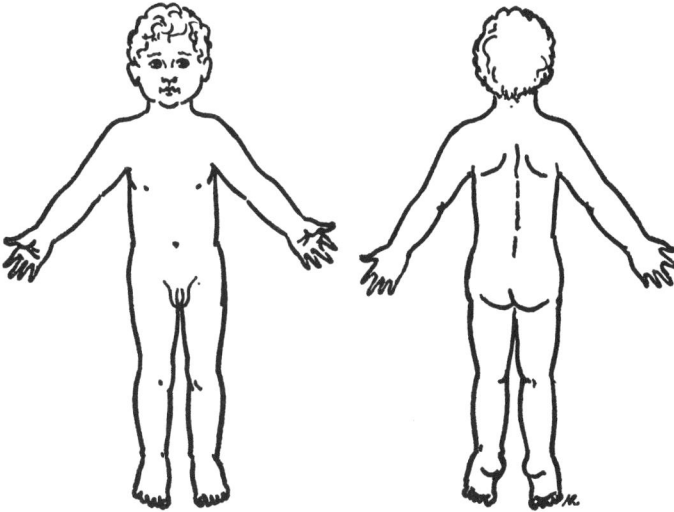

Fig. 52. 'Rules of Nine' for assessing the skin area involved by burn. (Figures indicate percentage of body surface area).

Head and neck	9%
Trunk—front	18%
Trunk—back	18%
Each arm	9% (+9%)
Each upper leg	9% (+9%)
Each lower leg	9% (+9%)
Perineum	1%
	100%

The proportions of a child's body are changed by normal growth so that the values of certain areas alter with size. The size of a child's hand is approximately 1% of his skin area. Any child who has a burn greater than ten times his hand size requires plasma replacement to prevent shock. Estimation of the packed cell volume (the relative proportion of red blood cells to plasma—haematocrit) at frequent intervals allows for a more accurate estimation of fluid and plasma requirement. An adequate urine output is usually an indication of adequate hydration.

The extensively burned child loses a great deal of protein. Body protein and weight loss are considerable unless a diet high in protein, kilocalories and vitamins is given. Full or supplementary tube feeding may be required, using milk, eggs, Complan and Casilan mixtures. Blood transfusions may be necessary to control anaemia.

Local Care of the Burned Area

The burned area is sterile until contaminated with micro-organisms. As a first aid measure and until such time as the child's shocked state is under control, the area is covered with sterile towels or freshly laundered cloth. Auto-infection from the child's own hands, nose and throat and cross-infection from other patients or staff, either through direct contact or by airborne transmission of nose and throat exhalations, is minimized by carrying out a strict aseptic technique in an air conditioned room with all participants wearing caps, gowns, masks and sterile gloves. The child must have hand restraint unless co-operation is forthcoming.

The area is cleansed with mild antiseptic, e.g. chlorhexidine with cetrimide (Savlon 1%), the large blisters punctured to allow release of plasma and the dead skin may be cut away. The area is then treated by either the closed or exposure method.

CLOSED METHOD

The closed method may be used following initial cleansing or to soften resistant slough (eschar) following a period of exposure. The principle involved is to cover the burn completely to protect it from contamination by micro-organisms. Only areas of the body which can be satisfactorily covered are treated by this method, the face, buttocks and perineum being most unsuitable. Circumferential burns of the limbs are usually treated by the closed method to prevent venous constriction by contracting dry slough.

Dressings must have high absorptive properties to accommodate the large quantity of serum exuding during the first few days of treatment. The inner dressing must be non-adherent to prevent disturbance to the healing tissues and painful removal. An antiseptic or antibiotic preparation may be prescribed as an anti-bacterial barrier and this is spread on the inner layer of gauze.

Non-adherent tulle gras is frequently used to cover the raw area. Many layers of highly absorptive gauze are covered with cotton wool and the dressings secured with a firm crêpe bandage and zinc oxide plaster. The first dressing is left intact for two to three days. Micro-organisms will invade the area and reach the burn if exudation is allowed to penetrate to the outside bandage. If this has occurred, a further pad of sterile wool is applied over the area and bandaged into place.

The second dressing entails removal of all dressings and application of further tulle gras, gauze, cotton wool and crêpe bandage. This dressing can be left intact for seven to ten days unless it becomes dampened or the child shows signs of infection, i.e. a rise in temperature or local pain or smell. By the third week, superficial burns show signs of healing and infrequent dressings are necessary until healing is complete. Burns involving destruction of the whole skin then require surgical excision or daily dressings of agents to encourage separation of slough in preparation for grafting.

Dressings must be carried out gently with as little physical and psychological trauma as possible. An anaesthetic may be necessary in the early days but analgesics are usually adequate later. A poor dressing technique may cause a superficial lesion to involve the full skin depth and, of course, introduction of micro-organisms must be avoided at all costs. The area is best kept dry unless encouraging separation of slough from a deep burn when lotions and saline baths may be used.

EXPOSURE METHOD

The principle involved is to allow the exudate to dry and form a hard impervious crust unfavourable for multiplication of micro-organisms. The area is exposed, clear of all possible contact, in a light, cool room (temperature 24°C or 75°F). A low relative humidity speeds the drying process. The child may be nursed on a sterile polyurethane mattress covering a nylon mesh frame to allow circulation of air around the trunk. Antibiotic or antiseptic powders may be used to prevent bacterial contamination and to aid the drying process. Strict barrier nursing precautions are necessary until healing is complete. An isolator tent may be used in severe cases.

With the use of this method, painful, tiresome dressings are avoided and nutrition is not interrupted by repeated anaesthetics. Limb restraint is frequently necessary to prevent interference and subsequent deformity.

A dry slough forms within forty-eight hours or so and superficial burns heal under its cover. Healing is usually complete within fourteen days and the slough separates spontaneously, or may require gentle lifting at the edges and snipping away, daily. If skin destruction is complete, as in deep burns, the slough is slow to separate to reveal granulation tissue. This may be removed by surgical excision, or with daily dressings of equal parts liquid paraffin and EUSOL, or other chemical or enzyme agents to encourage separation and preparation for skin grafting.

SKIN GRAFTS

Deep (full thickness) burns require skin grafts to prevent disfigurement. These may be applied within forty-eight hours of injury or following some healing by granulation and separation or excision of the slough. Split skin (Thiersch) grafts may be autografts (taken from the patient) or homografts (taken from another person). Homografts are rejected after about three weeks, but not until they have provided a valuable living-cover while awaiting regeneration of patient–donor sites.

The recipient area is prepared by excision of necrotic tissue and cleansing the fresh, young, pink granulations. The Thiersch graft is cut and spread on to tulle gras to make handling easier. It is then cut into strips or squares and placed edge to edge on to the raw area. The grafts are then secured in place by tulle gras, gauze, wool dressings, crêpe bandage and possibly plaster of Paris, and the site is elevated if possible to minimize oedema. This dressing is left intact for seven to ten days as instructed by the surgeon. The healthy graft acquires a blood supply from the recipient area and becomes stable within ten to twelve days. Infection, a collection of fluid under the graft and movement cause death of the graft. The donor site, covered with tulle gras, gauze, cotton wool and a firm crêpe bandage, is left undisturbed for seven to ten days. Re-packing may prove necessary. Further split skin grafts can be taken from the same site fourteen days following the first donation.

Full thickness (Wolfe) grafts, flaps and pedicles may be used for later repair of deformities. Scarring of both the recipient and donor sites is inevitable.

Complications

There are three main complications of burns:
1 Shock.
2 Sepsis.
3 Scarring.

SHOCK

Oligaemic shock is prevented or overcome by careful assessment and replacement of plasma loss until the leaking capillaries have been sealed off by natural processes. This process takes twenty-four to forty-eight hours. Pain is an aggravating factor, but is not usually severe. If more than 50% of the skin is destroyed, the mortality rate is high, even with the best of medical and nursing care.

The effect the accident has on the child as an individual may take months or years to overcome. Initially, the child is numbed by the event, but as he returns to reality the impact of the injury unfolds. He may experience terrifying nightmares and be constantly haunted, day and night. Separation from his familiar home environment adds to his distress, and frequent contact with his parents is of vital importance. Feelings of guilt by either the child or his parents increase distress and anxiety which separation will not improve.

Once the parents have overcome the shock, the mother should be encouraged to assist in the care and amusement of her child, thus reducing the necessity for sedation and restraint.

SEPSIS

All burns are sterile initially, despite the necrosis. Subsequent infection with staphylococci, pseudomonas pyocyaneus, coliforms and proteus is uncommon. Septicaemia and toxic absorption may cause death. Infection with haemolytic streptococci is of particular danger, contra-indicating the use of skin grafts.

The healing area must be kept as dry as possible and the dressings are carried out away from the general ward environment. Wound swabs, taken at intervals, detect early infection so that appropriate treatment can be commenced. Scratching and picking of annoying lesions are a temptation to all and especially to a small child. The child may have to be restrained to prevent him introducing infection and delaying the healing process, although diversional therapy and company are preferable.

SCARRING

Gross disfigurement scars the personality and lowers morale. Contractures involve particularly the flexor surfaces of joints—fingers, elbows, knees, axillae and groins. Application of skin grafts within three weeks of burning helps to prevent contractures. Physiotherapy is necessary throughout treatment to prevent and correct contractures. Splints may be applied for the same reason. Once healing is complete, either by spontaneous epithelization or by grafts, the skin should be treated with lanolin based cream to render it soft and supple.

For Further Reading

ELISON NASH D. F. (1969). *The Principles and Practice of Surgery for Nurses and Allied Professions*, 4th edition. Edward Arnold (Publishers) Ltd.
ELLSWORTH LAING J. and HARVEY J. (1967). *The Management and Nursing of Burns*, 1st edition. The English Universities Press Ltd.

CHAPTER FOURTEEN

Pre- and Post-Operative Care

Basic pre- and post-operative care is described in the first part of this chapter. This is essentially care of a child before and following general anaesthesia and applies to any operation, examination or investigation demanding a general anaesthetic. There is little place for the use of local anaesthesia in paediatric work, although this may be used for performing minor surgery when general anaesthesia is contra-indicated by the child's poor condition or at the wish of the anaesthetist.

The second part relates to suggested specific pre-operative preparation and post-operative care. Details of some related procedures are included in this chapter; the reader is asked to refer to the index for procedures included elsewhere.

Basic Pre-Operative Care

Children admitted for minor elective surgery have a very short stay in hospital with minimal pre-operative preparation. Those children with conditions necessitating major surgery require a much longer pre-operative stay to enable investigations and preparations to be adequately completed during the settling-in period. Others are admitted for emergency surgery when there is time for only minimal preparation.

Psychological Preparation

To avoid unnecessary psychological trauma, non-urgent elective surgery is avoided during the second and third years of life. A small child does not experience the fear of operation, anaesthesia and possible death which are natural typical fears of the adult, but his greatest fear is separation from his mother in an unfamiliar environment with inability to understand the reason for his hunger and for the strange activities centred around him. Underlying anxiety is often revealed in the careful questioning of an older apprehensive child, but a simple truthful explanation is invariably accepted if all pre-operative preparations are directed towards 'getting him better'. If the operation is likely to result in temporary pain, a period of immobility or confinement to an oxygen tent, the child should be suitably prepared.

The parents must be seen by the surgeon and the nature of their child's operation explained. Their written consent is obtained allowing the surgeon to perform the operation and to give the child a blood transfusion, if necessary.

Physical Preparation

From the time of admission, the child should be carefully observed for signs contra-indicating surgery. He should be accurately weighed (and measured if requested) and a record of his temperature, pulse and respiration (and blood pressure) maintained. A specimen of urine is collected for routine ward testing. If he has a tendency to constipation, this is best relieved by administration of a mild aperient thirty-six hours before operation. Routine bowel preparation is not required unless the child is to undergo bowel surgery.

Blood is taken for haemoglobin estimation, grouping and cross-matching if a blood transfusion is anticipated.

General cleanliness of the child is important. The hair should be inspected for the presence of nits and lice and treated as necessary as part of the routine admission procedure. Dirty hair should be washed, particularly if it is close to the operation site. A bath is given on admission, if necessary, and on the day of operation. Special attention should be paid to the cleanliness of the umbilicus— an area often grossly neglected—ears, and finger and toe nails. The use of talcum powder is best avoided.

The operation site must be as free as possible from micro-organisms. Any local hair is removed as appropriate, i.e. the pubic area prior to abdominal surgery, axillae for thoracic surgery, scalp for neurosurgery and the appropriate limb prior to orthopaedic surgery.

Shaving

An electric razor may be used, otherwise the following requirements are necessary:

REQUIREMENTS
Razor and blade in a receiver.
Talcum powder or soap and warm water.
Medical wipes or cotton wool balls.
Protection for the bed.
Receptacle for used swabs.

METHOD

The bedclothes are protected. Small areas of hair can be carefully removed using a razor and talcum powder, but a good soap lather applied to larger hairy areas facilitates the procedure. Cuts in the skin are painful and liable to infection and must be avoided. A bath following the procedure removes any loose hairs.

Skin Preparation

Routine skin preparation in the ward is no longer the accepted practice in most hospitals. With the exception of some orthopaedic and neuro-surgery, most surgeons now rely on general cleanliness of the patient and their preparation of the operation site in theatre, to avoid sepsis.

REQUIREMENTS

The basic trolley is prepared as described on page 258, with the addition of the following equipment:
Sterile towels to drape the area.
Open-weave bandage or Tubegauz.
Appropriate lotions.

METHOD

Using a strict aseptic technique as for dressing procedure, skin toilet is carried out by systematically cleansing a wide area with the recommended lotion(s). The area is allowed to dry before covering with a sterile towel which is secured in position with a cotton bandage or Tubegauz.

Immediate Pre-Operative Care

An empty stomach is necessary to avoid the risk of aspiration of vomitus if a general anaesthetic is to be administered. Prolonged starvation in childhood is badly tolerated, the blood sugar falling quickly to a low level. The fear of surgery and anaesthesia is not apparent in the small child so that gastric emptying is not delayed. A child can, therefore, take light food to within six hours, and fluids to within four hours, of the time of operation. An infant is given a clear fluid feed instead of milk for the last feed before operation. An older child is told that he must not eat anything and a notice to this effect should be fastened to his cot or bed. All food and fluid should be moved from his reach and he is best nursed away from the sight and sound of his fellow patients' eating activities.

After a bath has been given, he is dressed in an open-back operation gown and returned to his cot, which should have been made up with clean linen. Long hair is secured with a cotton bandage and all hair grips and jewellery are removed. The mouth should be inspected for the presence of loose teeth or an orthodontic plate. His identity band should be checked for legibility and he is encouraged to empty his bladder before being given his pre-medication.

Pre-medication, if prescribed by the anaesthetist, is given half to one hour prior to the time of operation, after which the child should be encouraged to sleep with his favourite toy in a quiet corner of the ward. A small dose of atropine is usually prescribed to inhibit the action of the vagus nerve. Atropine depresses the respiratory secretions and quickens the heart rate. A potent sedative given either orally or by the rectal route avoids the necessity for a second injection and ensures that a small child is at least very drowsy when he arrives in the operating theatre.

The child's notes, written consent for operation, charts and X-ray films are collected together so that all is ready for the ward nurse to take him to the operating theatre and stay with him until he is anaesthetized.

Basic Post-Operative Care

During the child's absence in the operating theatre, his bed is prepared for his return. The top bedclothes are folded into a pack and the head end of the mattress is covered with waterproof protection. Warming of the bed is contra-indicated unless specially requested by the surgeon. Cot-sides, pillows and other accessories are placed nearby. A suction apparatus (page 301) and post-anaesthetic tray are made available for use, if necessary, in maintaining a clear airway.

POST-ANAESTHETIC TRAY
Tongue depressor.
Mouth-gag.
Tongue forceps.
Sponge-holding forceps.
Gauze swabs.

The child does not leave the operating theatre until the anaesthetist is satisfied that his condition is satisfactory. With the use of modern anaesthesia, consciousness is quickly regained. A clear airway is maintained by placing the child in the semi-prone position and by the use of an airway which is ejected on return to consciousness. Forward support of the lower jaw directs the tongue away from the air-passages.

The child is best returned to a warm recovery area where he will not be seen by other children awaiting operation. He should remain under constant observation until consciousness is regained, his airway, colour, state of his skin, pulse and respiration rates being carefully observed. Particulars of the operation performed and instructions regarding post-operative care are collected by the ward nurse returning the child to his ward. Restlessness and complaints of pain on regaining consciousness should be reported and relieved by analgesics prescribed by the doctor.

As soon as his condition allows, the child's hands and face should be washed, his operation gown exchanged for his own nightclothes and his hair combed. His temperature should be recorded, his dressing inspected and a mouth-wash given. Unless contra-indicated, he should be allowed to adopt a comfortable position in which he will probably fall asleep.

Routine observations of pulse and blood pressure, if necessary, are recorded until such time as they are satisfactory. Small quantities of clear fluid can usually be offered within the first four hours following operation if the child does not vomit and a normal diet is resumed the following day. Post-operative urinary retention is rare in childhood. Early ambulation is encouraged, but creates little problem in the younger age group who are usually only too willing to resume their boisterous activities. Some restriction may prove necessary.

The sutures are removed as requested by the surgeon, and the child is discharged home as soon as his general condition permits. Arrangements are made with the family doctor, or for a return visit to the out-patients department, for removal of sutures, if necessary.

This is a very anxious time for the child's parents. Accurate information with maximum reassurance given by the ward sister or her deputy, and opportunity to be with their child as soon as possible following operation, will greatly help to relieve their anxiety.

Neonatal Surgery

Emergency major surgery during the first week of life is remarkably well tolerated by a mature infant who is well nourished and has a high level of circulating haemoglobin.

An infant's prospects of survival depend on:
i   the severity of his abnormality;
ii an early diagnosis;
iii the skill of the surgical team;
iv the meticulous nursing care given by an observant skilled paediatric nursing team.

PRE-OPERATIVE CARE
1   Maintenance of body temperature is of utmost importance. Chilling and excessive handling add to the hazards of surgery; pre-operative rest in an incubator or warm, humid environment is therefore a necessity. Infants travelling many miles to receive treatment in a neonatal surgical unit must be allowed to recover from their journey.
2   The infant is weighed.

3 The umbilical cord is attended to.

4 The haemoglobin level is estimated, and the blood grouped and cross-matched.

5 Drugs prescribed by the doctor are administered. Vitamin K is normally produced by the commensals of the large intestine and is essential for the formation of prothrombin necessary in the blood-clotting process. Newborn infants lack colonic commensals and therefore require an intramuscular injection of vitamin K_1.

6 Resistance to infection is poor, often justifying the use of wide-spectrum antibiotic prophylaxis.

7 The parents' wish regarding baptism is fulfilled.

Special Points

INTESTINAL OBSTRUCTION

1 A polyvinyl naso-gastric tube is passed to drain the gastric secretions. There is a danger that a small, weak infant may inhale vomitus.

2 Fluid and electrolyte balance is restored by intravenous infusion.

3 The serum electrolyte values are estimated.

OESOPHAGEAL ATRESIA WITH TRACHEO-OESOPHAGEAL-FISTULA

1 The infant is nursed on one side in a head-up position. This discourages regurgitation of gastric secretions through the fistula into the lungs.

2 Frequent suction to the oesophageal pouch prevents inhalation of accumulations of saliva.

MYELOMENINGOCELE

1 The infant is nursed prone or in a sling (FIG. 17, page 99).

2 Sterile saline soaks or non-adherent, non-greasy Nusan B squares are applied to the exposed nerves and meninges to inhibit infection and prevent drying of the vital structures.

OMPHALOCOELE AND EXOMPHALOS

1 The exposed abdominal contents are covered as above.

POST-OPERATIVE CARE

1 The infant is returned to a warmed cot or incubator and allowed to rest while under constant observation.

2 Overhydration could well prove a real problem unless the doctor's instructions are carefully followed.

3 Unless the abnormality is gastro-intestinal in nature, routine feeding is usually commenced three to four hours following operation.

Reconstructive Surgery

Examples: Cleft lip and palate.
Skin grafts (page 271).
Hypospadias (page 297).

Cleft Lip

A cleft lip is usually repaired at the age of three months following pre-operative measures to align the alveoli with the use of an orthodontic plate.

PRE-OPERATIVE CARE
1   The infant is nursed in isolation and the attending staff wear masks. These measures are taken to avoid respiratory infections.
2   Local sepsis of the upper respiratory passages is excluded—throat and nasal swabs are sent for laboratory examination.
3   The haemoglobin level is estimated and the blood grouped and cross-matched.
4   A photograph is often taken.
5   The infant is fed by cup and spoon and all feeds are followed by a small quantity of clear fluid.

POST-OPERATIVE CARE
1   The tongue stitch is removed on recovery to full consciousness.
2   Elbow restraint is applied.
3   A clear fluid spoon feed is offered about four hours post-operatively, followed three to four hours later by one half-strength feed, then return to normal feeds. Adequate nourishment is necessary to avoid undue fretfulness. All feeds are followed by a small quantity of clear fluid.
4   The suture-line is kept clean and dry by cleansing with sterile water and cotton wool buds following each feed.
5   Sedatives may be necessary, e.g. chloral hydrate, to avoid restlessness.
6   The sutures are removed as requested by the surgeon, usually on the sixth day. This is an exacting task, demanding considerable skill on the part of the nurse, time, patience, adequate lighting, fine pointed scissors and a heavily sedated, restrained infant. A Logan's bow, if used, is removed at the same time.
7   Bottle feeding is resumed when the sutures have been removed.

Cleft Palate

A cleft palate is usually repaired between the ages of fourteen and eighteen months.

PRE-OPERATIVE CARE

1 The toddler may be nursed in isolation to avoid the risk of respiratory infections.

2 and 3 As for cleft lip.

4 Self-feeding is avoided in the post-operative period by the use of elbow splints which may be introduced to the active toddler pre-operatively. This measure invariably proves distressing and frustrating and is probably best delayed until the operation has been performed.

5 A suppository may be given if post-operative hydration is to be complemented via the rectal route.

POST-OPERATIVE CARE

1 The tongue stitch is removed on recovery to full consciousness.

2 Elbow restraint is applied.

3 Sedatives, e.g. papavaretum and later chloral hydrate, are given as prescribed by the doctor to control restlessness.

4 The mouth is extremely sore. Spoon feeding should be established by an experienced nurse. Small quantities of bland fluid may be offered at two hourly intervals, followed by a small amount of clear fluid commencing three to four hours following operation.

5 Six-hourly rectal saline infusions may be given to complement a poor oral fluid intake.

6 Soft diet is introduced over a period of several days, all foods being followed by a small quantity of water.

7 Damage to the repaired palate is prevented by choosing suitable toys, and excluding sweets and hard foods from the diet.

8 The palate is usually healed by the tenth to fourteenth post-operative day when the elbow restraint is removed and the child goes home.

Gastric Surgery

Example: Rammstedt's operation for congenital hypertrophic pyloric stenosis. This is the most common paediatric disorder requiring surgery.

PRE-OPERATIVE CARE

1 Fluid and electrolyte balance is restored by intravenous infusion, or subcutaneous infusion and/or oral clear fluids, the route depending on the severity of the condition.

2 A gastric washout is performed two to four hours prior to operation.

3 A naso-gastric tube is passed.

4 Vitamins K_1 and C supplements are administered if prescribed by the doctor.

5 If a local anaesthetic is to be used a sedative is given and crucifix restraint applied.

POST-OPERATIVE CARE

1   Oral feeding is commenced two to four hours post-operatively. Small quantities are offered initially, the quantity and the quality of the feeds being increased according to the infant's progress.

Example: Schedule feeds suitable for a six-week-old infant who weighed 2700g at birth.

Birth weight   = 2700g

Expected weight gain   800g (6 − 2 × 200g)

Therefore   Expected weight   = 3500g

Fluid requirement   =   150ml × 3·5 = 525ml/day.

Day 0 and 1—Schedule feeds for the first 36 hours.

Full cream milk mixture		15ml	20ml	25ml	30ml	45ml	
5% sugar in N/5 Saline	30ml	15ml	15ml	15ml	15ml	15ml	
Volume	30ml	30ml	35ml	40ml	45ml	60ml	= 660ml
Number of feeds (2 hourly feeding)	× 1	× 3	× 3	× 3	× 3	× 3	

Day 2—Full cream milk mixture: 60ml, 3 hourly for 8 feeds (480ml)
Day 3—Full cream milk mixture: 75ml, 3 hourly × 7 (525ml)
Day 4—Full cream milk mixture: 90ml, 3 hourly × 6 (540ml)
Day 5—Full cream milk mixture: 105ml, 4 hourly × 5 (525ml).

2   The infant's fluid requirement for the day of operation—150ml/kg (2½oz/lb) —can be complemented by administration of rectal saline.

Gastric Washout (Lavage)

A stomach washout is necessary:

1   To clear the stomach of curds and mucus prior to surgical relief of pyloric stenosis (Rammstedt's operation).

2   To remove the contents of the stomach following ingestion of most poisons.

REQUIREMENTS

Sterilized equipment is required for an infant. For an older child it is sufficient for the equipment to be clean, and sterilized after use.

TROLLEY

Top shelf:

Measuring jug containing boiled water, normal saline or weak sodium bicarbonate solution (depending on medical instructions) temperature 38°C (100°F).

Lotion thermometer.

Graduated cylindrical funnel.

Short length of tubing and straight connection.

Oesophageal tube—size depending on the size of the child, but not less than 18 F.G. (10 E.G.)

Small container of warm water.

Graduated jug for residue.

Split pressure tubing 10cm (4 inches) long.

Bottom shelf:

Large jug of solution, temperature 40°C (105°F).

Floor protection.

Bucket.

Treatment blanket.

Bath towel.

(Vomit bowl and cover.)

METHOD

Two nurses are essential for this procedure, one to perform the gastric washout and the second nurse to support and restrain the child. The passage of a stomach tube is a most unpleasant experience to the conscious small child, and co-operation is rarely forthcoming. Explanation should be given to obtain co-operation from an older child. A younger child is securely restrained in the treatment blanket, and sat upright on the nurse's knees facing the operator (FIG. 53). A bath towel placed around the neck and chest protects the child's clothing. If the gastric washout is being carried out to remove ingested poison,

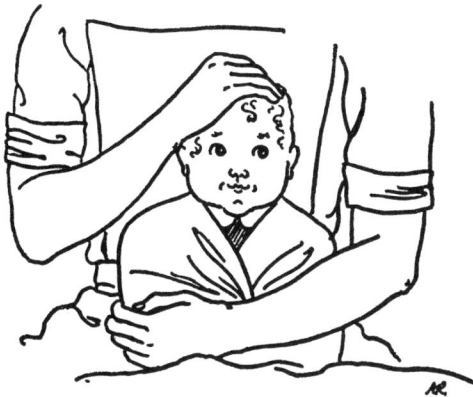

FIG. 53. Method of restraint that can be adapted for most procedures related to the ear, nose and throat and for a gastric lavage on a conscious infant.

the restrained child is placed in a head low prone or lateral position and the procedure carried out by a member of the medical or senior nursing staff (FIG. 54).

A bucket is placed on the protected floor. The apparatus is assembled and the length of tube to be passed is measured from the xiphisternum to the bridge of the nose. An older child may attempt to bite through the tube. A mouth-gag may be used to separate the upper and lower molar teeth or the stomach tube is passed through a piece of split pressure tubing on which the child can safely bite. The tube is moistened, passed over the back of the tongue into the oropharynx and advanced slowly and gently into the oesophagus and stomach for the assessed length. An echo can be heard in the funnel as the oesophageal tube enters the stomach and on lowering the funnel, the gastric residue can be drained into a graduated jug.

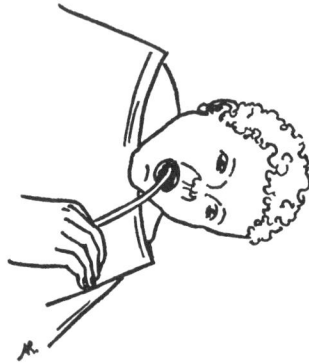

FIG. 54. Position of an unconscious child for gastric washout.

Once in position, the tube is held in place by the assisting nurse. The temperature of the solution is checked, the tubing kinked and a quantity of solution is poured into the flask. The amount of fluid used for each cycle varies with the size and age of the child, 60ml (2oz) being used for a small infant, increasing in amount to 200ml (6oz) for a ten-year-old child. The funnel is held 15cm (6 inches) above the child's head and the fluid is allowed to flow by gravity into the stomach. When almost empty the funnel is lowered in an upright position until the equivalent amount of fluid has been syphoned. The tubing is kinked and the funnel inverted so that its contents are emptied into the bucket. The procedure is repeated until the returned fluid is clear.

When satisfied that all fluid has been returned and that the stomach lining is clean, the tube is kinked and withdrawn swiftly but smoothly. The child is made comfortable in his bed and allowed to rest.

The equipment is washed, rinsed and boiled or disposed of, as appropriate. The washings are retained for inspection or examination and the result is recorded.

Elective Surgery of the Lower Alimentary Tract

Examples: Hemicolectomy.
Colonic transplant for oesophageal replacement.
Construction of an ileal conduit.
Recto-sigmoidectomy for Hirschsprung's disease.

PRE-OPERATIVE CARE
1   A low residue diet is given for five days prior to surgery.
2   Clear fluid only is given for twenty-four hours prior to surgery.
3   An enema followed by a rectal washout is given daily for four days and twice on the day prior to operation. No washout is performed within four hours of surgery.
4   Bowel antiseptics such as neomycin or phthalylsulphathiazole are frequently prescribed for five days prior to operation to reduce the intestinal flora.

POST-OPERATIVE CARE
1   A strict fluid balance chart is maintained.
2   Intravenous therapy   ⎫ are continued until return of normal
3   Naso-gastric intubation and drainage⎭ bowel function.
4   Routine oral toilet is carried out two to four-hourly.
5   Commencement of oral fluids and eventual bowel management depend on the child's progress.
6   Analgesics are given to relieve pain and to rest the bowel.

Gastric Drainage

The gastric contents are drained by an indwelling naso-gastric tube to prevent exhaustive vomiting, with its associated risk of inhalation of vomitus in a weak, ill child suffering from mechanical intestinal obstruction or paralytic ileus.

Passage of the naso-gastric tube is as for naso-gastric intubation (page 111). A Ryle's tube is used for older children, a polyvinyl feeding tube is used for infants. The gastric contents are aspirated by gentle suction created by a 5 or 10ml syringe and the tube is left open to allow free escape of intestinal gas and fluid. Intermittent aspiration of the gastric contents at hourly intervals ensures that the stomach remains empty. For small children, the naso-gastric tube is inevitably of narrow bore and readily becomes blocked. 1–2ml of water injected prior to aspiration confirms patency of the tube (and the volume of fluid injected is deducted from the total aspirate). Alternatively, if the aspirate is excessive in amount, the open end of the tube may be attached to a low powered Roberts type suction pump supplemented by intermittent aspiration.

Rectal Washout (Lavage)

A rectal washout may be ordered prior to examinations such as barium studies and proctoscopy and sigmoidoscopy, and prior to rectal surgery. An evacuant enema is necessary to clear the rectum of solid matter prior to a rectal washout being given.

REQUIREMENTS

Top shelf:

Measuring jug of solution 0·9% sodium chloride, one 5ml spoonful to 540ml water, temperature 38°C (100°F).

Lotion thermometer.

Funnel, 45cm (or 18 inches) tubing, straight connection.

Jacques catheter or rectal tube size 15–24 F.G. (8–14 E.G.)

Lubricant.

Medical wipes.

Receptacle for soiled apparatus.

Receptacle for disposable articles.

Bottom shelf:

Bucket.

Large jug containing additional saline solution.

Waterproof protection for the bed.

Waterproof protection for the nurse.

Waterproof protection for the floor.

METHOD

Careful and adequate preparation of the child is of utmost importance as this procedure may be prolonged and require repeating daily to ensure adequate cleansing of the bowel.

The bucket is placed on the protected floor at the bedside and the child is placed in the left lateral position. The terminal 5–10cm (2–4 inches) of the catheter or rectal tube is lubricated and inserted 5–10cm (2–4 inches) through the anus into the rectum to release any flatus. The temperature of the isotonic solution is checked and the assembled apparatus is filled to displace the air. The tubing is kinked and the connection inserted into the catheter.

The fluid in the funnel is allowed to flow slowly into the rectum. The amount of solution used in each cycle depends on the size and age of the child. As little as 60ml (2oz) may be used for each cycle during infancy, increasing to 300ml (10oz) for a ten-year-old. When almost empty, the funnel is lowered to floor level in an upright position until the full amount of fluid has been syphoned. The tubing is then kinked, the funnel inverted to empty the contents, and the funnel replenished with a further supply of saline solution before being raised

30cm or 12 inches or so above mattress level. The procedure is repeated until the returned fluid is clear. The catheter is withdrawn through a medical wipe placed over the anus, while the funnel is held at a low level. This allows for any retained fluid to be syphoned. The whole apparatus is placed in the receptacle for later cleansing and disinfection.

The child is left clean, dry and comfortable in a warm bed and his co-operation is acknowledged. A temporary desire to defaecate may follow which is best treated by a visit to the lavatory and sympathetic reassurance.

The whole apparatus is thoroughly washed and disinfected after use. The bucket content is examined, measured and disposed of and the result recorded. The bucket is subsequently suitably disinfected.

Colonic Washout (Lavage)

The procedure ordered by the doctor is essentially as for rectal washout, with the following exceptions:
1 Larger volumes of isotonic solution are necessary.
2 The catheter or rectal tube is inserted for a greater distance, for 20–30cm (or 8–12 inches).
3 Irrigation and syphonage is performed with the child in the right as well as left lateral and supine positions.

INDICATIONS FOR USE
1 Prior to colonic surgery.
2 In Hirschsprung's disease.

Use of a Flatus Tube

A flatus tube differs from a catheter in that the opening is at the end and not to one side of the tube. Its passage into the rectum allows release of uncomfortable abdominal distension due to flatus (wind).

REQUIREMENTS
Tray.
Bowl of water.
Flatus tube or rectal tube size 15–24 F.G. (8–14 E.G.) (depending on the age).
Lubricant.
Medical wipe.
Protection for the bed.
Receptacle for soiled swab.

METHOD
The child is reassured and prepared as given above. The lubricated flatus tube is inserted to beyond the internal sphincter (or aganglionic section of rectum

in an infant with Hirschsprung's disease)—usually 5–10cm (2–4 inches)—while the free end of the tube is placed under the water level in the bowl. Escaping flatus will be seen to bubble through the water.

Following withdrawal of the tube, the anal area is cleansed with a medical wipe which is then discarded. The abdomen is often much softer with relief of abdominal discomfort.

Colostomy and Colostomy Care

A temporary (loop or spur) colostomy may have to be performed during the early neonatal period as a life-saving measure in infants suffering from imperforate anus or Hirschsprung's disease. By the age of two years, most of these children have dispensed with the colostomy following an abdomino-anal pull-through operation. A permanent (terminal) colostomy is fortunately rarely necessary in childhood, but may prove preferable to incontinence or an unreliable anal sphincter in an older child.

Ileostomy is also uncommon and is confined to a child of any age requiring

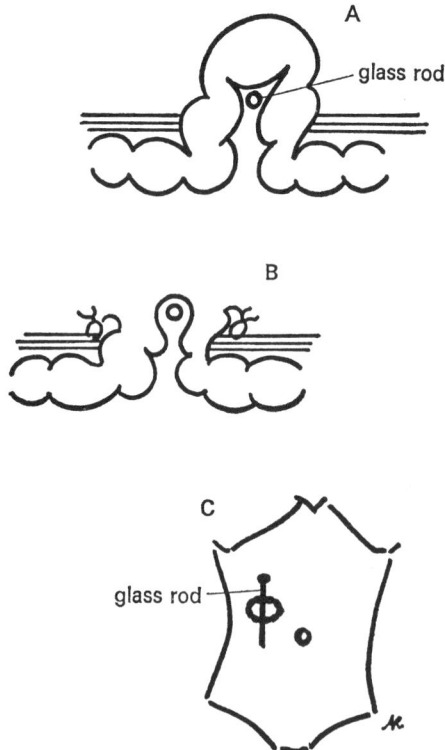

FIG. 55. Loop colostomy. A = Closed. B = Open. C = Showing position on the abdomen. A glass rod prevents regression of the loop.

temporary rest of an ulcerated colon and is occasionally necessary if the entire colon is aganglionic in extensive Hirschsprung's disease. Fluid and electrolyte loss is excessive and continuous, demanding great care with fluid and electrolyte balance and protection of the skin surrounding the stoma from the proteolytic enzymes present in the fluid excretion. Topical calamine lotion or Karaya powder applied to the skin is covered with a double sided adhesive square. The flange of a water-tight appliance, basically similar in design and use to those used for urinary diversion, is then applied (FIG. 66, page 323).

An artificial opening into the alimentary tract is made at a distal point in a mobile portion of gut. A colostomy is made into the transverse or pelvic colon and an ileostomy at a point close to the ileo-caecal valve. In the immediate post-operative period, a glass rod is passed through a small hole in the mesentery to prevent the loop of gut slipping into the abdominal cavity. A loop of rubber tubing connects the ends of the rod until it is removed, as requested by the surgeon (FIG. 55). If it is necessary to open a temporary colostomy at the time of operation, the surgeon may prevent contamination of the healing wound by securing a special right-angled glass tube into the colon, using a catgut purse-string suture. Paul's tubing attached to the exposed end of the tube drains the faecal matter into a closed container at the child's bedside. The catgut dissolves four to five days later, releasing the glass tube from the colon (FIG. 56). Alternatively, a Chiron type colostomy bag may be applied. This water-tight seal

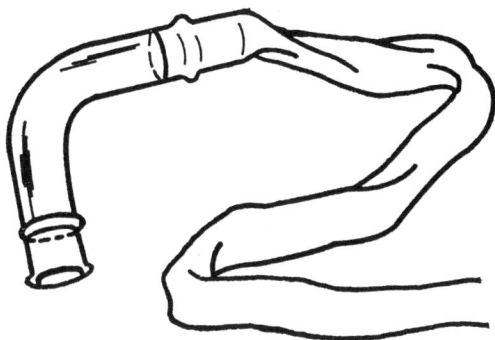

FIG. 56. Paul's tubing

prevents contamination of the healing abdominal incision and provides a transparent covering through which the stoma can be readily seen.

The healthy stoma is bright red in colour and its delicate insensitive mucous surface is liable to damage. A purple discolouration must be reported immediately as this is a sign of strangulation. Slight bleeding is not uncommon in the early days and must be reported if it is not controlled by pressure or application of a gauze swab soaked in adrenalin solution 1 : 1000. Prolapse and regression of the loop must also be reported.

Until such time as the wound is healed and the sutures removed, the colostomy is cared for using an aseptic technique. Subsequent care involves the use of clean equipment. The skin surrounding the stoma is not accustomed to faecal contamination and may become sore. Excoriation is prevented by frequent, thorough cleansing with soap and water (or liquid paraffin if the skin is sore) and protecting the dried skin with silicone cream, Vaseline or zinc paste. Each time the colostomy is dressed it should be covered with tulle gras or some other non-adherent dressing to prevent friction over the delicate surface. Absorptive dressings are then applied and secured in position with a bandage or Netelast.

Faecal matter produced by a colostomy is less solid than that produced by a normal bowel action. Adjustments to the diet and the administration of prescribed doses of methyl cellulose as Celevac between meals or feeds help to prevent diarrhoea and make the colostomy more acceptable and manageable. With care, the bowel of an older child can be regulated to produce a semi-formed stool once or twice a day. During infancy, however, this is more difficult. Children with a permanent colostomy are fitted with a 'made-to-measure' colostomy belt and encouraged to independence as soon as possible.

When the parents have overcome the initial shock of their infant's abnormality, colostomy care is reasonably well accepted. The temporary nature of the faecal diversion helps in parental acceptance of the situation and most mothers readily respond to instruction in their child's care. Most infants are able to spend a period of time at home until old enough to undergo major surgery to correct their abnormality. With careful instruction and opportunity to carry out colostomy care under supervision while the infant is still in hospital, most mothers are confident to cope at home with the supportive help and advice of the family doctor and his nurse colleagues.

Colostomy Washout (Lavage)

Prior to subsequent surgery, the colon is prepared as described on page 285, the rectal washouts being substituted for colostomy washouts.

The principle, requirements and procedure are essentially as for rectal washout (page 286). The child is placed slightly towards the left and the lubricated soft catheter gently directed 5–8cm (2–3 inches) through the functioning opening. The colon is then irrigated with isotonic saline in 60ml (2oz) to 300ml (10oz) cycles according to age. As the child has no control of his colostomy, leakage around the catheter is inevitable. The nurse should anticipate this happening and protect the bed accordingly. A warm bath following this procedure gives the child some pleasure and ensures that he is clean and dry before re-dressing.

Irrigation of the non-functioning opening may be requested as a pre-operative measure. A soft, lubricated catheter is inserted for 2·5–5cm (1–2 inches) and the distal colon and rectum are irrigated with 60ml (2oz) of isotonic saline.

Thoracic Surgery

Examples: Lobectomy for bronchiectasis.
Repair of tracheo-oesophageal fistula.
Colonic transplant for oesophageal replacement.
Division of a persistent ductus arteriosus.

PRE-OPERATIVE CARE
1 Local sepsis of the upper respiratory passages is excluded—throat and nasal swabs are sent for laboratory examination. Topical antibiotic or antiseptic creams are prescribed as necessary. Dental sepsis is eradicated.
2 The child is taught some simple breathing exercises.
3. A plain X-ray film of the chest is taken; preliminary diagnostic X-ray procedures will have already confirmed the diagnosis.
4 The haemoglobin content is estimated and the blood grouped and cross-matched.
5 The child is introduced to oxygen therapy.

POST-OPERATIVE CARE
1 The child is turned at half to one-hourly intervals.
2 Physiotherapy is carried out at hourly intervals under the guidance of the physiotherapist.
3 Oxygen is administered by face mask or into a tent if required.
4 Quarter to half-hourly recordings of the pulse, respiration rate and depth, and blood pressure are made and the temperature is recorded at hourly intervals.
5 A plain X-ray film of the chest is taken on return from theatre and as demanded by the child's condition.

Cardio-Vascular Surgery using Cardio-Pulmonary By-Pass

Examples: Repair of septal defects.
Correction of Fallot's tetralogy.
Mustard's operation for transposition of the great vessels.
Valve replacement surgery.

PRE-OPERATIVE CARE

1, 2 and 3   As for thoracic surgery.

4   An electrocardiograph is recorded.

5   Blood investigations performed include estimation of haemoglobin content, prothrombin and bleeding times, packed cell volume, full blood count, grouping and cross-matching. The serum electrolyte and blood gas levels are also estimated.

6   The child is weighed and measured for calculation of surface area.

7   An antibiotic cover is commenced.

8   The child is introduced to oxygen therapy and to the staff of the recovery area.

IMMEDIATE POST-OPERATIVE CARE

1   The child is nursed by the experienced staff of a recovery area.

2   His lateral position is changed at hourly intervals.

3   Physiotherapy is carried out at hourly intervals under the guidance of the physiotherapist.

4   Oxygen is administered by face mask or into a tent. Alternatively, positive pressure ventilation may be used.

5   Small doses of analgesics may be given to help to achieve co-operation.

6   Physiological observations may be monitored continuously or recorded as described in Chapter 9. The electrocardiograph, pulse, systemic arterial blood pressure, central venous pressure, temperature and respiration rate may be recorded at quarter-hourly intervals initially, the time between observations being extended as the child's condition improves.

7   Restoration of fluid, electrolyte and blood balance.

8   Pleural, mediastinal and pericardial drainage is estimated and balanced at quarter-hourly intervals.

9   A naso-gastric tube is allowed free drainage.

10   Routine oral toilet is performed at two to four-hourly intervals.

11   An accurate record of urine output is maintained. A urine collection bag or urethral catheter may prove necessary.

12   The blood chemistry—Astrups and Po_2 (page 193), and electrolytes—are estimated on return to the ward and at six to twelve-hourly intervals until satisfactory.

13   A plain X-ray film of the chest is taken on return from theatre and as demanded by the child's condition.

14   Drugs are administered as prescribed by the doctor, e.g. antibiotics, digitalis and diuretics.

15   An early return to the main ward environment is made as soon as the child's general condition allows.

16   The psychological care of the child and his anxious parents should not be forgotten.

Closed Drainage of the Pleural Cavity

PRINCIPLE

Each lung is enveloped by a double layer of serous membrane; the visceral layer of pleura closely investing the elastic lungs and the parietal layer lining the thoracic walls and diaphragm. The potential space between the two layers is called the pleural cavity. The opposing forces of the muscles of respiration and the elastic recoil of the lungs maintain a constant sub-atmospheric or negative pressure within the pleural cavity.

On inspiration, the diaphragm flattens and the rib cage is lifted upwards and outwards, thus increasing the thoracic cavity in depth and circumference. The lungs are expanded because of their firm attachment to the thoracic walls by the two layers of pleura, separated by a thin film of fluid. Air is drawn into the expanded lungs to equalize the gas pressure. As the elastic lungs recoil, expiration takes place.

During inspiration, the intrapleural pressure becomes increasingly sub-atmospheric because of an increase in the opposing forces. If the normally intact pleural cavity is punctured, atmospheric air will rush in to equalize the gas pressures on either side of the thoracic wall. The elasticity of the lung tissue will cause it to collapse. When drainage of the pleural cavity is necessary, an under-water seal prevents air entry and at the same time encourages expansion of the lung and drainage of blood or exudate. Pleural drainage is used:

1 Routinely following thorocotomy for operation on the heart and great vessels, lungs or oesophagus to reveal bleeding or leakage and to allow the lungs to expand.

2 To relieve a pneumothorax $\Big\langle$ tension.
 spontaneous.

3 To drain an effusion which may be serous, pus (empyema) or blood (haemo-thorax).

REQUIREMENTS

All sterile

A sterile jar—a calibrated cylindrical jar is ideal.

A bung with two holes.

Polythene or glass tubing—one long, one short.

Length of non-kink tubing, sufficient to extend from the patient to the drainage bottle.

Straight-sided nylon connection.

Sterile distilled water.

METHOD

The surgeon inserts the catheter into a dependent part of the pleural cavity. The catheter is kept firmly occluded with two pairs of large haemostats until the under-water seal is attached (FIG. 57).

Using a strict aseptic technique, the apparatus is prepared for use. A known quantity of sterile distilled water is poured into the jar. The bung carrying the tubing is inserted, the long tube extending at least to 2·5cm (1 inch) below the water level. One end of the pressure tubing is attached to this tube. The connection is inserted into the other end and firmly driven home into the pleural catheter. The jar is placed on a tray on the floor. All connections are examined for leaks before the haemostats are removed.

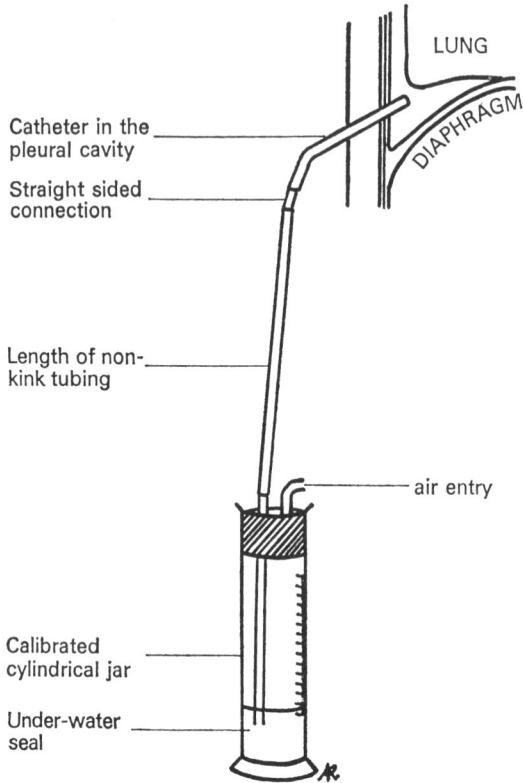

FIG. 57. Under-water seal drainage.

With respiratory effort, the column of water in the under-water seal is seen to rise and fall; the increased sub-atmospheric pressure during inspiration causes the column to rise and to fall as the negative pressure is reduced during expiration. Full lung expansion and blockage of the lumen of the apparatus will cause oscillation to cease. Any blood, serum or air in the pleural cavity drains down the tube into the jar. Blockage by blood clot can be prevented by milking the tubing at frequent intervals.

Suction created by a low pressure Roberts type suction pump may be applied to the short inlet tube following thoracic surgery. The negative pressure must be accurately controlled as excessive suction may prove harmful.

The child is comfortably positioned in such a way that there is no pull or kinking of the tubing. A large safety-pin inserted through the drawsheet on either side of the tubing allows for limited movement.

The jar is changed every twelve to twenty-four hours and at intervals between, depending on the amount of drainage. A deep under-water seal inhibits adequate lung expansion.

To change the jar, the apparatus is prepared as given above. The catheter is occluded with two haemostats positioned between the connection and the child's skin before the tubing is disconnected. The prepared apparatus is connected and the haemostats removed. The content of the drainage jar is inspected and the volume recorded (deducting the volume of water).

The jar must be maintained below chest level to prevent fluid from being sucked into the chest, and sterile water is used to avoid the risk of pleural irritation, should this occur. If the jar has to be raised for transport or movement of the child, then the tubing must be securely clamped. Should the jar be accidentally knocked over or broken, immediate occlusion of the tubing is essential to prevent lung collapse.

Removal of the Catheter

When the doctor is satisfied that drainage has ceased and that the lung is fully expanded, the catheter is removed. This is usually twenty-four to forty-eight hours post-operatively.

PRINCIPLES INVOLVED

1 The catheter is withdrawn during inspiration when the lungs are fully expanded. An older child may co-operate by holding a deep inspiration while the catheter is withdrawn. An opportune moment is chosen during an infant's cries.

2 To prevent air entering the pleural cavity, an occlusive dressing is applied over the fistula immediately following withdrawal of the catheter. It is, therefore, necessary to prepare the occlusive dressing before the anchoring skin sutures are released.

3 X-ray of the chest following removal of the catheter will show if there is air in the pleural cavity.

REQUIREMENTS

The basic trolley is prepared as described on page 258 with the addition of the following sterile equipment:

    1 pair of stitch scissors.

    Tulle gras.

METHOD

Removal of a pleural drain is an unpleasant, often frightening procedure to an apprehensive child. A sedative may be given.

The occlusive dressing is prepared by cutting a suitable length of Elastoplast. A small piece of gauze is placed in the centre of the strip allowing a 2–3cm or 1 inch seal all round. A square of tulle gras is folded into four and placed in the centre of the gauze (FIG. 58).

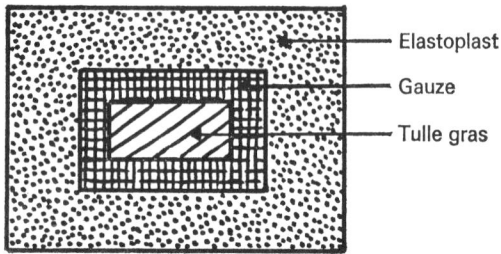

FIG. 58. Occlusive dressing for a chest wound.

The basic procedure is as for surgical dressing technique. The free ends of an occluding pursestring suture inserted at operation are drawn up and tied as the catheter is withdrawn, thus closing the wound, or the catheter is released by cutting the anchoring skin stitch between its knot and the catheter. The occlusive dressing is held to one side of the catheter as gentle traction allows the catheter to be withdrawn at an opportune moment. The fistula is immediately covered and the adhesive moulded into position.

Following removal of the catheter, healing is rapid unless infection is present. The occlusive dressing can be safely removed after twenty-four hours and the sutures five days later.

The drainage is measured and recorded.

Genito-Urinary Surgery

Examples: Nephrectomy.
          Pyeloplasty for hydronephrosis.

PRE-OPERATIVE PREPARATION

1   The necessary renal function tests and examinations are performed.

2   The blood urea is estimated.

3   Urinary infection is excluded—a mid-stream or clean-catch specimen is examined in the laboratory.

POST-OPERATIVE CARE

1   The child is initially nursed on his affected side to encourage drainage.

2   A drain to the kidney-bed is shortened daily from the second day.

3   A nephrostomy drain connected to a sterile closed drainage system is removed when urine flow through the T-tube is negligible—usually ten to fourteen days post-operatively.

4   Ample fluids are offered orally or administered intravenously to ensure an adequate urine flow.

5   A urethral catheter is connected to a sterile closed drainage system. Twice daily toilet of the genitalia should be given.

6   A urine specimen is obtained to exclude urinary infection forty-eight hours following removal of the urethral catheter.

Hypospadias

In hypospadias, the urethral meatus terminates at some point on the under-surface of the penis or scrotum. Usually the defect is corrected in two stages so that the boy is able to pass urine in the proper manner before he goes to school. The first stage operation aims at correcting the chordee (ventral flexion of the penis). The special points related to a second stage Denis Browne type operation are given below.

POST-OPERATIVE CARE

1   The bladder is drained via a perineal urethrostomy for ten to fourteen days to allow a buried strip of penile skin to form a urethra, extending the full length of the penis. The catheter is connected to a sterile closed drainage system.

2   Double-stop tension-relieving sutures are used. Beads and crushed metal cylinders secure the suture in position and reduce the tension on the suture-line (FIG. 59). These are removed by releasing the crushed metal tube and gently withdrawing the suture.

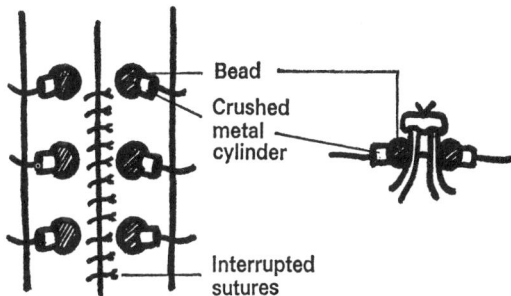

FIG. 59. Double-stop tension-relieving sutures.

3   A gentle sterile dressing technique is achieved by the use of sterile gloves rather than cumbersome forceps.

4   The success of this operation depends to a large extent on patient co-operation. Diversional therapy is encouraged.

Bladder Drainage

When a urethral catheter is to remain in the bladder for a period of time, a self-retaining balloon-type catheter is attached to a sterile closed drainage system.

REQUIREMENTS

As for catheterization of the urinary bladder (page 361).

Additional requirements:
Balloon catheter of suitable size.
5ml syringe.
5ml ampoule of sterile water.
No. 1 hypodermic needle.
Adhesive tape.
Sterile continuous bladder drainage bag or bottle and tubing.
Safety-pin.

METHOD

The procedure is as described for catheterization. The catheter is inserted for an additional 2cm ($\frac{3}{4}$ inch) to allow the balloon portion to be in the bladder. The required amount of water is inserted into the balloon via the diaphragm (the quantity of fluid necessary is shown on the catheter) and the catheter is attached to the sterile closed drainage system.

Prophylactic urinary antiseptics or antibiotics are usually prescribed, and twice daily catheter toilet is performed to promote comfort and reduce the risk of ascending urinary tract infection. Bladder irrigations are avoided unless drainage is unsatisfactory. Extra fluids are given to ensure a good urine flow and an accurate fluid balance chart is maintained.

The connection between the catheter and the tubing should be straight-sided, not tapered, to allow for free drainage. The non-kink drainage tubing should be secured to the drawsheet and be of sufficient length to allow free movement. Both drainage bottle/bag and tubing should be changed for sterile renewals at least once daily. Satisfactory drainage of urine can be observed if the drainage reservoir is left uncovered.

Toilet of the Genitalia

Toilet of the genitalia is necessary when both boys and girls have an indwelling catheter on continuous bladder drainage.

1 FEMALE-VULVAL TOILET

With the girl in a semi-recumbent position, the vulva is swabbed as for catheterization (page 362). Alternatively, the girl may be sat on a bedpan and a small quantity of warmed lotion contained in a jug used to irrigate the vulva. Whichever method is used, care must be taken to ensure that all parts of the vulva are dried with sterile cotton wool balls before turning the child on to her side to dry the anal area.

2 MALE

In the male child, the foreskin is gently retracted, the area surrounding the urethral meatus gently cleansed with cotton wool balls moistened in sterile water or antiseptic lotion and the area dried well with sterile swabs.

Bladder Irrigation

Routine bladder irrigations during continuous bladder drainage are now the exception rather than the rule. A strict aseptic technique is necessary to avoid introduction of micro-organisms into the bladder.

REQUIREMENTS

The basic dressing trolley is prepared as described on page 258, with the addition of the following sterile equipment:
Measuring jug containing lotion, i.e.:
  Normal saline
  Chlorhexidine 0·01%
  Acriflavine 1 : 1000
Disposable balloon-type syringe.
Receiver.
Waterproof protection.

METHOD

The lotion is prepared to a temperature of 38°C or 100°F.

The procedure is essentially as for any aseptic technique. After thoroughly washing and drying her hands, the nurse places a sterile towel between the child's thighs and using two pairs of forceps, separates the catheter from the connection. The open end of the catheter is placed on the sterile towel and the forceps are discarded.

The syringe is filled with lotion by first releasing, then compressing the bulb while the open end is in the jug of solution. Using gentle pressure, the solution is slowly injected into the bladder. Gentle release of compression should remove all the injected fluid from the bladder.

Gentle withdrawal is essential if damage to the delicate transitional epithelial lining of the bladder is to be prevented. Over-distension of the bladder is avoided by the use of small quantities of solution, i.e. 30–60ml for each cycle.

On completion of the irrigation, the catheter is connected to a further sterile closed drainage system and the child is left dry and comfortable.

Neurosurgery

Operations on the brain demand a large proportion of the scalp to be shaved. Parental consent must be obtained prior to careful shaving of the scalp. To facilitate removal, resistant scurf can be softened twenty-four hours prior to preparing the head; salicylic acid and sulphur ointment is effective for this purpose. The use of an electric razor will reduce the risk of breaking the skin, with subsequent discomfort and low grade infection, and the child should be given opportunity to become accustomed to its noise before putting the razor to use. An older girl will naturally be very upset at losing her hair. She must be assured that a wig can be worn until her own hair has grown again.

If requested by the surgeon, the shave is followed by antiseptic preparation of the scalp.

The special post-operative care is related to the operation performed. Following a craniotomy, for example, the care is essentially as for care and observation of an unconscious child.

For Further Reading

DENNISON W. W. (1967). *Surgery of Infancy and Childhood*, 2nd edition. E. & S. Livingstone, Edinburgh.

ELISON NASH D. F. (1969). *The Principles and Practice of Surgery for Nurses and Allied Professions*, 4th edition. Edward Arnold (Publishers) Ltd., London.

FARROW R. and FORREST D. (1968). *The Surgery of Childhood for Nurses*, 3rd edition. E. & S. Livingstone, Edinburgh.

NIXON H. H. and O'DONNELL B. (1966). *The Essentials of Paediatric Surgery*, 2nd edition. William Heinemann (Medical Books) Ltd., London.

RICKMAN P. P. and JOHNSTON J. H. (1969). *Neonatal Surgery*, 1st edition. Butterworths, London.

CHAPTER FIFTEEN

Emergency and Resuscitative Measures

Maintenance of a Clear Airway

A suction unit should be a standard piece of equipment in any acute ward. This may be a simple, disposable mucus extractor for use with newborn infants, or a more complex apparatus attached to a vacuum pipeline, or electrically, foot or gas powered. All machines are capable of producing a fairly wide range of negative pressure and the nurse must be familiar with the performance of the particular apparatus in use. Considerable damage to the delicate mucosal lining of the upper respiratory passages can result if too much power is exerted.

Unless the apparatus is confined to the use of one child, cross-infection could prove a problem. The suction jar should be changed for another jar as necessary, and at least daily, when the tubing should also be re-sterilized.

Pharyngeal Suction

Infants and small children suffering from respiratory infections, the unconscious, and children with palatal paralysis require frequent aspiration of secretions from the upper respiratory passages in order to maintain a clear airway.

REQUIREMENTS
Suction unit, pressure tubing and tapered or Y-shaped connection.
Sterile atraumatic suction catheters of suitable size.
Sterile disposable gloves.
Receptacle containing water.
Receptacle for disposable items.

METHOD
Unless the child is deeply unconscious or securely restrained, two nurses are necessary for this procedure. The child is placed in a supine or lateral position with the neck extended.

A non-touch technique is used. A sterile catheter is attached to the connection. After washing and drying her hands, the nurse puts a sterile glove on to her right hand, and withdraws the catheter from its protective bag. The suction unit is turned on with the ungloved hand. The uncontaminated catheter is kinked while being passed into the mouth and oro-pharynx. The secretions are aspirated by rotating the catheter as it is gently withdrawn. The catheter is cleansed by aspirating a small quantity of water and the procedure is repeated if necessary. (For use of the Y-shaped connection, see page 306).

At the end of the procedure, the suction unit is turned off and the sterile glove and catheter are discarded.

Tracheostomy

A tracheostomy is the surgical construction of a temporary, artificial airway in the trachea through which a suitable sized tracheostomy tube is inserted. The operation is usually performed as a life-saving measure.

A variety of silver, polyvinyl and rubber tracheostomy tubes are available. All require a suitable length of narrow tape securely attached to each side of the flange (page 306). A silver tube consists of three parts, an outer tube with a key to lock the inner tube in position, and an introducer. For long term use, pre-sterilized polyvinyl tubes are preferable to those made of rubber. An inflatable cuffed tracheostomy tube is used to achieve an air-tight seal when prolonged positive pressure ventilation is used to maintain the life of a paralysed child. Deflation of the cuff at one to two-hourly intervals ensures that the tracheal tissues do not become devitalized.

Reasons for Performing a Tracheostomy

1   Obstruction of the nose and naso-pharynx due to:
    i   a foreign body;
    ii   Inflammation due to:
       acute laryngo-tracheo-bronchitis
       trauma—following intubation
             burns—chemical
                   physical;
    iii   congenital laryngeal stridor due to:
       small larynx
       tumour
       laryngeal web
       laxity of sub-glottic tissue
    iv   extra-tracheal pressure due to, for example, a cystic hygroma.

2 In respiratory insufficiency:
  i to aid liquefication and aspiration of tenacious pulmonary secretions from the trachea and bronchi;
  ii to reduce the anatomical dead space.*
3 To prevent aspiration of saliva and vomitus by isolating the respiratory passages of a child in deep coma.
4 To allow positive pressure ventilation:
  i to obviate the need for respiratory effort following major cardiac surgery;
  ii in respiratory paralysis due to the effects of tubocurarine in the control of tetanic spasms, and in poliomyelitis and myasthenia gravis.

Post-Operative Care

The constant observation of a 'special nurse' is essential to ensure that an adequate airway is maintained. The child will be very frightened when he discovers that speech is impossible and the constant presence of a sympathetic nurse will help to allay his anxiety. Temporary restraint of the hands or elbows may be necessary until the child becomes accustomed to his change of airway.

Post-operative observations include half-hourly recordings of the pulse rate (which may be high if respiratory distress is evident), respiratory rate, depth, rhythm and effort, and the colour and general behaviour of the child. Temporary inco-ordination of swallowing may be sufficient to demand feeding via a naso-gastric tube for the first few post-operative days, particularly in a small infant. The use of pliant polyvinyl tracheostomy tubes has reduced the incidence of dysphagia (difficulty in swallowing), but care with feeding is still necessary during the first few days. An older child may be offered oral fluids as long as his general condition is satisfactory.

REQUIREMENTS AT THE BEDSIDE
Good lighting is essential.
1 For removal of secretions:
  Suction unit, pressure tubing and Y-shaped connection.
  Sterile atraumatic suction catheters of suitable size.
  Sterile disposable gloves.
  Receptacle containing water.
  Receptacle for disposable items.
  Receiver containing a saturated solution of sodium bicarbonate for the reception of non-disposable catheters.

* When a child is experiencing respiratory difficulty, half or more of his respiratory effort is expended in ventilating the air passages (the anatomical dead space). In performing a tracheostomy, the volume of air contained in the dead space is halved, giving a greater alveolar ventilation without an increase in respiratory effort.

Pipe cleaners

Gallipot containing a saturated solution } for cleansing an inner silver tube.
   of sodium bicarbonate

2   For humidification, see page 236.
3   For local care of the stoma:
   Small sterile key-hole dressings.
   2 pairs of dressing forceps.
   Gallipot for cleansing lotion.
   Cotton wool balls.
4   For emergency use:
   Spare tracheostomy tube of same size as in use.
   Tracheal dilators.
   Laryngoscope.
   Endotracheal tube.
   Emergency bell.
5   For intermittent positive pressure inflation of the lungs:
   Oxygen or compressed air supply.
   Anaesthetic bag.
   Expiratory valve.
   Angled mount.
   Nosworthy union.

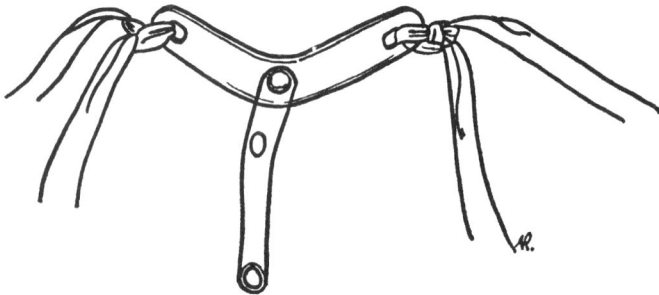

FIG. 60. Fenestrated polyvinyl tracheostomy tube with tapes.

Maintenance of a Clear Airway

1   POSITION OF THE CHILD

Unless unconscious, an older child is nursed in an upright position with the head adequately supported with pillows to prevent the chin blocking the tracheostomy tube opening. An infant is nursed on alternate sides with a rolled napkin placed under the shoulders to extend his short neck.

2   HUMIDIFICATION

The normal functions of the upper respiratory tract are lost when air is inspired through a tracheostomy. To aid aspiration and to prevent viscosity of respiratory secretions and formation of crusts, humidification of the surrounding environment or ventilating circuit is essential. Water saturation of the air is achieved by the use of a nebulizer, as in a Croupette or Humidaire tent, or by moist steam therapy, using a steam kettle and canopy. An ultrasonic nebulizer is included in the ventilating circuit of most modern ventilators. Alternatively, normal saline may be dripped slowly through a fine hypodermic needle inserted into the ventilating circuit, but only if requested by the doctor.

3 REMOVAL OF SECRETIONS

Regular efficient aspiration of the trachea and bronchi is the only satisfactory means of maintaining effortless, inaudible breathing in a child with a tracheostomy. Maintenance of a clear airway is assisted by regular changing of the tracheostomy tube and physiotherapy—chest wall percussion, voluntary or positive pressure inflation of the lungs, and coughing.

Tracheal toilet is required at the following times:

1 Every ten to fifteen minutes immediately post-operatively when secretions are excessive.
2 Every four hours for an established tracheostomy.
3 If respiration is audible or the child restless.
4 When requested by an older child.
5 Before and after changing the child's position.
6 In conjunction with physiotherapy.
7 Before feeding.
8 Before deflation of a cuffed tube when naso-pharyngeal aspiration is also necessary.

Principles of Tracheal Toilet

1 To prevent the introduction of micro-organisms, a non-touch technique is practised and the sterile atraumatic-tipped catheter used once only.
2 To facilitate aspiration, tenacious pulmonary secretions may be liquefied by inserting 1–2ml of sterile normal saline into the tracheostomy tube, during an inspiration, immediately prior to aspiration.
3 To prevent excessive withdrawal of residual alveolar air causing lobar collapse and hypoxaemia, the external diameter of the suction catheter should not exceed half the internal diameter of the tracheostomy tube. For the same reason, time for withdrawal of the catheter should not exceed ten seconds at a carefully controlled negative pressure.
4 To prevent an injury and to assist easy passage of the catheter, suction is not applied until the bifurcation of the trachea is reached—8–20cm or 3–8 inches. If a Y-shaped connection is not used, the catheter is kinked while being inserted.
5 If bronchial aspiration is requested, the catheter is inserted into the left

bronchus with the head turned to the right side. Similarly, the right bronchus is entered by turning the chin towards the left.

METHOD

Two nurses are essential for this procedure unless complete patient co-operation can be assured.

Wearing a mask, the nurse washes and dries her hands and puts a sterile glove on to her right hand. Using her left hand, the suction unit is turned on. A sterile catheter is attached to one limb of the Y-shaped connection, and withdrawn from its protective bag. The inner tube of a silver tracheostomy tube is unlocked, removed and placed in a receptacle of saturated sodium bicarbonate solution.

Held in the gloved right hand, the uncontaminated catheter is directed accuraltey into the lumen of the tube and gently advanced for the previously assessed length. A digit of the ungloved hand partially occludes the open limb of the Y-shaped connection and the secretions are aspirated by rotating the catheter as it is gently withdrawn. The catheter and glove are then discarded.

The Y-shaped connection and pressure tubing are cleansed by aspiration of a small quantity of water, and the suction unit is turned off.

The silver inner tube is freed of mucus by cleaning with pipe cleaners soaked in sodium bicarbonate solution, sterilized and re-inserted.

If requested by the doctor, the lungs may be manually inflated by attaching the connection of an inflated anaesthetic bag to the tracheostomy tube and compressing its contained gas into the lungs. The expiratory valve must be open to allow adequate expiration while the bag refills with a fresh supply of oxygen or air. An anaesthetic bag of appropriate size is essential to avoid the risk of over-inflation. Positive pressure inflation of the lungs relieves bronchial secretions before applying suction and reduces the possibility of segmental collapse following aspiration.

Changing and Securing the Tracheostomy Tube

The tracheostomy tube inserted at the time of operation is usually left in position five to seven days to allow adequate track formation. The slightly longer inner tube of a silver tracheostomy tube is cleansed, re-sterilized and re-inserted at each aspiration. Subsequently, a daily or weekly change of tracheostomy tube may be requested.

METHOD

A check is made that all the necessary equipment is at the bedside. The sterile tracheostomy tube is prepared for insertion. Two lengths of narrow tape are cut, the length required varying with the size of the child. One length is threaded through the opening on one side of the tube and secured in a reef knot, close to the flange; the second is similarly secured.

The child is placed in the supine position, restrained in a treatment blanket if necessary, with the shoulders raised on a rolled napkin or sandbag to extend the neck (Fig. 61). Tracheal aspiration is performed, the tapes securing the tube in position are cut, and the flange lifted while the area surrounding the stoma is cleansed. The tube is then removed.

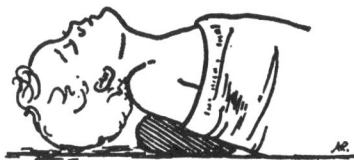

Fig. 61. Position of a child for change of tracheostomy tube. Note the position of the sandbag allowing for full extension of the neck.

To prevent the new tube entering the pre-tracheal tissues, its end is directed straight through the stoma before guiding the tube in a downward direction into the trachea.

The child is brought into a sitting position to allow slight flexion of the neck while each pair of tapes is securely tied in a reef knot on the posterior lateral aspect of the neck. The ends are trimmed to 1·5cm of each knot. This position

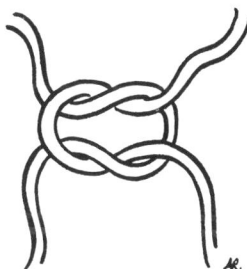

Fig. 62. Reef knot

of the knot does not cause discomfort and avoids the risk of confusing gown and bib tapes with the tapes securing the child's life-saving airway. Correct tension of the tapes is important. If the tapes are too loose, the tube is liable to become dislodged; if too tight, the child experiences discomfort.

Local Care of the Stoma

If the tracheostomy wound is clean, it need not be covered. Low grade infection of the area is not uncommon. A swab for bacteriological examination confirms the sensitivity of the micro-organism so that the appropriate antibiotics may be prescribed. A dry dressing may be placed under the flange and changed daily or more frequently as it becomes soiled. Following a Bjork flap-type tracheostomy, the sutures are removed as soon as the area is healed.

Extubation

Tracheostomy dependency is great, particularly in the first year of life. Early extubation is desirable, but can only be achieved when the reason for performing the tracheostomy has been satisfactorily overcome and the child has become accustomed to using his normal upper respiratory passages.

A fenestrated tube is introduced which has two possible air channels; out via the tracheostomy tube opening, or upwards to the larynx via a window cut into the tube at its elbow (FIG. 60). Insertion of a speaking valve encourages phonation and a certain amount of air control. Complete occlusion of the tracheostomy tube opening for increasing periods of time allows the child to re-adjust to normal breathing.

When the tracheostomy tube has been plugged for several days, the tube is finally removed while the child's attention is distracted by a familiar nurse. Adequate sedation may help to reduce fear of suffocation due to the increase in respiratory effort necessary to meet the increased resistance and to fill the now increased volume of the anatomical dead space.

The stoma is covered with an occlusive dressing. The fistula quickly closes, leaving a small scar.

Long Term Care of a Child with a Tracheostomy

Unless the reason for performing the tracheostomy can be quickly overcome, a child may have to retain an artificial airway for weeks, months or even years. The responsibility of the nursing staff is considerable, especially during the formative first years of the child's life. Of prime importance is maintenance of a clear airway at all times, so that continued supervision is desirable. Cross-infection is a constant hazard and respiratory infections are more common as the normal filtering mechanism of the upper respiratory passages has been by-passed.

With the necessary frequent change of the student population of the ward team, the emotional deprivation of such a child can be considerable. Sometimes it is possible for the child to be cared for at home under the close supervision of the family doctor and his nursing colleagues, but it is his mother who bears the biggest load. She needs explicit instructions and ample opportunity to care for her child in the hospital environment to give her the necessary confidence before taking him home.

Naso-Tracheal Intubation

To avoid tracheostomy dependency and difficulty in extubation of a small child or infant, a polyvinyl naso-tracheal Jackson Rees tube is used whenever possible (FIG. 63). It is of particular value in the care of small infants and for children with acute laryngo-tracheo-bronchitis requiring short term relief of inflammatory respiratory obstruction, and may be used as a means of providing temporary intermittent positive pressure ventilation (I.P.P.V.) of the lungs following cardio-pulmonary by-pass surgery.

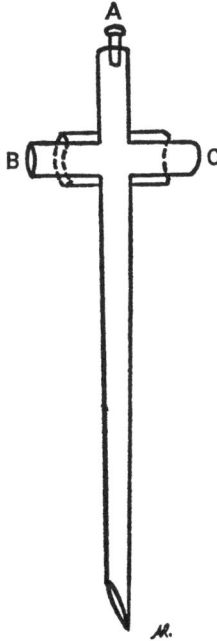

FIG. 63. Jackson Rees tube.

Care must be taken to see that the tube is held securely in position with non-allergic adhesive tape and/or a head harness, and that the three limbs do not become blocked. Occlusion of the suction limb (A) is essential when intermittent positive pressure ventilation is in use. The conscious child will require elbow restraint.

Maintenance of a clear airway is essentially as for care of a tracheostomy. The suction catheter is passed to a previously assessed distance just beyond the end of the tube before suction is applied. Placement and replacement of a naso-tracheal tube is beyond the scope of the nursing staff.

Intermittent Positive Pressure Ventilation (I.P.P.V.)

Normal spontaneous inspiration is initiated by an increase in the Pco_2 and a lowering of the Po_2 and pH of arterial blood. Subsequent contraction of the diaphragm and intercostal muscles causes expansion of the thoracic cavity in all dimensions. The elastic recoil of the lungs is expanded, creating an effective intrathoracic sub-atmospheric pressure, and air is drawn into the lungs from the atmosphere. Expiration is passive.

Respiratory effort is adequate if it results in removal of carbon dioxide from the blood and supplies sufficient oxygen to meet the needs of body metabolism. This depends on:

i   efficient respiratory effort;
ii sufficient and efficient functioning of alveolar membrane to allow gaseous exchange;
iii an adequate pulmonary circulation.

When a blood gas analysis confirms that respiratory effort is not fulfilling this criterion, intermittent positive pressure ventilation is instituted when there is good reason to believe that the child will recover. Rhythmic inflation and deflation of the child's lungs is made possible by delivery of a humidified air/oxygen mixture by way of a face mask or, more usually, by a polyvinyl naso-tracheal or tracheostomy tube. Use of an inflated tube prevents leakage of air and protects the lungs from aspiration of foreign material.

The anaesthetist or paediatrician is responsible for preparing a suitable ventilator for use by the child. Some machines are powered by electricity while others rely on a constant flow of compressed air or oxygen. Humidification of the gas is by the use of a nebulizer or water humidifier. The child's tidal volume (amount of air breathed in and out in a single respiration) is assessed according to his size and normal respiratory rate and the reading is adjusted to meet his particular need. Ventilators fall into three categories:

1   Pressure-cycled. Gas flows into the lungs until a certain pressure is reached, when the machine cuts the gas supply to allow for spontaneous relaxation of the chest wall (expiration).

2   Constant pressure ventilator. This time-cycled machine inflates the lungs at a constant pre-set pressure.

3   Volume-cycled. A constant pre-set volume of gas is delivered by the machine with each inflation, regardless of the resistance met.

It is possible to control a negative phase during the cycle on some machines to facilitate venous return to the heart. 'Patient-triggered' machines allow the small inspiratory effort created by the child to initiate full inflation of the lungs by machine.

It is imperative that the nursing staff caring for these children are fully informed and competent in the care of the child and the use and care of the special apparatus. Constant observation is essential. Children requiring intermittent positive pressure ventilation are best nursed in an intensive therapy unit together with other children requiring mechanical and electronic aid to support vital functions, and where the medical and nursing staff are trained in their special care and the intelligent use of the expensive equipment.

The child will need meticulous attention to nursing detail including care of the skin, hair, mouth, eyes, bowels and bladder, and maintenance of hydration and nutrition. Two-hourly turning prevents the occurrence of pressure sores and pulmonary congestion of the dependent lung, and four-hourly physiotherapy is essential both during the day and night. In addition, the child's special care involves care of the ventilator and of the tracheostomy.

Observations may be recorded at half, one or two-hourly intervals depending on the child's condition, and include:
1 Ventilation rate.
2 Tidal volume—recorded with a spirometer attached to the expiratory port.
3 Minute volume—ventilation rate multiplied by the tidal volume.
4 Ventilation pressure.
5 Blood pressure⎱ recorded to detect early hypercapnia (increase in P_{CO_2} of
6 Pulse   ⎰ blood).
7 Maintenance of a fluid balance chart.

It is most important that nurses working with critically ill children in an intensive therapy unit are able to support the parents in their anxiety. The parents must be suitably prepared for their first visit to the unit, and the appearance of their critically ill child. Some may wish to remain at their child's bedside, though he remains unconscious, while others are content to pay frequent, brief visits. Although the child may appear unconscious, conversation between members of the staff, and staff and parents, should be cautious at all times, and especially when the child is paralyzed by the effects of tubocurarine, but not unconscious. A child may appreciate a familiar short story read by his mother and will certainly like to hear her tell him little 'tit-bits' about his home, pets and school friends.

As soon as the child has been weaned from the need for intensive therapy, he should be returned to the more relaxed atmosphere of his familiar children's ward. His critical condition has demanded much time and effort on the part of the unit staff and this is frequently manifested as a temporary over-demanding attitude on return to the ward. To a greater or lesser extent, this pattern of behaviour is typical of most children once on the road to recovery after a severe illness, but is probably at no time more obvious than in those discharged from an intensive therapy unit.

Sudden Collapse of a Child

As it is the nursing staff who are with the children all the time, it is usually a nurse who is attracted by a sudden deterioration in a child's condition. Resuscitation is often most successful when the person making the diagnosis of arrest institutes treatment. All the staff of wards and departments, therefore, should be conversant with the routine adopted for this emergency and location of the resuscitation box or trolley. Resuscitation should be commenced as soon as the diagnosis of circulatory arrest has been made (unless the medical staff have decided that prolonging life is not in the interests of the child) as irreversible brain damage occurs approximately three minutes from the cessation of circulation.

Signs of Circulatory Arrest

1 Absence of a pulse in the carotid or femoral arteries.
2 Absence of respiration (apnoea).
3 Abrupt unconsciousness.
4 Dilating pupils.

Treatment

The aim of treatment is to create an effective circulation of oxygenated blood by means of external cardiac massage and artificial respiration until arrival of the resuscitation team. Both can be performed simultaneously if two people are available, but if the nurse is on her own, she must alternate between the two in the ratio of one respiratory ventilation to six cardiac compressions.

METHOD
1 Once diagnosis has been made, another nurse is called to make the hospital 'resuscitation call' and to return immediately to assist with the procedure.
2 The bed is screened and the time noted.
3 Either a board is put under the child's chest or the child is placed on the floor. An infant is lifted from his incubator on to a flat surface. An intravenous infusion is preserved if possible.

4 ARTIFICIAL RESPIRATION
 i The head and neck are hyperextended and the jaw pulled forward to clear the tongue from the back of the mouth (FIG. 61, page 307). Suction or a finger is used to clear the airway of mucus, blood or vomit.
 ii The lungs are filled by positive pressure ventilation using mouth to mouth ventilation unless an Ambu (re-breathing) bag or Brook airway (for older children) is available. For instituting mouth to mouth ventilation, the nurse places her mouth over the open mouth of the child (mouth and nose of an infant or toddler) and prevents loss of air through the nostrils during inflation of the lungs by pinching the nose. Whichever method is used, the seal must be air-tight.
 iii The nurse uses her expired air to inflate the child's lungs. The amount of air used varies from little more than a puff for an infant to complete ex-

piration of air to give adequate inflation of the lungs for an older child. The child must be allowed to exhale completely between inflations. Artificial ventilation is carried out sixteen to twenty times per minute for a child, and twenty-five to thirty per minute for an infant.

The effectiveness of artificial ventilation can be seen with adequate expansion of the chest with each inflation and with an improvement in the child's colour.

5 EXTERNAL CARDIAC MASSAGE
 i The sternum is located and the nurse places the heel of one hand over the lower half of the sternum, avoiding the ribs, and the other hand is placed on top of the first.
 ii Keeping her arms straight, the sternum is quickly but firmly depressed 2·5cm–3·75cm (1–1½ inches). The rib cage of a small child is pliable and considerably less pressure is required to depress the sternum for the required distance. A thumb over the lower half of the sternum may be used to produce effective cardiac compression in an infant.

The heart is compressed between the sternum and the vertebral column, forcing its contained blood into the great vessels (pulmonary artery and aorta). The chest is allowed to expand after each compression to allow the venous return to enter the heart. The venous return may also be encouraged by raising the legs.

External cardiac compression is carried out seventy to 100 times per minute, depending on the age of the child and is effective if a carotid or femoral pulse is produced with each compression. As the result of oxygenated blood reaching the brain, the pupils become less dilated.

This routine in most circumstances will maintain an adequate circulation of oxygenated blood until the arrival of the resuscitation team. The nurse is then relieved of her responsibility and she assists the medical staff with further treatment.

SUBSEQUENT CARE
1 An endotracheal tube will be passed for more effective and less exhausting positive pressure ventilation to be instituted.
2 An intravenous infusion will be commenced so that drugs may be administered:
    i Sodium bicarbonate to correct the metabolic acidosis which is the inevitable result of circulatory arrest.
    ii Adrenaline 1–10,000 ⎫ to increase the tone of the heart muscle
       Calcium chloride 2% ⎭ (myocardium).
    iii Lignocaine 1% ⎫
       Potassium chloride ⎭ to depress irritability of the myocardium.

3 Electrocardiograph leads will be attached to the child to monitor the activities of the heart.

4 When cardiac arrest has been due to ventricular fibrillation, an electric shock from an electrical defibrillator is applied to the heart through the chest wall. This causes the heart to stop its ineffective contractions with restoration of normal myocardial activity.

Fire

Hospitals have a responsibility to provide instruction in their fire routine to all grades of staff. This should include the siting of fire escapes and the location and use of the extinguishers and hose-reels.

In the event of fire, the fire-alarm must be promptly sounded so that the whole hospital is aware of the situation. With some automatic fire warning devices, both the hospital switchboard and the local fire station are informed. If this system is not in operation, the switchboard operator must be told the exact location of the fire and he will inform the necessary personnel.

Until the fire appliances arrive, the staff of the ward should remain calm while making every effort to extinguish the flames and to confine the fire by closing all windows and doors. The person in charge of the ward is responsible for the safety of her patients and it is she who will organize their evacuation should this be necessary. Each child should be wrapped in a blanket and carried or directed to safety. All exits should be kept clear of beds and other furniture to allow for a speedy evacuation.

For Further Reading

EDWARDS J. M. and ROBERTS K. D. (1971). *Paediatric Intensive Care*, 1st edition. Blackwell Scientific Publications, Oxford.
CLEMENT A. J. 'The Treatment of Cardiac Arrest'. *Nursing Times*, 5.11.65.
FELDMAN S. A. (1967). *Tracheostomy and Artificial Ventilation in the Treatment of Respiratory Failure*, 1st edition. Edward Arnold (Publishers) Ltd., London.
GILSON A. 'Cardiac Resuscitation'. *Nursing Mirror Reprint*, June 1967.

CHAPTER SIXTEEN

Meeting Specific Needs

Care of the Febrile Child

Normal body temperature is 'thermostatically' controlled within its limited range, 36·3–37·2°C (97·4–99°F), by the hypothalamus.

When the body is overheated, vasodilatation of the superficial blood vessels leads to cooling by convection, conduction and radiation of the heat from the blood circulating through the skin, and increased production of sweat which cools the body by evaporation.

When the body temperature falls, peripheral vasoconstriction reduces the blood flow to the skin and sweat production is diminished. Involuntary contraction of the erector pilores muscles produce more heat in the body and erection of the cutaneous hairs (shivering). Trapped warmed air, an insulating layer of subcutaneous fat and vasoconstriction help to conserve body heat.

In many infections, the 'thermostat' of the heat-regulating centre is set higher. The child looks pale, feels cold and may shiver. Once the temperature has reached its new level, vasodilatation and sweating occur. In a small child, the onset of fever may be heralded by a convulsion.

A febrile child feels hot and clammy, looks flushed, and is generally anorectic, fractious and irritable. Urine output is diminished in volume and concentrated, and he may be constipated. The pulse and respiration rates are increased in order to maintain a higher metabolic rate.

Symptomatic treatment of the febrile child calls for good bedside nursing care and thought.

1 The child is nursed in a well ventilated but draught-free area. A guarded fan may be used to encourage greater circulation of air.

2 Most of his bedclothes should be removed and the linen changed whenever it is damp. Few children are happy with no bed coverings, but a covering sheet is often sufficient. Excessive exposure causes shivering which increases the body temperature.

3 Frequent sponging of the hands and face and twice daily bed baths will make the child feel more comfortable and encourage rest and sleep.

4   Long periods of rest and sleep should be encouraged. A sedative or analgesic may be prescribed by the doctor.

5   Because of his increased fluid loss and inevitable thirst, large amounts of cool fluids should be given. Added glucose helps to meet the body's need for extra kilocalories, thus reducing ketosis. Four-hourly oral care will prevent cracking of the mucous membrane.

6   Anti-pyretic drugs containing aspirin may be prescribed. These reduce the temperature by re-setting the 'thermostat' to a lower level. Heat is then lost from the body by sweating. Aspirin is also a mild analgesic.

7   If the body temperature remains high, the doctor may ask for the child to be given a tepid sponging.

Tepid Sponging

This procedure may be ordered by the doctor when the temperature of the body reaches a high level—usually above 39·5°C or 103°F.

PRINCIPLE

The aim of this procedure is to reduce the body temperature not more than 1·5°C or 2°F by allowing water to evaporate from the skin surface. Water maintained at a temperature of 30°C or 85°F is used and the procedure carried out systematically over a period of twenty minutes. Shivering will cause the body temperature to rise and should be avoided.

REQUIREMENTS

Trolley.

Top shelf:

Clinical thermometer.

Washing bowl of water, temperature 30°C or 85°F.

Bath thermometer.

Bowl of iced water.

6 sponges or flannels.

Face flannel and towel.

Lint for cold compress.

Talcum powder.

Hair brush and comb.

Bottom shelf:

Clean bed linen.

Clean personal clothes.

Additional requirements:

Linen carrier for soiled linen.

METHOD

An older child is offered a bedpan or urinal. A simple explanation is given. The top bedclothes and personal clothing are removed, a wet drawsheet pulled through or removed and the child left covered with the top sheet.

The face is sponged and dried and a cold compress is applied to the forehead. This is soothing and is renewed as required during the procedure.

The sponges are soaked in the washing bowl of water and excess moisture is removed. One sponge is placed in each axilla and one in each groin. In these flexures where two skin surfaces are in close contact, rapid cooling takes place as vessels conveying the blood to and from the limbs lie near to the skin surface. These sponges are changed three to four times during the procedure by first placing them in the bowl of iced water and removing the excess moisture before soaking them in the washing bowl of water. This measure is taken to avoid heat from the sponges removed from warm areas of the body increasing the temperature of the water in the washing bowl.

Using the two remaining sponges alternatively, a thin film of water is left over the surface of the skin. The upper extremities are treated first; long, sweeping movements being made from the shoulder to finger-tips, the sponge being sufficiently moist to leave small beads of moisture on the skin surface. The nurse's hand holding the sponge should be relaxed to avoid water running from the limb on to the bed.

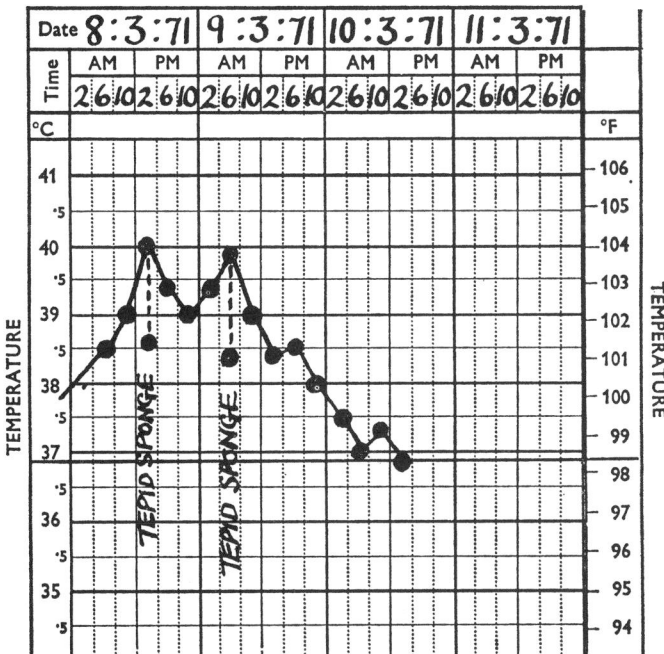

FIG. 64.

The arms are placed by the side of the child's trunk. The chest and abdomen are similarly treated, but the long sweeping strokes used for the arms are replaced by circular movements, as these are less disturbing to the child. The lower extremities are treated as for the arms, the long sweeping strokes extending from the groins to the toes. Special attention should be given to particularly warm areas of the lower limbs, such as the groins, between the thighs, and the popliteal spaces (flexures of the knees). The child is then turned on to his side, and long sweeping strokes are made slowly from the nape of the neck to the buttocks.

Talcum powder is applied to the skin of the back after ensuring that the film of water has evaporated. Barrier cream is applied to the buttocks if necessary and a clean bottom sheet and drawsheet are placed in position. The child is then turned on to his back and the bottom sheet and drawsheet are tucked in. The pillow case is changed and the child dressed in light cotton clothing. The body temperature is then recorded (FIG. 64).

The hair is combed to help to refresh the child and to avoid tangles which readily occur in febrile, restless children unless frequent care is given. Clean, light top bedclothes are positioned and the child is left comfortable. A cool drink may be appreciated.

The general condition of the child should be observed throughout the procedure, although untoward effects are not usual. Weakness or irregularity of the pulse, pallor or cyanosis, undue restlessness and shivering are signs indicating that the procedure should be discontinued until a doctor has been consulted.

Care of the Unconscious Child

Basic nursing care and observation of a very high standard are necessary for the survival of an unconscious child, unable to communicate his needs to the nurse.

Maintenance of a Clear Airway

A good airway is essential if anoxaemia is to be prevented.

POSITION OF THE PATIENT
The child is nursed in the lateral or semi-prone position with no pillow. In this position, accumulated mucus will drain from the side of the child's mouth and will not be inhaled. An artificial airway may be used to keep the tongue in position.

ATTENTION TO THE CHILD'S AIRWAY
Frequent naso- and oro-pharyngeal suction will clear the air passages of accumulated mucus. Physiotherapy accompanied by suction will ensure that the lower respiratory passages and lungs are kept clear.

ADMINISTRATION OF OXYGEN

Only when the air passages have been cleared is administration of oxygen of value. Cyanosis, should it occur, may be due to blockage of the air passages.

General Nursing Care

Meticulous nursing care aims at preventing complications to which the unconscious child is prone. Although for all other purposes the child is unconscious, cautious conversation is necessary in his presence. Hearing is the last sensation to be lost and the first to be regained and the child's conscious level may be just at this crucial point.

CLEANLINESS

General cleanliness is essential. A daily bed bath and frequent spongings ensure that the skin surface is kept fresh. Special attention is paid to the skin over pressure areas and to areas of the body where two skin surfaces are in close apposition. Silicone cream applied to the buttocks helps to preserve the skin which is frequently moistened by urine. With every change, the area should be washed and dried and a small quantity of cream applied. Frequent brushing of the hair will prevent formation of tangles, and long hair should be plaited or tied back.

CHANGE OF POSITION

A change of position at two-hourly intervals relieves areas of pressure, encourages equal expansion of the lungs and discourages stagnation of urine. Passive exercises encourage venous return to the heart and help to reduce muscle wastage. Correct positioning of the limbs is important. Foot-drop and hyperextension of joints can be prevented by the use of a bed-cradle, foot-board and splints and by placing the limbs in the optimum position.

CARE OF THE BLADDER AND BOWEL

Urinary incontinence is inevitable. Continuous bladder drainage via an indwelling urinary catheter may prove necessary if maceration of the skin is causing soreness, or if there is retention of urine detected by suprapubic palpation. Paul's tubing attached to the penis allows urine to drain into a receptacle at the side of the bed, obviating the need for catheterization. Constipation is avoided by insertion of a Dulcolax or glycerin suppository every second or third day.

FEEDING AND FLUID BALANCE

If the child is unconscious for a prolonged period of time, a naso-gastric tube is passed and a fluid diet of suitable quantity and quality is given. Alternatively, the doctor may decide that gastrostomy feeding is preferable. Meticulous care of the mouth is necessary to prevent complications.

CARE OF THE EYES

The unconscious child tends to lie with his eyes partly open and as the blink and corneal reflexes are usually absent, the surface becomes dry. Corneal ulcers may develop, resulting possibly in blindness. Four-hourly insertion of oily drops and/or covering the closed lids with tulle gras prevents this tragedy occurring.

Observation

Only by constant observation can the welfare of an unconscious child be guaranteed. Recording of clinical observations vary with the reason for loss of consciousness. For example, if the child has sustained a recent severe blow on the head, quarter to half-hourly recordings of his pulse and respiration rates, blood pressure, conscious level and pupil reactions would be maintained to help the doctor to make an assessment of his condition. Conversely, four-hourly recordings of temperature, pulse and respiration rates would be adequate for the child nearing the terminal stages of cerebral disease. A strict fluid balance record is necessary for all unconscious patients.

Care of the Paralyzed Child

Paralysis is loss of muscular power, with or without accompanying loss of sensation. Paralysis may be spastic, when the pyramidal or motor pathway from the cerebral hemisphere to the anterior horn cell is affected (upper motor neurones), or flaccid, when injury or disease involve the lower motor pathway, i.e. from the anterior horn cell to the peripheral motor unit (FIG. 65). Paresis is the term used to describe partial loss of muscle power.

The increasing number of children surviving with spina bifida and those suffering from cerebral palsy form a large proportion of the physically handicapped children requiring special care, treatment and education.

Spina Bifida

Spina bifida occurs about once in every 300 births. The sight of bedridden, grossly hydrocephalic, mentally retarded, paraplegic, incontinent children, creating increasing nursing problems as their head circumference increases, has been almost entirely replaced by the sight and sound of happy, mobile children of normal intellect, the majority of whom have come to terms with their disability in a sheltered environment. To the young student nurse the inevitable question 'is it worth it?' must come to mind as she prepares the distorted body of yet another newborn sufferer for the first of many operations. Only experience in a large unit will give her the answer she is seeking. A mere existence can now be made into a life worth living for those who respond well to treatment.

With the myelomeningocele repaired in the first hours of life, followed by early drainage of a developing hydrocephalus, the neurosurgical problems are usually controlled and frequently resolved in the first year of life. The problem of paraplegia, however, persists throughout life.

The function of the spinal cord is two-fold, simple reflex action and to convey nerve impulses to and from the brain. A myelomeningocele sited at the lumbar region results in loss of sensation and flaccid paralysis or paresis of the muscles of both legs. This may not be symmetrical and only involve some muscle groups.

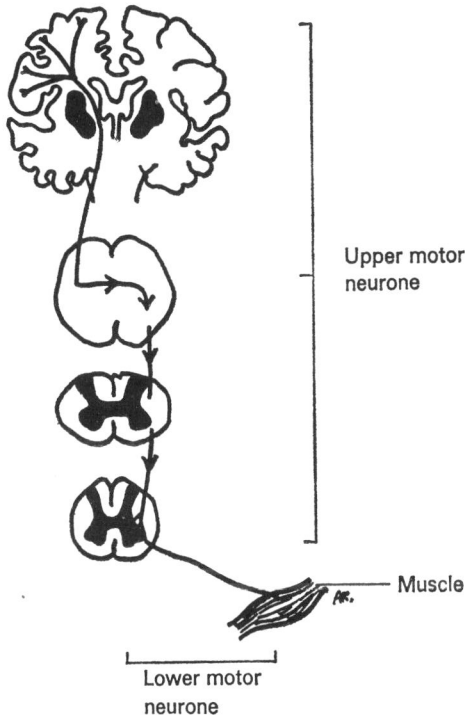

FIG. 65. The pathway for voluntary movement.

The unopposed pull of the unaffected muscle groups accounts for the characteristic flexor deformity of the hips and dislocation of the hip joints. Inactivity discourages calcification of the bones of the leg and painless fractures of the osteoporotic bones are not uncommon. The deformed legs and feet are usually wasted, cold and blue due to a diminished circulation and lack of activity. Loss of sensation may be partial or complete. The special care of these limbs involves care in handling, and avoiding pressure, application of heat and friction over rough surfaces.

Although paraplegic, there is no reason why these children should be confined to bed once they are convalescent. Even quite small children can be taught to manipulate a Chailey chariot, and older children should be supplied with a wheel chair of suitable size. Until the dislocated hip joints are reduced and the flexion deformity of the hips corrected, calipers and other walking-aids cannot be fitted. Bilaterai ilio-psoas muscle transplants are performed so that the non-affected flexor muscles of the hips are put to the more useful function of extending the legs. Further operative procedures may be necessary to stabilize the other joints of the lower limbs. Considerable care is necessary to ensure that walking appliances are well fitting, or painless pressure sores may develop.

Obesity greatly limits mobility and should be avoided by restricting unnecessary carbohydrate intake. Although the child may appear quite large as he sits up in bed, his legs are wasted and inactive, thus reducing his need for energy foods. A high fluid intake is encouraged to maintain a good flow of urine.

An equal, if not greater problem involves urinary incontinence and the risk of recurrent and persistent infection, resulting in permanent dilatation and damage to the kidneys. Careful observation should enable a nurse to answer the following questions:

i   Is urine passed as a continuous dribble?
ii   Does the infant have dry periods?
iii   Is the bladder palpable?
iv   Does gentle suprapubic pressure result in passage of a stream of urine?

Infants with a lumbar-sacral myelomeningocele constantly dribble urine from a toneless bladder via an incompetent urethral sphincter. Others with a slightly higher defect are able to retain urine in the toneless bladder as their urethral sphincter has some function. These children are in particular danger as the retained urine is only released as overflow and in states of stress, for example, when crying. The residual urine in either case is liable to infection, particularly in girls, and there is the added risk of cysto-ureteric reflux and inevitable kidney damage.

Most infants require expression of urine at regular, frequent intervals to prevent subsequent renal damage. At each feed-time, or two to four-hourly for older children, suprapubic pressure is applied by placing one or two hands over the lower abdomen. Little resistance is met as the abdominal muscles are invariably weak. The contained urine is thus expressed from the bladder by downward, backward pressure. The insensitive skin surrounding the genitalia requires meticulous care to prevent excoriation and ulceration.

Urinary tract diversions are performed on some of these children to safeguard the kidneys and to increase the child's confidence and social acceptance. A V-Y plasty of the bladder neck performed on some boys allows for free drainage of urine from the bladder into a penile appliance. For girls and some boys, the bladder is completely by-passed by construction of a double-barrelled cutaneous ureterostomy or transplanting the ureters into a resected loop of ileum opening on to the abdominal wall (ileal conduit). As long as a well-fitting appliance is firmly adhered round a well-positioned stoma, these children can experience freedom of activity and gain confidence for life in the community. An older child should be instructed in self-care and the parents of all children should be taught to care for the stoma and appliance. Basically, this is simple and is quickly mastered by the intelligent and well-initiated.

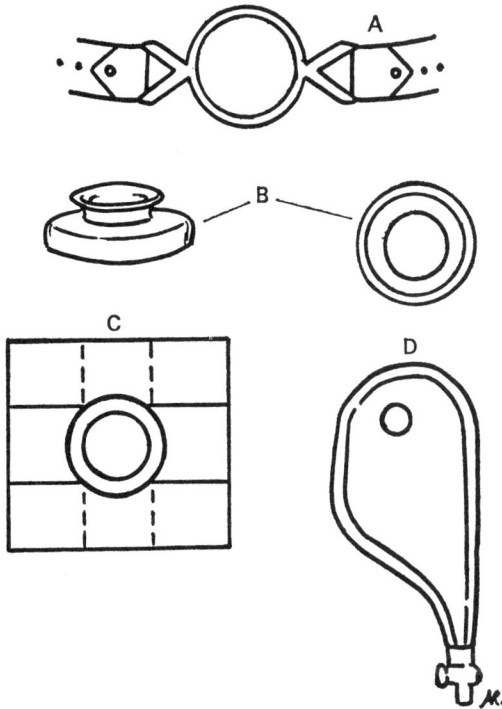

FIG. 66. Appliance for use with ileal conduit. A = Retaining ring and belt. B = Flange side-view and from above. C = Lengths of adhesive securing the flange in position. D = Rubber bag with tap.

A wide variety of appliances in a full range of sizes is available and the most suitable one chosen for each child. Correct fitting is vital, or leakage will occur. The appliance consists of a double-sided adhesive flange, collecting bag (these may form one piece) and a retaining ring and belt. Non-adhesive appliances have little place in paediatric work.

The skin surrounding the stoma must be clean and dry and may be painted with tincture of benzoin compound before attempting to apply the adhesive. Drainage from the stoma is continuous and, unless protected, may readily foul the area. Following application of the flange over the stoma, additional adhesive is applied in the form of lengths of waterproof adhesive tape. The collecting bag is fitted over the rim, the retaining ring threaded over the bag, and the belt adjusted (FIG. 66).

The bag should be emptied four-hourly to prevent detachment from the flange and changed each morning when the urine flow is minimal. The whole appliance is renewed as necessary and at least at weekly intervals to allow for skin care. The flange is removed from the skin with the liberal use of adhesive solvent and the area thoroughly washed with soap and water and dried before re-application is attempted.

With care, latex rubber collecting bags can be used for months. They should be washed well with soap and warm water while turned inside out, and dried. Odour can be eliminated by the use of a mild Milton solution 1:80, followed by thorough rinsing. Before storage, the bag should be sprinkled with talcum powder.

Fortunately, management of the bowel imposes less of a problem once a regular routine is established. The anal sphincter is incompetent, but as the rectum is also atonic, the child has a tendency to constipation. Faecal impaction is common and leads to soiling which makes life unpleasant and lowers morale. This can be prevented by the cautious use of aperients or suppositories. Manual evacuation of faeces may be necessary especially during infancy. Some older children can be taught to apply suprapubic pressure while sitting on the lavatory, following a hot meal or drink.

This is but a brief outline of the problems and management of spina bifida today, but it is sufficient to pose the following questions (which every nurse should be able to answer) concerning each individual child in her care.

1 Has he a valve?
2 Where does normal sensation end?
3 How extensive is his paraplegia?
4 What care does his bladder require:
    i   expression—at what intervals;
    ii urinary antiseptics;
    iii does he wear an appliance—what care does this require?
5 How is his bowel controlled:
    i   by diet alone;
    ii automatic daily evacuation;
    iii by the use of aperients;
    iv by the use of suppositories;
    v   manual evacuation?
6 What mobility aids has the child:
    i   walking aids;
    ii Chailey chariot;
    iii wheel chair?

Cerebral Palsy

Cerebral palsy affects about one child in 200 due to damage to the upper motor pathways of a developing brain, before, during or following birth. The affected limbs are usually spastic; one (monoplegia) or both limbs on the same side (hemiplegia) and in severe cases all limbs are paralysed (quadraplegia). Repetitive, slow, involuntary, writhing movements (athetosis) and inco-ordination of voluntary muscle activity (ataxia) are alternative or additional handicaps, due to damage to the basal ganglia and cerebellum respectively. The more severely affected experience frequent convulsions. Voluntary movement, posture and balance are all affected, delaying normal locomotor developmental progress. Sensation in the paralysed limbs is usually unaffected.

Cerebral palsy can usually be prevented but not cured. Careful observation and follow-up of 'at risk' infants ensures an early diagnosis and initiation of treatment. If behaviour is abnormal or the milestones of growth and development are not achieved within normal limits, brain damage producing cerebral palsy and/or mental retardation may well prove to be the cause. Infants and children who fall into one of the following categories are at particular risk. A large number, however, do not fall into any of these groups.

1 Those with a family history of congenital abnormality of the brain.
2 Those born following an assisted delivery or an abnormal presentation.
3 Those who were slow to respond to resuscitative measures at birth.
4 Those of low birth weight because they are more prone to:
    i   birth injury—cerebral haemorrhage;
    ii   cerebral anoxaemia;
    iii   hypoglycaemia;
    iv   severe and prolonged physiological jaundice.
5 Those who had Rhesus incompatibility. With prompt treatment, bile staining of the basal ganglia, due to hyperbilirubinaemia (kernicterus), is rarely seen today.
6 Those who have experienced metabolic disturbance, such as hypoglycaemia and phenylketonuria.
7 Those who have suffered from infections such as meningitis.

With physiotherapy and release of soft tissue deformity in selected cases, the child is taught to control and use his disabled limbs.

It is during admissions to hospital for routine dental and other minor surgery or orthopaedic procedures that the student nurse is likely to be confronted with a spastic child. The mother may feel able to spend most of the day with her child during his short stay in hospital, although this may prove an excellent opportunity for her to have a well-earned rest. The child is rarely in hospital long enough for an understanding nurse–patient relationship to be established.

The education of these children aims at achieving total independence. Equipment adapted to meet each individual child's needs assists in achieving this aim.

In a busy acute ward, time is precious and a young nurse will find that she can save time by attending to the child's nutritional and toilet needs herself, rather than awaiting his slow efforts. This may be to the advantage of the nurse, but to the utter humiliation of an intelligent spastic child. Opportunities for play and conversation are more important to the cerebral palsied child than to others who are contented and able to play with each other. Many of these children are of normal or superior intelligence despite their outward appearance and behaviour. Enunciation is frequently slow and expulsive, and outbursts of temper are provoked by sheer frustration at not being understood.

Listed below are a few questions which every nurse should be able to answer concerning each cerebral palsied child in her care. The list is by no means complete and parents and staff who have the care of these children will find helpful advice in the books listed at the end of this section.

1 How does he communicate—with words, gestures or sounds?
2 Can he sit unsupported?
3 In what position is it best to dress him—prone, supine or lateral?
4 Are there any feeding difficulties?
    i Is he able to take a normal diet for his age?
    ii In what position does he feed?
    iii Is he able to feed himself?
    iv Does he need modified cutlery and non-slip plates?
5 Has he control of bladder and bowel?
    i How frequently does he pass urine?
    ii Can he manage the lavatory unaided?
    iii Does he need special adjustments to the lavatory?
6 What mobility aids has he—boots, T-strap and iron, special chair with cut-out table and groin support?
7 Does he wear a hearing aid—does it work?
8 Does he wear spectacles—are they clean?
9 How does he like to amuse himself?

Acquired Paralysis

Unlike the cerebral palsied child, one who is paralyzed as the result of a head injury, encephalitis or poliomyelitis has had normal locomotor development interrupted.

As long as the spinal pathways remain intact, injury to the brain causes paralysis of the opposite side arm and/or leg and automatic reflex contraction of the muscles, with absence of co-ordinated voluntary movement. In poliomyelitis, the virus affects and may destroy the cell bodies of lower motor neurones—the anterior horn cells. Although sensation remains normal, the limb is hypotonic, wasted and motionless (flaccid paralysis).

Paralysed limbs are vulnerable to injury due to faulty positioning and pressure, both of which can be readily prevented by good nursing care and physio-therapy.

Care of the Child with Malignant Disease

Malignant disease is fortunately relatively uncommon in childhood, but never-theless accounts for a high number of deaths after the first year of life. Almost half of these children suffer from acute leukaemia; neuroblastoma (malignancy of autonomic nervous tissue), brain tumours—particularly medulloblastoma, nephroblastoma (Wilm's tumour) and teratomas arising from primitive tissues, account for most of the remainder. Childhood malignancy is particularly dis-tressing. Convincing the parents of their child's condition can naturally prove very difficult. Although the outlook is invariably gloomy, parents must be assured that everything possible will be done to relieve the condition and to make their child's remaining life as comfortable and happy as possible. Only on past experience will the doctor be able to answer the inevitable question—'how long will he live?' With the greater use of an increasing range of cytotoxic drugs, life may well be prolonged above his cautious expectation.

It is very important that the entire ward staff are aware of the exact informa-tion given by the doctor to the parents. Many questions will inevitably be asked of all grades of staff in an endeavour to obtain some ray of hope, and it is essential that mutual trust prevails. Fortunately, young patients rarely realize their predicament, but anxiety in the mother is quickly interpreted that all is not well. As near a normal life as possible should be encouraged, and over-indulgence avoided.

As in the adult field, paediatric malignant neoplasms may be treated by one, or combination of two, or all three of the following:

1 Wide surgical excision of the primary growth.
2 Radiotherapy.
3 Cytotoxic drug therapy.

Radiotherapy

Treatment in a radiotherapy unit demands a choice of alternatives, each child being individually assessed:

1 The child may receive his nursing care in a paediatric hospital and travel to the unit for his daily exposure. This may prove very satisfactory for com-paratively well children, but utterly exhausting to a weak, ill child.
2 An ideal situation is where the child is nursed in a paediatric unit of a district general hospital which has a radiotherapy unit.
3 Very few children may be cared for at home and visit the unit for daily exposure.

Each child has a carefully calculated amount of treatment divided between ten to twenty sessions. A fixation shell may be made for immobilizing the child and a strong sedative, e.g. rectal thiopentone may be prescribed to ensure that a small or unco-operative child remains still while exposed to the rays.

Beam direction therapy may be given as:

1 Deep X-ray.

2 Rays from a radio-active cobalt source (Orbitron).

3 Electrically generated X-rays of megavoltage range using a linear accelerator.

GENERAL EFFECTS OF RADIATION

The first few treatments may make the child appear less well, thus taxing the parents decision to accept the treatment advised. For their child to benefit, a full course of treatment must be given and the parents supported during the anxious early days.

1 Malaise and anorexia are common and are best overcome by rest. Visitors should sit quietly at the bedside rather than actively participate in diversional therapy. Extra nourishing fluids should be encouraged.

2 Nausea and vomiting may require anti-emetic drug relief.

3 Diarrhoea is common if the therapy is directed on the abdominal organs. Kaolin, prescribed for its soothing, constipating effect, is helpful.

4 A frequent blood cell count is made. Radiation depression of the bone marrow will result in a degree of anaemia, a reduced white cell count (leucopenia) and a low platelet level (thrombocytopenia).

LOCAL EFFECTS OF RADIATION

Apart from local transient early erythema, skin reactions are not seen. No real skin reactions are seen with use of the Orbitron or linear accelerator, but the radiotherapist's instructions regarding any special skin care should be carefully observed. Children undergoing deep X-ray therapy require special local skin care. The area should be kept dry and free from irritating clothing and other forms of irritation, as for example, sunlight. Starch (note, not zinc and starch) powder applied two or three times daily is comforting. The special care of the skin should continue for a further four weeks on completion of treatment.

Alopecia is inevitable if the brain is irradiated. This may prove most distressing to both parents and child, in spite of having been forewarned. They should be assured that the hair will grow again and a wig may be provided when the child goes home.

Cytotoxic Drug Therapy

Cytotoxic drugs cause malaise and anorexia, depression of the bone marrow and alopecia, demanding sympathetic nursing care and treatment as described above. The child may have to be isolated and barrier nursed for a short period of time while the white cell count is dangerously low.

On completion of treatment, and indeed before if his condition will allow, early discharge into the home environment is encouraged and willingly accepted by most parents.

Care of the Child with a Skin Disorder

Unfortunately, there is no rapid cure for the more common skin affections of childhood such as eczema and psoriasis, but much can be done to prevent exacerbation of symptoms. Prolonged preventive and curative treatment can prove tedious, and the parents of these children need much help and encouragement to continue the treatment ordered by the dermatologist.

General Care of the Child

Irritation may be intense and measures must be adopted to reduce irritation and to break the 'scratching cycle'.

1   Extremes of temperature should be avoided, especially over-heating. The child should sleep in a well-ventilated room with adequate, but not excessive light bedclothes.

2   Clothing should be light and non-irritating. A cotton shirt worn next to the skin is soothing. In cold weather a jumper can be worn over a long sleeve shirt so that the shirt collar covers the woollen neck of the jumper. At night, cotton pyjamas are preferable to nightdresses, especially if the pyjama legs are extended to include the feet.

3   A small child will use every available means to relieve his irritation, and only effective restraint will prevent him reducing his skin to a raw surface. Finger nails must be kept short and clean and cotton mittens worn, especially at night. Elbow restraint may have to be used.

4   During the acute stages of illness, it is necessary in some cases to ensure rest and sleep by means of sedatives, especially at night. Promethazine hydrochloride (Phenergan) may be prescribed for its anti-pruritic and sedative action.

5   Diversional therapy is essential. A bored child has nothing better to do than to relieve his irritation by scratching. Diversion is preferable to punishment, although bribery or reward for not scratching are best avoided as a young child may well use scratching as an attention-seeking device.

The majority of children with skin affections are not infectious, but are most susceptible to cross-infection. For this reason, the child may well be nursed in an isolation unit or in a special ward reserved for such patients when confinement to hospital proves necessary. Skin infections are highly contagious and require observance of strict isolation precautions.

Local Care of the Skin

Topical treatment ordered by the dermatologist is carried out by the nursing staff whose responsibility it is to educate the parents before their child goes home. Specific treatment in the form of medicated baths, lotions, creams, ointments, pastes or powders, may be prescribed containing antiseptic, antibiotic, fungicidal, anti-pruritic, anti-inflammatory or astringent medicaments.

1 *Baths.* Soap is irritating and should never be used. Bath water containing the prescribed solution, such as bath-oil, emulsifying ointment or antiseptic, should be of sufficient depth to cover the skin lesions and be just comfortably warm. Baths are given daily, or twice daily, as prescribed by the doctor, and the skin is patted dry, not rubbed.

2 *Hair care.* Hair should be kept as short as possible to make management easier. The hair is washed daily and rinsed thoroughly to ensure that all the prescribed shampoo is removed. The hair is then combed with a metal tooth comb to remove scales and crusts.

3 *Lotions* are medicaments in water or water and spirit, and are used on acutely inflamed areas for their anti-pruritic and soothing effect. They may be applied as wet dressings, or dabbed on to the skin lesions, as for example, calamine lotion in the treatment of sunburn and nettle-rash.

4 *Creams*, ointments and pastes should be applied gently and evenly with the fingers whenever possible. Contamination of the container is avoided by removing the mixture with a spatula. Creams are medicaments in an aqueous or oily base and are prescribed for use on less inflamed skin. To increase their effectiveness, the cream (usually containing a steroid) may be applied fairly liberally and then covered with a close-fitting occlusive polythene cover which is maintained in position and made airtight with Sellotape strips. Subsequent maceration of the skin results in greater penetration of the drug.

5 *Ointments* consist of medicaments in a thick, greasy base. Absorption is more limited than in either lotions or creams and their use is confined to the treatment of chronic inflammatory disorders where the skin is thick, dry and cracked.

6 *Pastes* are thicker and provide a protective layer on the skin, whilst remaining more porous than ointment. Zinc oxide or coal tar pastes may be prescribed as medicated cotton bandages. These are particularly useful in the treatment of eczema where they are maintained in position with Tubegauz and changed once or twice a week. The occlusive nature of the dressings discourages scratching and provides a valuable means of breaking the 'scratching cycle'.

7 *Powders* are a useful means of applying medications to intertriginous areas—groins and axillae—and may be applied with an insufflator or perforated carton.

8 *Poultices.* A starch poultice is still one of the most effective methods for removal of dried crusts in such conditions as impetigo.

Starch Poultice

The starch is prepared to a soft consistency and applied to the affected area where it sets as a jelly surrounding and softening the crusts, so making them easier to remove.

REQUIREMENTS
Tray.
Starch.
Cold water.
Boiling water.
Measure.
Tablespoon.
Teaspoon.
Wooden spoon.
Mixing bowl.
Poultice board.
Palette knife or metal spatula.
Old linen or lint.
Cotton wool.
Bandage or Tubegauz.
Vaseline.
Scissors.

PREPARATION
To make a poultice for application to the scalp, 1 rounded tablespoon of starch is mixed to a smooth paste with 30–60ml of cold water. Approximately 400ml of boiling water is poured on to the paste as it is slowly stirred. The starch will be seen to thicken and the white paste changes to a 'dirty' opacity of thicker consistency. Thickening of the mixture will proceed as the starch molecules burst. Boiling water is poured slowly on to the starch, while stirring briskly until the mixture is of soft consistency.

The old linen or lint is cut to the required size and moistened to encourage the starch mixture to adhere. Using the palette knife or spatula, the starch is spread evenly over the surface of the material to the required thickness. The thickness of the poultice depends on the depth of the scabs, which should be completely surrounded and covered by the starch when the poultice is in position. This usually means that the poultice is spread to 1–2cm ($\frac{1}{2}$–$\frac{3}{4}$ inch) of thickness. The poultice is allowed to cool and applied to the affected area when almost cold.

APPLICATION
Vaseline is applied to the perimeter of the affected area to prevent discomfort from the drying starch. The poultice is applied and covered with a thin layer of

cotton wool to absorb excess moisture from the poultice. The poultice is held in place for six to twelve hours by a cotton bandage or Tubegauz.

REMOVAL

The poultice is removed very gently and slowly, easing the loose scabs with sterile dissecting forceps so that as many as possible are removed with the poultice. Any bleeding points are mopped with wool swabs.

For Further Reading

BLENCOWE S. M. (1969). *Cerebral Palsy and the Young Child*, 1st edition. E. & S. Livingstone, Edinburgh.

BOWLEY A. H. and GARDNER L. (1968). *The Young Handicapped Child*, 2nd edition. E. & S. Livingstone, Edinburgh.

FINNIE N. R. (1968). *Handling the Young Cerebral Palsied Child at Home*, 1st edition. William Heinemann (Medical Books) Ltd., London.

LORBER J. *Your Child with Spina Bifida. Your Child with Hydrocephalus.* Published on behalf of the Association for Spina Bifida and Hydrocephalus.

CHAPTER SEVENTEEN

Orthopaedic Nursing

Some understanding of the more common devices used in the treatment of disorders of the locomotor system is necessary if the learner is to benefit from a period of time spent in an orthopaedic unit.

Orthopaedic devices are used:

1   In the prevention of bony and soft tissue deformity.
2   To correct congenital or acquired bony, soft tissue or joint deformity.
3   To immobilize an area:
     i   for the fixation of broken bone ends while allowing for free movement elsewhere;
    ii   to rest a diseased or painful bone or joint;
   iii   for elbow restraint;
   iv   for post-operative fixation;
    v   to maintain a joint in position, e.g. the hip joint in the treatment of congenital dislocation.
4   To restore function by gradual encouragement of joint movement.

Immobilization may be achieved by the use of:

   i   plaster of Paris and Plastazote (Smith & Nephew Ltd.) casts and splints;
  ii   traction devices;
 iii   splints;
 iv   internal fixation.

Plaster of Paris

Commercially produced calcium sulphate (gypsum) impregnated open-weave cloth is available in bandages of various widths and as slabs. These must be stored in a dry area. On wetting, a chemical reaction takes place (producing heat) and the powder sets and hardens as a strong, durable homogenous mass to fulfil the function for which it was intended without being excessively cumbersome.

Application of Plaster of Paris

REQUIREMENTS
Trolley.
Plaster bandages and slabs as required.
Tubegauz or stockinet.
Wool bandages.
Orthopaedic felt.
Waterproof protection for the
    bed.
    operator.
    floor.
Bucket of tepid water.
Flannel and towel.
Scissors.
Plaster knife.

METHOD
Unless the limb is injured, it should be washed with soap and water, dried, and talcum powder applied. A wool bandage is applied to an injured limb, otherwise it is ensheathed in a single layer of Tubegauz. Bony prominences are protected with orthopaedic felt or wool bandage. It is important that the area is retained in the desired position while the plaster of Paris is applied, otherwise the plaster will crack and disintegrate, or crease and cause pressure sores.

Each plaster bandage is immersed in the bucket of water until all bubbles have ceased to rise. On removal, surplus water is expressed and the wet bandage is applied smoothly and evenly. A slab of four to six layers is usually applied first and secured in position with simple spirals of plaster bandage, the redundant folds being moulded into the plaster slab. Before the final layer is put on, the ends of the Tubegauz or wool bandage are turned over at top and bottom to neaten the edges and to avoid chafing. Finally, the cast is rubbed over to give a smooth polished finish. Plaster drips are removed from the child's skin. When the cast is dry, shellac varnish may be applied to the napkin area of the plaster to help to prolong its useful life.

IMMEDIATE AFTER CARE
Although plaster of Paris sets within a few minutes of application, it takes twenty-four to forty-eight hours to dry. During this time, the cast should be exposed to the air and the child turned four-hourly. No artificial means of heat should be used. Cracks and dents in the plaster must be prevented by careful turning of the child in a hip spica and supporting a plastered lower limb on a pillow to raise the heel off the bed. To avoid dents, a wet plaster should be held in the palm of the hand and not the finger tips.

Exposed extremities of the plastered limb—fingers and toes—should be carefully observed for signs of impairment of the circulation:

1 *Colour*. The nail normally blanches on pressure and the colour quickly returns when pressure is released. If the venous return is obstructed, return of colour is slow.

2 *Swelling* of a temporary nature is common following injury or surgery. Elevation of the limb may help to reduce congestion, i.e. the foot of the bed may be elevated if a lower limb is affected, or an upper limb may be suspended in a roller-towel hung on an infusion stand placed in a convenient position at the side of the bed (FIG. 67). Swelling associated with discolouration of the extremity is highly suggestive of venous obstruction.

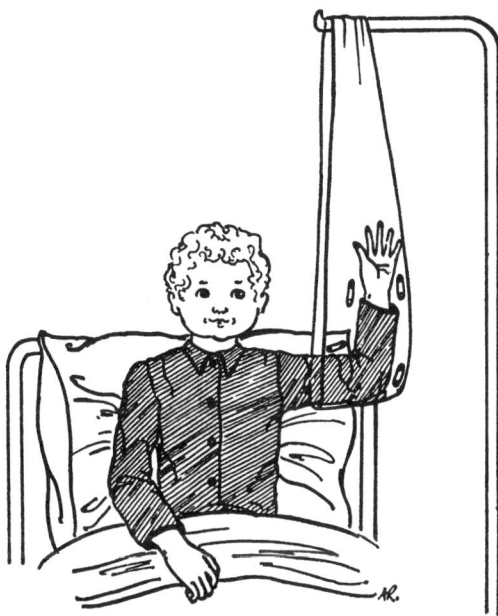

FIG. 67. Elevation of an arm with the use of a roller-towel, safety-pins and infusion stand.

3 *Pain*. Numbness or 'pins and needles' are due to nerve pressure or circulatory obstruction.

4 *Temperature*. The exposed digits may often feel cold. Gentle massage and exercise may improve the circulation and a sock or mitten may be worn. Presence of a cold, white extremity with a poor response to digital pressure is very serious as the arterial blood supply is obstructed.

If any of the above signs of circulatory impairment are found, the doctor must be informed *immediately* and preparations should be made for him to split (bi-valve) the plaster.

SUBSEQUENT CARE

The plaster should be kept dry and inspected daily for softening and cracks. No complaint of pain or discomfort should be ignored; a pressure sore may be developing and the doctor will decide either to cut a window or to remove the plaster to investigate and treat the underlying cause. Foreign bodies, either intentionally or accidentally pushed between the plaster cast and the skin, produce pressure sores, causing much discomfort. The child should be encouraged to exercise all joints above and below the cast.

ADVICE GIVEN TO THE PARENTS

Written instructions should be given to the mother before taking her child home following plaster application. She must be told to allow the plaster to dry naturally, not to let the child sit in front of the fire, and to avoid denting a new cast by disallowing her child to stand on a foot plaster for at least two days. The plaster must be kept dry. She must be instructed to bring her child back to the hospital immediately should the fingers or toes become discoloured, painful or swollen, or if he complains of pain or the cast becomes soft or cracked.

REMOVING A PLASTER CAST

Plaster of Paris may be removed using special plaster shears or an electric plaster saw with an oscillating cutting edge. Both instruments are frightening to the small child, and much tact and reassurance is necessary to obtain co-operation, even from a bigger child.

Using plaster shears. The plaster should be cut over soft tissues, the longer, shallow lower blade being advanced slowly as the shorter, upper blade takes small bites with each cut.

Using a plaster saw. As a precaution, a metal strip may be advanced under the plaster down the line of division and the plaster bi-valved over soft tissues, thus avoiding the bony prominences.

Following removal of the cast, the limb should be gently washed and dried and desquamation (peeling) treated by the local application of olive oil.

Plastazote is a comparatively new splinting material made of polyethylene foam. When pre-heated according to the manufacturer's recommendations, the sheets of foam can be moulded to fit the contours of the body to provide a light-weight splint.

Traction

Traction means 'pull, draw or haul' and to pull or apply traction effectively there must be something to pull against—this is called counter-traction.

Although traction can be exerted through bone and pulp, skin traction is used almost exclusively in childhood.

In this method adhesive (Elastoplast extension plaster with a crosswise, but not lengthwise stretch) or Ventfoam material is applied to the skin surface, then a pull is exerted down the long axis of the material. This pull is transmitted from the material and skin to the underlying soft structures and bone.

The amount of pull that can be applied using skin traction is limited. Skeletal traction may, therefore, be used to overcome the greater muscular spasm of adults.

Application of Skin Traction

REQUIREMENTS
Trolley.

FOR PREPARATION OF THE LIMB
Tray.
Razor and blade in a receiver.
Soap and warm water.
Gauze swabs.
Dressing forceps in a receiver.
Gallipot for tincture of benzoin compound.
Protection for the bed.
Receptacle for soiled swabs.

FOR APPLICATION OF SKIN TRACTION
Tape measure.
Elastoplast extension plaster 5cm (2 inches) or 7·5cm (3 inches) wide.
Lampwick webbing ⎱ or wooden spreader and extension cord.
Needle and strong thread ⎰
Scissors.
Felt strip(s) 4cm or 1½ inches wide.
Crêpe bandages.
Narrow adhesive tape.

Alternatively, skin traction kits are available which greatly simplify both preparation and application of skin traction. These consist of a length of extension plaster incorporating a spreader and cords. The central portion is lined with soft plastic foam for protection of the malleoli and the adhesive surfaces are covered with plastic protective backing, making handling easier.

ADDITIONAL REQUIREMENTS

FOR APPLICATION OF A THOMAS'S SPLINT
Thomas's splint of correct size.

Lengths of flannel for slings.
Safety-pins.
Cotton wool.
Crêpe bandages 10cm (4 inches), 15cm (6 inches) wide.
Frame on which to rest distal end of splint, *or*
Additional cord
Bed-blocks } for fixation to bed end, *or*
Additional cord
Pulleys
Weight } for suspending immobilized limb.
Bed-elevator

FOR TRACTION ON AN ABDUCTION FRAME
Special frame or splint.
Additional crêpe bandages 10cm (4 inches)/15cm (6 inches) wide.

FOR GALLOWS TRACTION
Additional cord.
Overhead beam with cross bar.

FOR PUGH TRACTION
Additional cord.
Pulley attachment at end of the bed.
Weights.
Bed-elevator.

FOR HAMILTON RUSSELL TRACTION
Overhead beam.
Spreader with pulley attachment.
Additional cord, pulleys and weights.
Flannel sling.
Bed-elevator.

Preparation of Skin Traction

USING LAMPWICK
A suitable width of Elastoplast extension plaster is chosen according to the size of the limb; the skin extensions are applied to the medial and lateral aspects of the limb with no overlap. Two lengths are prepared; the length for the lateral aspect of the leg must extend from the lateral malleolus to the greater trochanter,

and for the medial extension, from the medial malleolus to the adductor tendon in the groin.

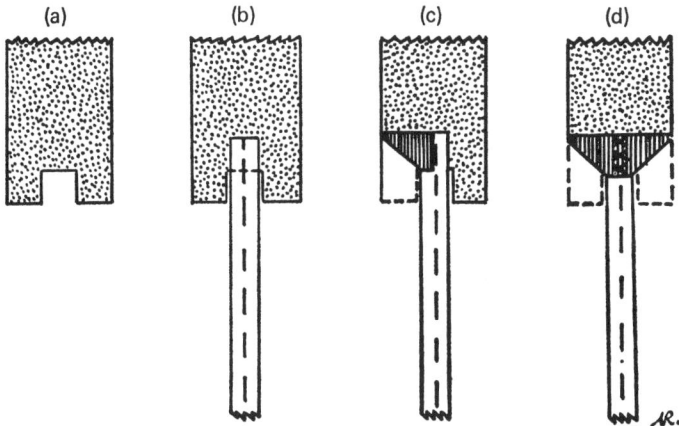

FIG. 68. Insertion of lampwick webbing into extension Elastoplast.

For each extension, a small postage stamp sized square is cut out from the centre of the free-end (a) and a 30–45cm or 12–18 inches length of lampwick is placed with 4cm or 1½ inches of its length lying on the adhesive surface (b). The Elastoplast is turned over to enclose the lampwick (c) which is firmly secured by means of centrally inserted cross-stitches penetrating all layers (d) (FIG. 68).

USING A WOODEN SPREADER

A suitable width of Elastoplast extension plaster is chosen according to the size of the limb. One continuous length is necessary to extend from the greater trochanter laterally to the adductor tendon in the groin medially. As the length must allow for inclusion of the spreader and for full plantar flexion at the ankle joint, 10–20cm or 4–8 inches is added to the length of both the medial and lateral skin extensions given above.

The estimated length of extension plaster is unrolled on to a long, clean surface (a). The wooden spreader is placed in a central position with its two holes along the long axis of the plaster (b). A second shorter length of extension plaster is cut to line the loop which is to extend beyond the child's foot (c). This should be of sufficient length to protect the malleoli at either side of the free loop. The two adhesive surfaces are then stuck together (FIG. 69).

A length of sash cord is threaded through the holes made through the extension plaster covering the spreader. The skin extension is ready for use and care must be taken to see that the long lengths of adhesive surface do not become stuck together.

(a)

(b)

(c)

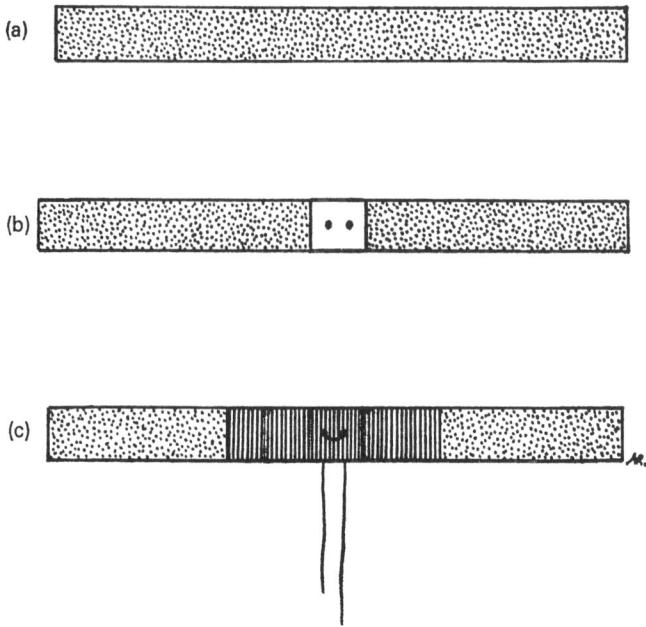

FIG. 69. Preparation of Elastoplast skin traction with the use of a wooden spreader.

PREPARATION OF THE CHILD

The co-operation of an older child is sought by simple explanation of the procedure. Most bigger children, unless ill, are intrigued by the whole procedure. A sedative is necessary for a small child.

The bedclothes are protected while the medial and lateral aspects of the limb are shaved, if necessary, and painted or sprayed with protective tincture of benzoin compound. A second nurse is necessary to support the limb until the lotion is dry. The malleoli are protected from any friction which may occur by securing a strip of felt neatly around the ankle.

Application of Skin Traction

Two nurses are necessary for this procedure, one supports the child's elevated leg while her colleague carefully applies the prepared skin extensions.

ELASTOPLAST SKIN TRACTION

The prepared extension for the lateral aspect of the limb is applied down an imaginary line between the external malleolus and the greater trochanter of the femur. The plaster is stretched sideways to mould to the contours of the limb, avoiding creases and folds. If the skin extension will not lie flat at the knee joint, small oblique downward directed 'nicks' will facilitate moulding. If a single length of extension plaster is being applied, the second nurse holds the spreader parallel to the sole of the foot while the medial skin extension is similarly applied between the internal malleolus and the adductor tendon of the groin, avoiding overlap at the back or front of the leg. The limb is then bandaged, a simple spiral and figure-of-eight method being used, leaving the patella exposed. The bandage ends are secured by stitching or with lengths of adhesive tape.

VENTFOAM SKIN TRACTION

This method is suitable for temporary traction and where there is allergy to adhesives. No prior preparation of the limb is necessary. The ventilated cotton-backed foam rubber extension strip is laid on either side of the limb, leaving a loop of 10–15cm or 4–6 inches beyond the sole of the foot. The extension is then secured to the limb, using crêpe bandages. The bandage is begun by making three turns around the ankle before catching the Ventfoam in the following turn. The bandage is continued up the leg, leaving the patella exposed. The metal spreader is then placed at the end of the free loop so that it is parallel with the sole of the foot.

Fixing the Traction

Traction may be fixed or balanced.
i Fixed traction is exerted on an area lying between two fixed points. A typical example is in the use of a Thomas's splint—the tapes secured to the distal W-shaped end of the splint exert traction, while counter-traction is exerted by the pressure of the padded ring on the prominent ischial tuberosity of the innominate bone.
ii For balanced or sliding traction, there must be two opposing forces which balance and are mobile. In order to achieve this balance, the two forces must be separated by a raised structure. The foot of the bed is therefore elevated. The weight hanging on a cord running over a pulley attached to the end of the bed exerts traction, while the child's tendency to slide towards the bed head exerts counter-traction.

APPLICATION OF A THOMAS'S SPLINT

This splint is used extensively to exert fixed traction to the leg. The child must be carefully measured as it is essential that a splint of correct size is used; if the ring is too small, much discomfort and pressure will result; if too large, immobilization will not be achieved. To estimate the size of ring required, a tape-measure is placed obliquely around the thigh, using the adductor tendon in the groin, the greater trochanter of the femur and the lower border of the ischial tuberosity of the innominate bone as landmarks. The necessary length is measured from the greater trochanter to the base of the heel laterally, and from the adductor tendon to the base of the heel medially. An additional 15–30cm or 6–12 inches is added to each length to allow for full plantar flexion.

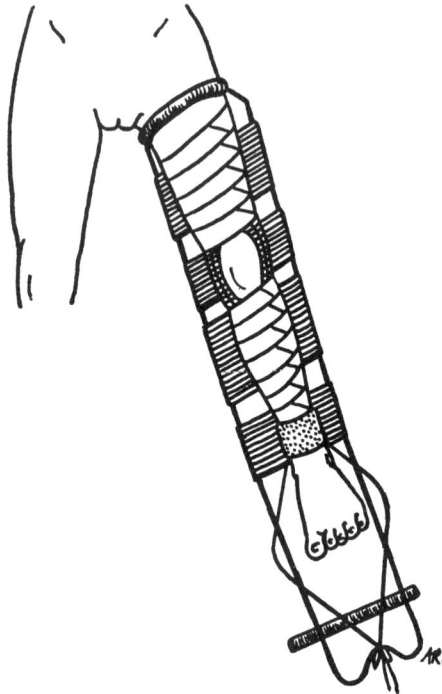

FIG. 70. Fixed skin traction using a Thomas's splint. Note the neutral position of the limb, exposure of the patella and slight abduction of the hip joint.

Four flannel slings are placed along the medial bar before the prepared limb is gently slid through the ring of the Thomas's splint. After checking that the ring fits snugly against the ischial tuberosity posteriorly and is not pressing hard into the groin, the slings are secured in position. One is placed under the knee; a pad of cotton wool allows for a 5° flexion of the knee joint. A second is placed beneath the ankle, a third supports the calf, and a fourth is placed beneath the fracture site. Cotton wool may be placed under the fracture site to achieve normal anterior bowing of the femur. All the slings are secured to allow the limb to be comfortably cradled. The extension tapes or cords are then tied securely to the W-shaped end of the Thomas's splint, which is then rested on a small bed-block.

Before securing the leg to the splint with a crêpe bandage, it must be checked to ensure:

i   that the ring is not pressing too hard into the groin;

ii that the slings have maintained their position;

iii that the leg is lying in neutral rotation with the patella and toes pointing directly upwards.

If instructed by the doctor, the traction tapes or cords may be tightened by rotating a metal or strong wooden windlass from medial to lateral bars, thus twisting and tightening the tapes to achieve the required traction (FIG. 70).

The splint end may be maintained on a bed-block to prevent the heel resting on the bed, or it may be secured to the end of the bed and the foot of the bed elevated, or additional cord attached to the W-shaped end is passed over a pulley attached to the elevated bed-end and a weight secured. The last two methods have the advantage that groin pressure can be relieved as the child slides away from the continual ring pressure. Whichever method is used, the affected hip should be moderately abducted to assist essential toilet procedures.

A bed-cradle is used to support the weight of the bedclothes and the child is allowed to adopt a sitting position during the day. Nursing the child in a recumbent position at night discourages flexion deformity of the hip.

FOR TRACTION ON AN ABDUCTION FRAME

An abduction frame is used in the treatment of a dislocated hip, to abduct the limbs gradually from the neutral position until each hip is abducted 90°, prior to plaster fixation.

Skin extensions are applied to both limbs and the extension cords or tapes secured to the W-shaped metal ends of the leg splints before securing each leg to the splint using crêpe bandages.

GALLOWS TRACTION

This is a simple, effective means of achieving balanced traction for a small child with a fractured shaft of femur. It has additional uses:

i   to elevate the legs to aid reduction of an incarcerated inguinal hernia;

ii to temporarily relieve a sacral pressure sore;

iii to allow a burn of the buttocks to heal.

Skin extensions are applied to both legs and the extension cords secured to an overhead cross-bar, so that the legs are maintained in neutral rotation and at right angles to the trunk with the buttocks clear of the mattress. If traction is to be maintained, the buttocks must be well clear of the mattress at all times (FIG. 71). This method of traction is, therefore, limited to the 'napkin age group' as resting a child on a bedpan, even for a short period of time, defeats the purpose of the traction.

Too much bulky material between the legs should be avoided and the child is kept warm by securing a soft blanket around his legs.

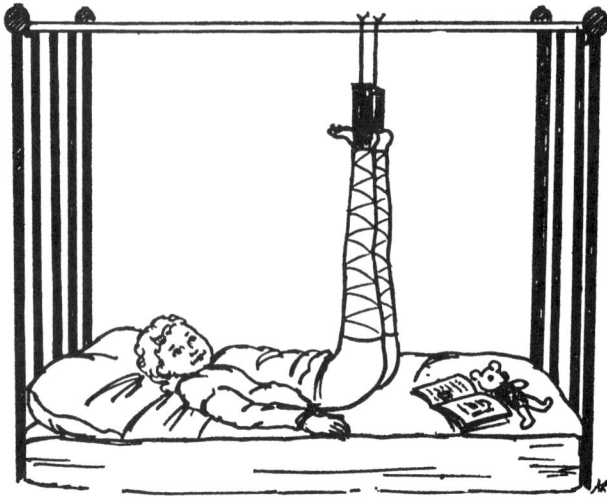

FIG. 71. Gallows traction.

PUGH TRACTION

This is a simple form of balanced traction for one or both legs and is a useful method of resting a painful hip and reducing muscular spasm in the hip region.

Skin extensions are applied to one or both legs. A length of extension cord fixed to a spreader is passed over a pulley attached to the elevated bed-end, and a weight is secured.

Balanced traction is only maintained by free-hanging of the weights counterbalanced by the recumbent position adopted by the child. If either is reduced, the balance is upset.

HAMILTON RUSSELL TRACTION

This is a more complicated form of balanced traction necessitating one length of cord passing over four freely moving pulleys. A weight is secured to the cord at the end of the bed (FIG. 72).

One end of the cord is placed through the eyelets of a flannel sling placed beneath the knee joint. The cord is then passed over a pulley placed directly above the patella and so to a second pulley on the bed-end, lying in line with the long axis of the leg. The cord is then passed around the pulley attached to the spreader and back to a second pulley positioned immediately below the first on the bed-end. The weight ordered by the doctor is attached to the free-end of the cord and the bed is elevated. The child can be nursed on several pillows without upsetting the balance.

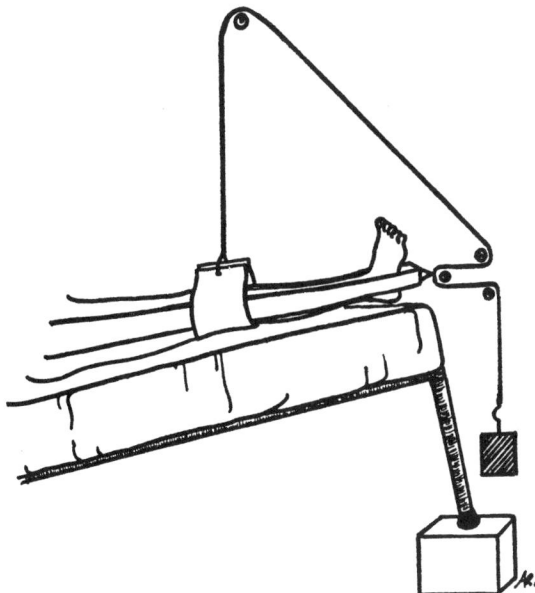

Fig. 72. Hamilton Russell balanced traction.

Removing Skin Traction

Traction on the skin reduces its vitality, consequently, great care should be taken in removing the plaster to prevent the delicate skin surface being torn. Adhesive remover is used on a cotton wool ball and the skin is gently released from the adhesive tape. The exposed leg is gently washed and dried and olive oil is applied to restore the normal texture of the skin.

Inspection and Maintenance of Traction

Only by frequent inspection of the splinted limb will complications be prevented. Each time the child's toilet needs are attended to, the limb should be inspected and foot exercises encouraged. Each day the bandages should be removed to allow a detailed inspection of the limb.

The foot must be inspected for discolouration and the presence of oedema and tested for sensation and tone. If the bandages are too tightly applied, circulation may be impeded. Pressure applied to the lateral popliteal nerve will cause tingling, loss of sensation and subsequent foot-drop.

The limb should remain in neutral rotation and be inspected for signs of pressure, especially under the ring of a Thomas's splint and over the Achilles tendon and malleoli. Irritation under the skin extension should not be ignored. This may be due to wrinkling or loosening of the adhesive, or to an allergic response to adhesive. If all is satisfactory, the limb is bandaged, using fresh bandages as necessary.

Balanced traction should be checked to ensure that the balance is maintained and all members of the ward team should be instructed in the necessity for this. A squeaking pulley is annoying and easily remedied with a little oil. Worn extension cord may be renewed while traction is maintained by a second person.

To reduce muscle wasting during immobilization, the child is taught to do static contraction of the quadriceps muscle. After removal of the skin traction, formal exercises are given by the physiotherapist until near normal activity is attained. Between the physiotherapist's visits, the nursing staff must encourage the child within his limited capacity. Small children need little rehabilitation.

Splints

Splints may be made of plaster of Paris, Plastazote, polyvinyl or chamois leather covered metal. Few splints are reserved exclusively for complete body restraint, the majority immobilizing just one or two joints. The two methods of immobilization already mentioned are concerned mainly with restricting a child's activities; splints, however, often immobilize to encourage mobility. A walking caliper is an excellent example of this.

Detail regarding application of the wide variety of splints is beyond the scope of this textbook and the student is advised to refer to books listed at the end of this chapter. Nursing care is essentially as for other forms of immobilization, with emphasis on the prevention of pressure sores and chafing. Appliances should be checked daily for wear and tear.

Nursing Care of the Immobilized Child

The nursing care of an immobilized child is basically the same whether he is immobilized in plaster of Paris, on traction, or splinted. An appreciation of the special needs of children on long-term immobilization is necessary.

A children's orthopaedic ward resounds with the chatter and clatter of reasonably healthy children, and ideally such children should be nursed away from an acute surgical ward where a rapid turnover of short-stay patients, or a preponderance of ill children, makes great demands on the ward staff. Team work is essential, the doctors and nurses, school teachers, occupational therapists, and 'playladies' working together to ensure that each child's physical, mental, social and educational needs are fully met.

A child quickly adapts to the inconvenient position in which he may find himself. Carefully positioned mirrors will allow him to watch the activities of others. Independence should be encouraged and some method can usually be found to overcome feeding and toilet difficulties. Food should be nourishing and digestible and excessive amounts of carbohydrate should be avoided. A good fluid intake will help to discourage constipation and encourage a good urine output, thus preventing consequent pooling of calcium in the pelvis of the kidney and the formation of stones.

Soiling or contamination of bandages, plaster or splints with urine can usually be avoided by taking care in the administration and removal of bedpans and urinals. Constant supervision is necessary until an older child learns how to cope with this difficulty.

All basic nursing care is necessary, with special attention paid to pressure areas. These need frequent attention and must be inspected at least every four hours for signs of pressure and for gentle massage. To encourage a restful night, the bed requires re-making at the end of the day's activities. This may be made up over a bed-cradle or divided into two packs. Nightwear is best changed for day clothes each morning (if at all possible) and the lower trunk protected with divided pants.

Special occasions call for celebration and help to maintain the high morale of these immobilized children.

For Further Reading

ASTON J. N. (1967). *A Short Textbook of Orthopaedics and Traumatology*, 1st edition. The English Universities Press Ltd., London.
FISK G. R. and WILKINSON M. C., (1966). *Orthopaedics for Nurses*, 2nd edition, Faber and Faber.
NICHOLL K. B. 'Understanding Traction'. *Nursing Times Reprint*, 1963.
POWELL, M. (1968). *Orthopaedic Nursing*, 6th edition. E. and S. Livingstone, Edinburgh.

CHAPTER EIGHTEEN

Caring for Children with Mental Disorders

Illness.
A state of disordered mentality
in an apparently previously
normal child, often amenable
to curative treatment.

Subnormality.
A state of arrested or incomplete
development of the mind of such
a degree that the child will
respond to medical treatment or
special care and training.
    I.Q. 55–70

Severe Subnormality.
A state of arrested or incomplete
development of the mind of such
a degree that the child will be
incapable of living an independent
life or of guarding himself
against serious exploitation.
    I.Q. Below 55

Fig. 73. Classification of Mental Disorder.

Care of the Emotionally Disturbed Child

contributed by Frances M. Wheeler, S.R.N., R.S.C.N.

This section aims at introducing some of the basic principles of child psychiatric nursing and is concluded with two patient care studies to demonstrate application of these principles:

1 Establishment of relationships.
2 Definition of the child's needs.
3 Meeting his needs.
4 Involvement of the staff in the recognition that management is determined by the child's needs and not their own.

Because this type of nursing is arduous, it is essential that the tensions which arise in a working team are minimized by good communication between all

348

members, promoted by frequent ward meetings attended by the whole team—psychiatrists, psychologists, psychiatric social workers, nurses and school teachers.

To increase the understanding of the discipline and to help the child, it is necessary to regard the child as an organism, developing in biological, psychological and social areas.

Biological. A detailed history is taken and a full physical examination is carried out and the findings assessed, bearing in mind the details of pregnancy, labour and birth as given by the mother. An examination of the central nervous system may reveal a degree of brain damage often associated with a clinical picture of a slow and clumsy or overactive child whose mother says 'he never stays still for a moment'.

Psychological. This area deals with the child's personality and intelligence. There are many tests to assess the intelligence of a child and where discrepancies occur, further tests may clarify areas in which the child may be malfunctioning. For instance, a child of average intelligence may have specific reading difficulties associated with behavioural difficulties in school and often these have generalized to other areas. Also under this heading comes an important area of function which includes the child's way of dealing with, and reacting to, people and problems. For example, a child who has been overprotected will not have learned how to accept frustration of wishes, and faced with a situation with which he cannot deal, may react in a way which makes him socially unacceptable—by temper tantrums, aggressive behaviour or withdrawal from the situation.

Social. The social history covers the child's family and upbringing and the educational environment. One may affect the other and a child coming from an inadequately functioning family may experience increasing difficulty coping in an educational environment more socially demanding of the child. It is important when obtaining the family history to see where the patient comes in the family, how many siblings there are, whether the pregnancy was wanted, how the child gets on with other members of the family and with his parents and how they function as a family. The child's friendships outside the family also indicate his level of function.

The most common reason for admission to hospital is when the child is behaving in such a way that the family or society—usually school—can no longer contain him. Following admission, the aim of the staff is to assess his biological, social and psychological functioning so that a plan of management and treatment for the child and his parents can be established.

The child should be shown round the ward to be introduced to the other children and the ward routine. If it is possible, one of the other children may be better at helping with this. Initially, he should not be left alone or with a group of children unless the staff are sure that he will not find the situation too frightening. When there is severe separation anxiety, drugs such as chlorpromazine may be prescribed, providing that a member of the staff stays with him until he is more settled. Such an experience often helps the child to form his initial ward relationship.

Having altered the child's environment by admission, he may lose his symptoms for a week or two. He should be encouraged to establish relationships with the staff whose individual observations are important. Behaviour is in response to particular people and it is important that these individual observations are shared. A nurse may hesitate to say, for instance, that she is experiencing difficulty with one particular child when she knows that her colleagues are not having similar difficulties. The informality of ward meetings helps to overcome such hesitancy, thus increasing the value of group observations.

Many disturbed children have a deep distrust or fear of adults and other children which may be the result of inadequate early relationships with their parents. This difficulty is continued into school and by the time a child is admitted to hospital, his distrust is longstanding. He no longer wants to please, and is fearful of adults. This may become evident in many ways. He may avoid people whenever possible, be hostile when spoken to, and rude or cheeky in his replies. Many children have received inconsistent, excessive punishment and when a child has been so treated over a long period of time, punishment has very little beneficial effect. Only through the repeated experience of consistent care will a child learn to accept and respect the staff, and wish to please them. It may take many weeks to establish this short of positive relationship, but much more controlled behaviour results.

The feelings of individual nurses towards the child are extremely important as they often indicate general feelings towards the child and reactions to his behaviour in the outside world. These feelings, however, should not be allowed to determine his treatment and management. For example, a charming child may often get comment from people and be the centre of attention, whereas an unattractive child is passed unnoticed. A brain-damaged, over-active child may cause great exasperation to his parents, school teacher and ward staff. The task of caring for this child proves less tiring when the nurses are able to share the time spent with him. Staff meetings help the staff to express their feelings towards individual children and then the reason for the response may be apparent and often a way is found to help the child obtain more gratifying responses.

Children who are mentally disturbed are often unable to tolerate physical stress and it is important whenever possible to delay investigations until the child has established at least one positive relationship. The nurse then adopts a supportive role and investigations cause the minimal amount of distress. When investigation or treatment are likely to cause much discomfort or anxiety, sedation should be given and the nurse with whom the child has the greatest positive relationship should be present to comfort him.

CONTROL AND MODIFICATION OF BEHAVIOUR

It is easier to modify unacceptable behaviour if a child is distracted from, rather than reprimanded for, negative behaviour. For example, instead of saying 'don't do that', an alternative task is offered—'will you help me to . . .'. Should the child refuse, he can be offered a more acceptable alternative and the nurse has not lost face. All children have a need to be contained and feel safe, therefore, it is important that children requiring correction are not challenged beyond their limit.

When there is aggressive behaviour, this should ideally be contained by the staff, thus increasing the child's responsibility for his own behaviour and his ability to deal with situations himself. Drugs may be used, but these diminish the child's responsibility for his behaviour. If help is given by the staff, this increases the child's responsibility for his own behaviour and his ability to deal with situations himself.

When holding a physically aggressive child there are two important rules to observe: the child should be held for the minimum amount of time required for him to regain self-control and not be hurt in the process, and secondly, the staff should not be hurt as any harm done may cause considerable guilt and distress to the child.

ATTITUDE TO PARENTS

Often the parents of disturbed children have unknowingly behaved in a way inappropriate to the needs of their children. It is important to bear in mind that this is rarely intentional and that they themselves are often in much need of help, perhaps having had a deprived childhood. The psychiatric social worker may be able to help them to understand and deal with their problems. It is easy to criticize the parents, not realizing that they are in as much need of care and concern as their child.

The parents often feel guilty at their child's admission for psychiatric treatment. They feel that they have failed in their care and often they may be hostile towards the staff. They may have difficulty in accepting that they may be a part of their child's difficulties, and expect a rapid cure in a child following, for example, an appendicectomy. They may be critical of their child's care or resent the fact that the child talks to the staff, whereas at home they cannot get him to communicate.

Patient Care Studies

1 ANDREW

Andrew, a four-year-old, adopted child, was first seen in the out-patients department where he had been referred by his general practitioner with a history of destructive behaviour, clumsiness, over-activity and verbal abusiveness. He was self-destructive, and because he would not sleep, had to be 'tied up' at night.

His adoptive mother had never had good health and had recurrent periods of depression. She was unable to tolerate Andrew's behaviour, and this extra tension increased her anxiety and decreased her ability to manage him. The adoptive father was more positive towards Andrew, but his main concern was for his wife's health and although he was able to recognize Andrew's need, his wife's needs took priority. Since adopting Andrew, the parents had had a child, now aged three years, and who was said to be no problem. Observation showed Susan to be an outgoing child—always neatly dressed, with a personality similar to that of Andrew. As the parents did not find her a problem, it was thought that Andrew carried the blame for her misdeeds.

The diagnosis was made of a brain damaged child with over-activity directed to obtaining the parental love of which he was deprived.

When Andrew was admitted he was found to be moderately over-active, clumsy and euphoric. He possessed an instant charm which made management difficult because it would have been so easy to respond to his charm and not his needs, i.e. to spoil him. Drugs were used to modify his behaviour and to help him to become more acceptable to his parents. Nursing care was aimed at helping him to channel his own activity more usefully and so become less destructive. He was encouraged to help with small jobs and errands. For a long time repeated requests and encouragement were needed to accomplish these tasks. Initially, he was unable to sit through a meal on the ward and it was many weeks before he was able to eat at a socially acceptable rate rather than at a great speed. His attention span was extended through play and stories, and he was encouraged to be independent. Andrew was encouraged to think positively about his parents by talking about them and he looked forward to daily visits from his mother. He was given the physical love and affection for which he craved and encouraged to look to his parents for this rather than to strangers. His mother was encouraged to visit daily and to bring Susan to play with him. She was very critical of his care while on the ward. She would not let him wear his own clothes for fear they would be lost, yet was angry if he was not well dressed when she visited. It was not always easy for the staff to accept these criticisms without evoking further hostility, but the psychiatric social worker saw both parents and as much of mother as was possible and her depression was helped with drugs.

The problems in the care of Andrew were twofold—Andrew, and his adoptive parents. Andrew was an appealing child and evoked a response of liking and pity. Because of these responses, there was a danger that he would receive much handling from the staff generally and that he would be deprived of consistent control. Student nurses in particular were at risk of behaving in this way, and recognition of these feelings at ward meetings helped prevent them being acted out. The parents' inappropriate reactions to Andrew's needs often provoked aggressive feelings in staff which, if expressed, could have led to a state of mutual antagonism between staff and parents. Recognition of the need of the parents for acceptance and approval helped the staff to control angry and rejecting feelings.

Andrew spent each week-end at home and when finally discharged from hospital, the parent/child relationship was greatly improved and his parents were more able to give him the love for which he craved.

2 IAN

Ian was first seen at the child guidance clinic and subsequently admitted to hospital. He was a lad of thirteen years with an eight year history of soiling and enuresis, school refusal and intolerance to maternal discipline. The youngest of five children, he had an elder brother and sister each of whom was married and living away from home. Another sister of eighteen years was living at home and was deaf since suffering meningitis in early infancy. Another boy had died in infancy. Ian's mother was a deaf Scots lady of fifty-one years. Father was a carefree fifty-year-old who had worked as an engineer since his discharge from the navy ten years previously. There were longstanding marital difficulties, and the marriage had drifted for many years. Ian and his father shared a bedroom, and apart from this he had little to do with him, other than infrequent rides on his motor cycle.

Ian was born in hospital after an uneventful pregnancy and delivery and weighed 7½lb. Speech was late in developing and he had a stammer for six months. This had been thought to be due to having a deaf older sister. The main complaint was of soiling intermittently from five years-of-age. Mother claimed this had followed an incident when another child had pushed him through a lavatory wall. He was playing truant from school and ignoring maternal discipline. There had also been intermittent reluctance to attend school since five years-of-age. Since attending secondary modern school, he had had more difficulty and was stated by the school, to be lazy and making no effort, although of average intelligence. Three months prior to admission he had started playing truant, returning home after mother had gone to work.

When Ian was first admitted, physical examination of the abdomen revealed a palpable mass in his descending colon, and rectal examination confirmed a diagnosis of impaction of faeces. Ian stated the reason for not attending school as being teased about soiling.

On admission, Ian settled very slowly. He was extremely distrustful of staff and slow to establish a relationship with anyone. He talked very little and answered only when approached directly. When he had settled a little he was treated with rectal saline washouts. Phenergan was given prior to these to lessen his anxiety and discomfort. Senokot was given orally and toilet training initiated. It took several weeks for Ian to become more confident with the staff. Gradually during his stay he was helped to become more self-confident and to face new

situations with less fear and anxiety. A slightly better relationship was established between Ian and his father, and he became more able to accept maternal
discipline after accepting discipline from the nursing staff.

Ian had great difficulty in coping with new situations. Often it was difficult
to see that this was due to fear. For example, when several attempts were made
to get him to a hostel he remained mute under the bedclothes. When attempts
to get him up were abandoned he would rise and enter into the ward activities
as if nothing had happened. It took many weeks to encourage and give enough
support to enable Ian to attempt new situations.

Ian's management presented a number of problems. After eight years of
soiling, he had much difficulty in overcoming the apprehension inherent in
establishing relationships. Once this was dealt with, the soiling ameliorated
rapidly, but the damage to his personality development made it difficult for him
to face the world—hence the hiding under the bedclothes. This behaviour could
have discouraged staff. Some staff saw Ian's behaviour as volitional, that is, he
would stay in bed rather than face the prospect of a hostel and more strangers.
The frustration inherent in trying to help Ian came out as antagonism between
staff groupings in ward meetings. It was thus diverted from Ian himself.

Care of the Mentally Subnormal Child

Probably in no other branch of nursing is constant, unfailing love and attention
so necessary as in the total care of those who have been deprived of their full
intellectual faculty.

Many of these unfortunate children are cared for at home by loving parents,
most of them attending a school for the educationally subnormal, or training
centre or local subnormality hospital for social training. Some of the more
severely handicapped are cared for in special units with others less severely
affected who cannot be cared for at home. The impact that a mentally subnormal child has on a family varies considerably. Some parents do not want to
accept that they have produced an imperfect child and only as his physical
growth supersedes his mental development do they appreciate the situation.
Others accept that the child is not normal and reject him in his early days, not
minding who cares for him as long as it is not them. Many devoted parents
deprive themselves of all pleasures so that they can direct their time, energy and
resources towards keeping their child at home. Only when he becomes too big,
noisy, badly behaved or a nuisance to the other children or neighbours will they
reluctantly consent to hospital care. Such parents benefit from help and moral
support shared with others faced with similar problems, and the National Society
for Mentally Handicapped Children does much in meeting this need at both
national and local level. (Appendix B).

The staff of an acute paediatric unit meet these children when they are admit-

Hereditary ⎡ Chromosomal abnormalities   e.g. Down's syndrome (Mongolism)
          ⎣ Genetic disorders: i. Inborn errors of metabolism:
                                        Phenylketonuria
                                        Lipidosis
                                        Leucoencephalopathy
                                        Mucopolysaccharidosis

                                  ii. Developmental abnormalities:
                                        Absence of thyroid gland–cretinism
                                        Hydrocephalus

Environmental ⎡ Prenatal: i. Infections–Rubella, Syphilis,
              │   Toxoplasmosis,
              │   Cytomegalic inclusion disease
              │   ii. Radiation
              │
              │ Natal: Brain damage, anoxaemia and haemorrhage
              │
              │
              ⎣ Post Natal: i. Physical: Head injury

                             ii.Chemical: Poisoning, e.g. lead
                             iii. Biological: Meningitis and encephalitis
                                        Hyperbilirubinaemia ⭢ kernicterus
                                        Hypoglycaemia

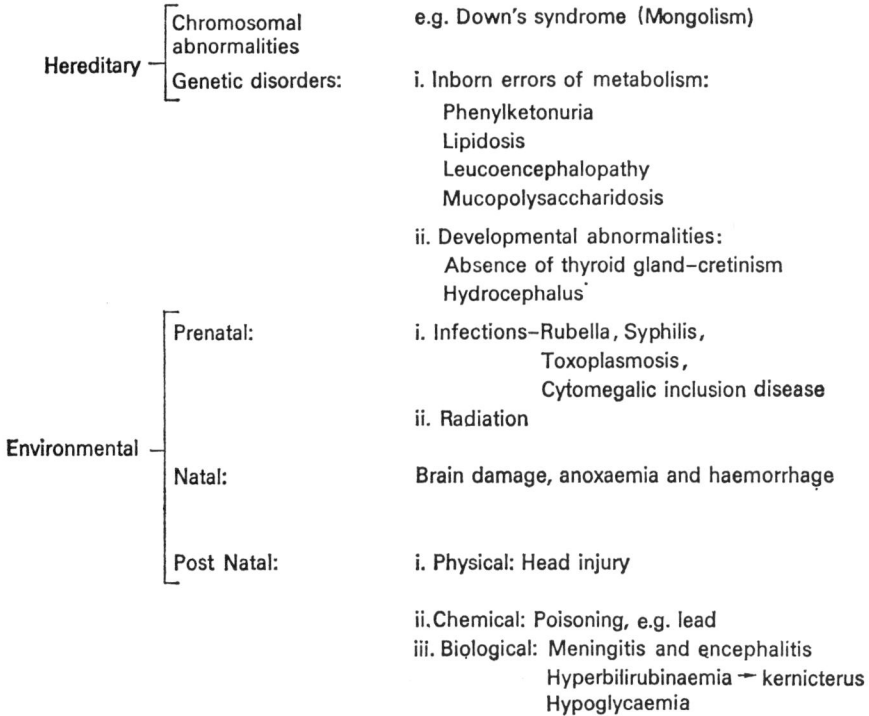

Fig. 74. Some causes of Mental Subnormality.

ted with intercurrent infections, or for surgery, or investigation. If the child is admitted from home, then his mother may feel able to spend most of the day with him, although this may prove an excellent opportunity for her to have a well-earned holiday. The mother will best understand her child who is rarely in hospital long enough for a good nurse–patient relationship to be established. Mentally subnormal children requiring long-term hospital care are best nursed in a specially designed unit where the staff are trained to meet their special need.

The main aims in nursing these children must be:

i to make the best of their limited minds—encouraging them to attain their innate potential.

ii to make them independent and socially acceptable to the community.

The popular concept 'to nurse' is only applicable in the care of the severely mentally subnormal patient whose basic needs the nurse must fulfil. To the less severely handicapped the emphasis is on teaching, leading and encouraging. Routine physical care is obviously necessary, but the child is taught and encouraged to carry out this care for himself. It is much quicker for the busy nurse to do these things for the child, but she must have patience while he strives towards independence. Teaching must be simple and repeated over and over again in exactly the same way. It may take many months for a child to learn a simple procedure, but what a goal to achieve!

Mentally subnormal children have likes and dislikes as normal children, but difficulty arises when they cannot express their feelings. Many emotional outbursts and displays of temper are caused by inability to express their feelings or frustration at not being understood. Most of their abnormal emotional reactions are an exaggeration of how normal children would behave in provoking circumstances.

Spontaneous play comes naturally to the normal developing child, but mentally subnormal children have to be taught how to play. Their natural love of water, colour, rhythmics and music is encouraged and their social training is confined to self-care in the early years. Academic attainments are out of reach of some and are the last to be considered. It is futile, for example, to teach a child to count even from one to five if he is incapable of feeding, washing and dressing himself. Teaching for social acceptance and independence takes priority; education for life in the community comes later.

The days of moulding a mentally subnormal child into passive acceptance of an institutional pattern are slowly slipping into the past. The emphasis now is on bringing the child to his full innate potential so that he is socially acceptable in a tolerant society. For the severely mentally subnormal child who may have associated spasticity, deafness or blindness or be subject to frequent convulsions, life is short, few living to attain adult stature.

For Further Reading

BOWLBY J. (1953). *Child Care and the Growth of Love*. Pelican Original.
CHESS, STELLA. (1969). *An Introduction to Child Psychiatry*. Grune and Stratton, New York and London.
HADFIELD J. A. (1962). *Childhood and Adolescence*. Pelican Original.
HALLAS C. H. (1970). *The Care and Training of the Mentally Subnormal*, 4th edition. John Wright and Sons Ltd.
LACEY P. R. (1969). *Life with the Mentally Sick Child*, 1st edition. Pergamon Press.

CHAPTER NINETEEN

Collecting Specimens

Specimens of urine, faeces, sputum, vomit, duodenal juice and discharges and, in some instances, blood for laboratory examination are collected by the nursing staff. Other body fluids and tissues are collected by the medical or technical staff and are included in Chapter 20.

Laboratory examination of specimens is necessary:

i to make a diagnosis;

ii to decide on an appropriate course of treatment;

iii to assess progress.

Specimens are examined in the appropriate hospital laboratory:

1 *Haematology*, where capillary and venous blood specimens are examined for content and function, and cross-matched with donor blood.

2 *Biochemistry*, where specimens of blood, urine, faeces, cerebrospinal and ascitic fluids are analyzed to assess the metabolic and chemical activities within the body.

3 *Microbiology* including both bacteriology and virology, where uncontaminated specimens of urine, faeces, sputum, cerebrospinal fluid and discharges are examined for the presence of pathogenic micro-organisms, and their sensitivity to chemotherapeutic agents assessed.

4 *Histology*, where the microscopic structure of living tissue is examined.

General Principles

1 Before Collection of a Specimen

i The nature of the specimen and the examination requested is ascertained from the doctor's request form.

ii The appropriate specimen container is chosen.

iii Particulars are entered on the label as requested.

Name (in full).

Age or date of birth.

Hospital registration number.

357

Ward.
Nature of specimen.
Date.
Time of collection (if relevant).

2 Collection of Specimen

i Most specimens deteriorate on standing, therefore, routine specimens should be collected during laboratory working hours.
ii Whenever practical, contamination of a specimen for bacteriological and/or viral studies is reduced by collecting the specimen straight into the sterile specimen container.
iii Contamination of the outside of the container should be avoided and the container securely sealed.

3 Following Collection of Specimen

i The date and time of collection is inserted on the request form.
ii The completed label is firmly attached to the body—not the lid—of the specimen container, which is maintained in an upright position.
iii The specimen and request form are dispatched to the laboratory without delay.
iv The written laboratory report is brought to the notice of the medical staff and retained in the patient's records.

Urine

Collection of an Uncontaminated Specimen of Urine for Bacteriological Examination

Various methods are used for obtaining a specimen of urine for bacteriological examination. Those included in the text are:
1 A mid-stream, or clean-catch, specimen of urine.
2 A 'bag' specimen, using a urine collecting bag.
3 A catheter specimen of urine.
4 Percutaneous puncture of the bladder.

REQUIREMENTS
Bowl or bath of hand hot water.
Toilet soap.
Clean bath towel.
Receptacle for used swabs.

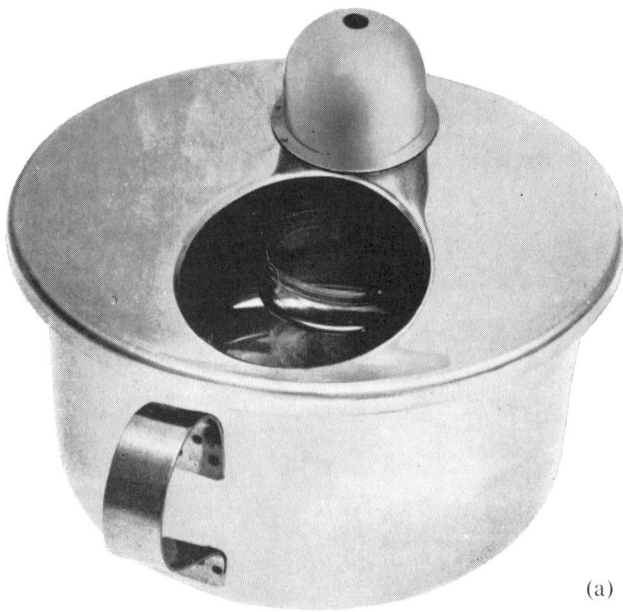

(a)

(b)

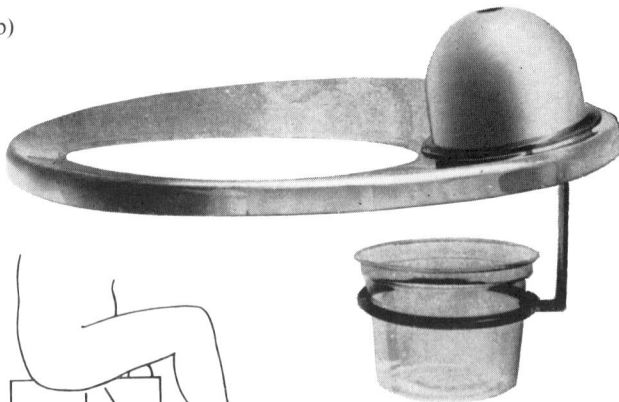

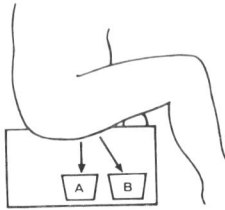

(c)

PLATE 12. A simple method for collecting a mid-stream specimen of urine from a girl.

(a) Pot for collecting specimen. (b) Seat of the pot showing position of the pommel and cup rack. (c) Diagram showing direction of the stream of urine.

Method The nurse confirms that the child has not passed urine recently. A sterile cup is placed in the cup rack. The girl sits on the pot, bent slightly forward, with the pommel between her thighs. As the result of gravity, the first and last part of the stream of urine fall straight down into cup A on the bottom of the pot. The velocity of mid–stream is higher as the result of greater pressure in the bladder, and flows into cup B. The urine collected in cup B is the required mid-stream specimen.

(Reproduced by kind permission of Dr. Paavo Mäkelä of Helsinki Children's Hospital, Orion Pharmaceutical Co., Helsinki, Finland and the Editor, The Lancet).

Completed laboratory form and label.
Sterile screw-cap laboratory container.

Sterile requirements:
Gallipot of warm sterile water.
Sterile cotton wool balls.

PREPARATION OF THE CHILD

i *Male*. Unless a bath has just been taken, the buttocks are cleansed and the groins, scrotum and penis washed with soap and water, rinsed and dried on the clean bath towel. The nurse washes and dries her hands. The genitalia is swabbed with sterile cotton wool balls moistened in sterile water, ensuring that the area surrounding the meatus is clean. The foreskin of an older child should be gently retracted and the glans cleansed. The area is carefully dried with dry sterile swabs.

ii *Female*. Unless a bath has just been taken, the buttocks are cleansed and the external genitalia and surrounding area are washed well with soap and water, rinsed and dried on the clean bath towel. The child is placed in a semi-recumbent position on the cot or bed. The nurse washes and dries her hands. The labia majora and minora are separated and cleansed with sterile cotton wool balls moistened in sterile water, swabbing from above, downwards, using the swabs once only (page 362). The area is dried thoroughly with dry sterile swabs.

METHODS

1 A MID-STREAM OR CLEAN-CATCH SPECIMEN OF URINE

This method for collection of a specimen of urine is only suitable for an older, co-operative child. The child is prepared as above and encouraged to pass urine into the lavatory, bedpan or urinal. After a small amount has been voided, the stream is diverted into a sterile, wide neck screw-cap laboratory container. The child then empties his bladder into the appropriate receptacle (see Plate 12).

2 A 'BAG' SPECIMEN—USING A URINE COLLECTING BAG

Additional requirements:
Urine collecting bag.
Scissors.
Requirements for leg restraint.

The small child is prepared as above. The hole in the urine collecting bag is shaped so that it fits snugly around the genitalia which should protrude into the bag—i.e. the penis and scrotum, or the labia majora. The hips are flexed and the thighs separated. The skin of the perineum is stretched laterally to make the groove as shallow as possible. The protective covering is removed from the adhesive and the lower end applied to the perineum, pressing firmly across the mid-line. The adhesive is eased from the anus and any excess cut away. The remaining adhesive is applied, working from below, upwards.

Restraint of the infant's feet may be necessary to prevent dislodgement of the collecting bag.

The urine contained in the bag may be transferred to the sterile laboratory container by either of the following methods:

i Removing the stopper from a specially-designed bag,

ii By inserting a sterile catheter into a hole made in the collecting bag and aspirating the contents with a sterile syringe.

The collecting bag is then gently eased from the adherent skin, using adhesive remover.

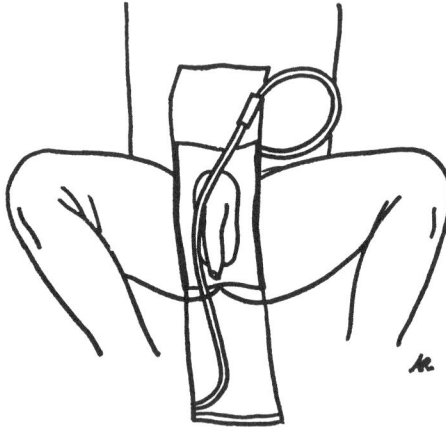

Fig. 75. A urine collecting bag in position. May be used for either boys or girls.

Catheterization of the Urinary Bladder

When alternative methods can be employed, catheterization of the urinary bladder is avoided. In spite of meticulous cleansing of the external genitalia, use of sterile equipment and practising a faultless aseptic technique, micro-organisms may be introduced into the urinary tract. The delicate urethral lining may be damaged if too large a catheter is passed, or a poor technique adopted.

REASONS FOR CATHETERIZATION

1 To relieve retention of urine:

     i following injury to the spinal nerves;

     ii caused by posterior urethral valves;

     iii in the immediate post-operative period—extremely rare in childhood.

2   As an aid to diagnosis:
    i   to obtain an uncontaminated specimen of urine for bacteriological examination;
    ii   prior to cysto-urethrography;
    iii to obtain a specimen of urine for testing when diabetes mellitus is suspected in a comatose child.

3   Continuous bladder drainage via an indwelling urethral catheter may be used:
    i   to protect a healing wound or burn from chemical irritation of urine;
    ii   if the child is unconscious:
         (a) to ensure adequate emptying of the bladder;
         (b) to avoid maceration of the skin predisposing to pressure sores;
    iii to maintain an accurate record of urine output.

4   To measure the residual urine. Following prolonged continuous bladder drainage, there is temporary hypotonia of the detrusor muscle. The child empties the bladder to the best of his/her ability, immediately followed by passage of a catheter to withdraw the residual urine.

5   prior to surgery or procedures:
    i   pelvic surgery;
    ii   abdominal paracentesis;
    iii peritoneal dialysis.

Catheterization of the Bladder—Female

This procedure is carried out by the nursing staff. Two nurses are essential and the co-operation of the child is sought. A mild sedative may be prescribed for a small or apprehensive older child.

REQUIREMENTS
The trolley is prepared as described on page 258, but using the following equipment:

Sterile requirements:
For top shelf of the trolley (these may be contained in a composite pack).
3 dressing towels.
10–12 wool balls.
Gallipot for warmed cleansing lotion.
Gallipot for warmed sterile water.
One pair of plain dissecting forceps.
2 Jacques catheters size 8–12 F.G. (3–6 E.G.) depending on size of the child.
Receiver.
Graduated jug.

Bottom shelf.

Cleansing lotion, e.g. aqueous solution of chlorhexidine 0·05%.

Sterile gloves ⎫
Mask   ⎬ for the nurse.

Sterile water.

Water soluble sterile lubricant, e.g. K.Y. jelly—if desired (single dose dispenser).

Sterile screw-cap laboratory container.

Completed laboratory form and label.

Waterproof protection for the bed.

Additional requirements:

Anglepoise lamp.

PREPARATION OF THE CHILD

Adequate privacy must be ensured. A simple explanation is given to the child, and her co-operation encouraged and praised. Unless a bath has just been taken, the genitalia, buttocks and thighs are washed well with soap and water, rinsed and dried with a clean bath towel.

The girl is placed in a supine position with the head resting on one low pillow. The top bedclothes are folded to the bottom of the bed and the trunk is protected by the treatment blanket. To give better access to the urethral orifice, the buttocks are raised on a folded napkin or sandbag. The waterproof protection is placed under the buttocks. The child's feet are drawn up to the buttocks and the thighs abducted to expose the genitalia. This position is maintained throughout the procedure. The anglepoise lamp is placed in position.

METHOD

The top of the trolley is prepared and glove pack opened. The nurse undertaking the procedure washes and dries her hands well and, on return to the bedside, puts on the sterile gloves.

The area is draped, using three sterile towels, one covering each leg and crossing over the abdomen, and the third is placed between the legs up to the perineum.

Using dressing forceps, the vulva is swabbed, dipping each swab into the lotion so that it is sufficiently moist, but not saturated. The swabs are used once only, from above, downwards:

> two for labia majora, which are then held apart with the first two fingers of the left hand to expose the labia minora;
> two for the labia minora which, when separated, reveal the vestibule;
> one centrally.

The vestibule is then similarly cleansed with the warmed sterile water and examined for the urethral orifice. This is seen as a small dimple, lying above the opening of the vagina.

The forceps are discarded.

The receiver containing one catheter, previously lubricated if desired, is placed on the sterile towel between the child's legs. Holding the catheter 2–3cm from its tip in her gloved right hand, the nurse slowly and carefully inserts it into the urethral meatus until urine flows. Should the catheter become contaminated during this procedure, it must be discarded and another catheter used.

The bladder is emptied and a specimen collected directly into the sterile laboratory container. The catheter is pinched and gently withdrawn. The towel drapes are removed, and the vulva and anal area dried. Although the bladder is empty, the child may feel she wants to pass urine, due to irritation of the urethral mucosa. A bedpan or pot should be offered and the child reassured and made comfortable.

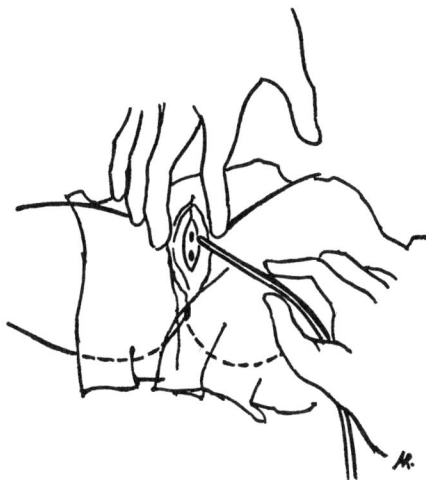

FIG. 76. Passing a catheter into the female urethra. Note that á non-touch technique is achieved with the use of sterile gloves.

Catheterization of the Urinary Bladder—Male

Although included in this chapter, this procedure is never used merely to collect a urine specimen. It is performed by a doctor with the help of an assisting nurse to reassure the child.

Requirements are as above, the Jacques catheters being substituted with Tiemann's catheters of a suitable size. A water soluble sterile lubricant or xylocaine gel is necessary

Collection of a Specimen of Urine from an Indwelling Catheter

REQUIREMENTS
Aqueous lotion.
Sterile water.

Gallipot.
Cotton wool balls.
Sterile receiver.
Completed laboratory form and label.
Sterile screw-cap laboratory container.

METHOD

The bladder is first allowed to fill by occluding the drainage tubing for two to four hours. The catheter is then disconnected from the drainage tubing and the end cleansed with the lotion and sterile water. The catheter is opened to allow a little urine to flow into the receiver. A mid-stream specimen is then collected directly into the sterile laboratory container. The catheter is cleansed, dried and reconnected.

Suprapubic Puncture

This procedure may be carried out by the doctor if other methods have given contaminated results, particularly in small female children.

REQUIREMENTS

The trolley is prepared as described on page 258 with the addition of the following equipment:

10ml syringe ⎫
No. 1 hypodermic needle ⎬ both sterile.

Sterile screw-cap laboratory container.
Completed laboratory form and label.

2ml syringe ⎫
Lignocaine 1% ⎬ for local anaesthetic, if required.
No. 12 hypodermic needle ⎭

METHOD

The nurse must confirm that the child has not passed urine recently. A mild sedative may be prescribed for a small or an apprehensive older child. The co-operation of an older child is achieved by a simple explanation and reassurance. He is placed in a semi-recumbent position, restrained if necessary, while the suprapubic area is cleansed and urine obtained from the bladder by a percutaneous approach.

Collection of Urine for Biochemical Analysis

An uncontaminated specimen is not necessary, but the urine must be free from faecal matter. Collection is usually over a period of time, i.e. one day, or sometimes longer, so that meticulous care must be taken to ensure that all urine is saved and that the collecting apparatus is free from leaks, while not causing too much distress or discomfort. Diversional therapy is important. Any leakage should be reported to the biochemistry department. A special bottle containing the appropriate preservative is obtained from the biochemistry department.

Twenty-four Hour Urine Collection

The child empties his bladder (at 08.00 hours) on the first day and the urine is discarded.

All urine is collected for the following twenty-four hours. The urine voided at 08.00 hours on the second day is saved and concludes the twenty-four hour urine collection.

A flexible arrangement is necessary for small children. The exact time is immaterial as long as it is recorded.

Methods Used for a Twenty-four Hour Collection of Urine from Small Children

1   Using a urine collecting bag.
2   Using a urine collecting bag with attached non-kink tubing.
3   Using Paul's tubing (male).

1   USING A URINE COLLECTING BAG

The urine collecting bag, used for either sex, is applied as described on page 359 and the legs are restrained. A catheter inserted through a small opening made in a top corner of the bag is secured in position with adhesive tape. A spigot is inserted into the catheter end. Frequent inspection of the dependent bag is necessary and the urine aspirated and placed in the laboratory collection bottle on each voiding. This is a useful method for collecting individual urine specimens for biochemical analysis.

2   USING A URINE COLLECTING BAG WITH ATTACHED NON-KINK TUBING

The urine collecting bag, used for either sex, is applied as described on page 359. The distal end of the tubing is secured into the neck of the bottle standing on a tray at the foot of the cot. To allow free drainage of voided urine, the collecting bag must be dependent. This can be satisfactorily achieved by nursing the child in a chair with the tubing passing through the opening in the seat to the bottle standing on the floor. The legs should be supported to prevent dependent oedema.

3   USING PAUL'S TUBING

This is a very satisfactory method for collection of urine from a small boy. The Paul's tubing should be of sufficient width to accommodate both the penis and scrotum, and be of sufficient length to extend from the child to the bottle which stands on a tray at the foot of the cot. The groins and scrotal area are cleansed of grease and powder and thoroughly dried. The scrotum and penis are placed within the lumen of the Paul's tubing and secured in position with lengths of adhesive tape. The distal end of the tubing is secured into the neck of the bottle. The legs are restrained and the child nursed in a semi-recumbent position. Slight elevation of the head of the bed encourages urine drainage into the bottle.

Alternative methods may have to be used, especially for small girls. The principles of collection are essentially the same, namely:

1   The collecting apparatus must fit snugly around the genitalia without causing discomfort.

2   The tubing must be of the non-kink variety.

3   Free drainage is assisted by elevation of the child or her cot.

4   Diversional therapy is important.

Faeces

1   SINGLE SPECIMEN

Using a wooden spatula, a small specimen is taken from the centre of the stool and firmly enclosed in an impervious, screw-cap laboratory container.

2   WHOLE STOOL

Occasionally, it is necessary for the whole stool to be sent to the laboratory for examination for evidence of intestinal infestation. The stool is collected into a polythene-lined bedpan, pot or napkin, and placed in a covered container for transfer to the laboratory for immediate examination.

3   FIVE DAY COLLECTION

A fat balance, carried out over a period of five days, is used to determine the fat content of faeces following ingestion of a known quantity of fat. A daily output in excess of 4–10% of the intake is indicative of steatorrhoea. It is important that the staff, the parents and the child are all aware that the diet must be adhered to and that all stools must be collected.

The diet, containing a known quantity of fat, is commenced forty-eight hours prior to commencement of the stool collection. A carmine marker is then given. Passage of the first pink stool marks commencement of the collection. This is discarded, and subsequent stools are collected in a covered container which is renewed every twenty-four hours. A second carmine marker is given five days after ingestion of the first. Passage of the second pink stool completes the collection, this stool being included in the collection.

During the test, rejected food and vomit must be retained for analysis and the results adjusted accordingly.

When the child is old enough to co-operate, he is asked to defaecate in a polythene-lined bedpan or pot, and the stool is transferred to the closed laboratory container. An infant may be nursed in a chair and the stools collected in a polythene-lined receptacle placed beneath his buttocks. Alternatively, he may have his napkin lined with polythene. There is a tendency for the buttocks to become very sore with the use of this latter method, so it is best avoided.

A urine collecting bag may be applied over the external genitalia to prevent dilution of the faeces with urine.

Sputum

Secretions produced by the respiratory passages are wafted by the cilia into the pharynx and either swallowed or expectorated. Small children cannot co-operate in producing a specimen of sputum. Their respiratory secretions are simply swallowed.

METHODS.

1 An older child is asked to cough and expectorate his sputum, not saliva, into a sterile laboratory container.

2 Gastric washings are taken from a small child. If examination is to be made for tubercle bacilli, the following procedure is repeated on three consecutive mornings on waking and before any food is taken.

Requirements and procedure are as for naso-gastric intubation (page 111). A sterile, screw-top laboratory container is required. The gastric residue is collected into the laboratory container. The stomach is gently irrigated with 10ml of sterile water and the aspirate added to the gastric residue. The occluded tube is then pinched and gently withdrawn.

3 Suction catheter. Following completion of an aseptic tracheal toilet (page 305) the suction catheter is placed in a suitable sterile laboratory container.

Duodenal Juice

The collection of duodenal juice for biochemical estimation is necessary in the investigation of children with cystic fibrosis, when the specimen would show diminished or complete absence of tryptic activity.

REQUIREMENTS

As for naso-gastric intubation (page 111).

A radio-opaque intestinal tube is used.

Additional requirements:

pH paper.

3 Universal containers.
Receptacle containing ice.

PREPARATION OF THE CHILD
This exacting procedure demands a contented infant, time and patience. Food and milk drinks are omitted for six hours, but 5% sugar in N/5 saline should be continued to within three hours of commencement. The infant may be given an occluded teat to suck. A sedative, if required, is given rectally.

METHOD
The naso-gastric tube is passed as described on page 111 and the gastric contents are aspirated and discarded. A further 5–10cm (2–4 inches) of tubing is passed, and the infant placed in the right lateral position to encourage passage of the tube through the pyloric sphincter. The tube is then secured to an immobile part of the face and closed with a spigot.

Fluid is aspirated at quarter-hourly intervals. The duodenal juice required is golden yellow in colour and its alkalinity is confirmed with pH paper (pH8). A doubtful position of the distal end of the tube may necessitate X-ray examination.

Three 5ml specimens of duodenal juice are collected into specimen bottles which are transported on ice to the laboratory immediately following collection. Only when the biochemist is satisfied that the specimens are suitable should the tube be removed and the infant given a feed.

Sweat Test

Children with cystic fibrosis have an increase in the sodium chloride content of their sweat. This test is carried out by a member of the laboratory staff with the help of a nurse or the infant's mother.

Localized sweating is induced on the forearm or thigh. After five minutes of stimulation, the area is washed with distilled water and dried. An accurately weighed filter paper is placed over the area with forceps and covered with a slightly larger polythene square, sealed to the skin with lengths of adhesive tape. This is maintained in position for half-an-hour. The polythene square is then carefully removed and the filter paper returned to its original container and sent without delay to the laboratory, where the sodium level is assessed. Values exceeding 60mEq sodium/litre are considered abnormal and indicative of cystic fibrosis.

Swabs

A sterile dressed applicator contained in a plugged tube is used to collect material for bacteriological examination from the body surface and from inside orifices.

General Principles

i The child should be restrained if unable to co-operate.

ii A good light is essential, particularly if an orifice is to be entered.

iii The swab should not touch any part except the site requiring investigation.

iv Skin, wound, nasal and eye swabs are collected before any antiseptic or antibiotic lotions or creams are applied.

v The swab is carefully returned to its sterile tube, sealed, labelled and dispatched immediately to the laboratory before becoming dry.

Throat Swab

The child, restrained if small, is sat comfortably facing the operator (FIG. 77). To open the mouth of an unco-operative child, a thumb is placed on the chin

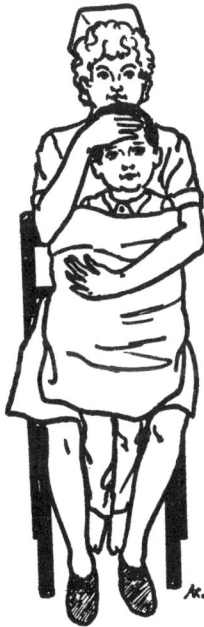

FIG. 77. Method of restraint that can be adapted for most procedures related to the ear, nose and throat and for a gastric washout on a conscious child.

and gently pressed downwards to lower the jaw. The tongue is depressed with a spatula placed towards the back of the tongue, while the swab is swiftly but accurately introduced, and the specimen collected from the tonsillar area.

Per-Nasal (Cough) Swab

This special swab on a flexible wire carrier, is introduced into one nostril and passed into the naso-pharynx. The child will inevitably cough, and the swab is withdrawn and replaced into its tube.

Ear Swab

An aural speculum of suitable size, a head mirror and light, or head light are necessary requirements. The child is either seated or placed in a lateral position. The speculum is inserted into the external auditory meatus and the pinna drawn upwards and backwards (just backwards in infancy). With the light directed in the orifice, the swab is gently introduced through the speculum, and the specimen obtained.

Rectal (Sleeve) Swab

When a stool specimen cannot be obtained, a rectal swab may be requested. The sterile dressed applicator lies inside a lubricated glass sheath contained in a plugged tube. The child is placed in the left lateral position, as for all rectal procedures, and the sheath is gently inserted through the anal sphincter for 1–2cm or $\frac{1}{2}$–$\frac{3}{4}$in. The dressed applicator is extended beyond the end of the sheath into the rectum and then withdrawn until it lies inside the sheath. The sheath containing the swab is withdrawn, and reinserted into the sterile tube.

Sellotape Slide

This simple test is used to confirm a diagnosis of threadworm infestation. During the night, the female threadworm migrates to the anal area to lay her eggs. On waking, a short length of Sellotape is placed, adhesive side down, over the anal area. The Sellotape is then stuck to a microscope slide, labelled and sent to the laboratory for microscopic examination for the presence of ova.

Blood

Blood specimens are, unfortunately, necessary for a wide range of routine and diagnostic tests carried out both in the in and out-patients departments. Children dislike this often frightening, painful procedure, and much ingenuity is necessary to distract the attention of a young child while an experienced doctor or technician obtains his specimen. Micro-techniques demanding as little as 0·1–1ml of capillary blood are carried out in the laboratories of most paediatric units. Collection of blood by venepuncture is now the exception rather than the rule.

A variety of tubes are used to receive blood specimens. They fall into two main groups:

1   Plain, or universal, tubes containing no anticoagulant. These are used when serum is required for the test, as the contained blood will coagulate, thus separating the cells from the serum.

2   When tests require whole blood specimens, the tube must contain an anti-coagulant such as heparin, oxalate or citrate which is thoroughly mixed with the blood specimen.

Capillary Blood

This is the method of choice for collecting small quantities of blood from children, especially when repeated collections are necessary.

REQUIREMENTS
Tray.
Sterile cotton wool balls.
Spirit lotion in a container.
Sterile disposable lancet.
Collection test tubes, capillary tubes, micro-pipette, paper, etc. as required.

SITES USED
1   Heel (but not the dorsum) is the site of choice for children under the age of two years.
2   The medial aspect of the terminal phalanx of the index finger for older children.

METHOD
To induce hyperaemia, the limb is warmed with an electric heat pad or by washing in warm water. After washing and drying her hands, the operator cleanses the dependent site with warm cleansing lotion which is allowed to dry.

The heel is controlled by dorsi-flexion of the foot and the index finger is grasped at the base of the terminal phalanx. The point of the lancet is forcefully introduced through the skin into the subcutaneous tissues and quickly removed. Using a dry sterile swab, the first drop of blood is removed and the specimen collected. Blood flow from an adequate incision is increased by compressing the calf or the base of the finger. Local squeezing causes dilution of blood with tissue fluid.

A dry swab is held firmly over the incision at the end of the procedure.

Venous Blood

Withdrawal of venous blood is performed by the doctor.

REQUIREMENTS
Tray.
Dry sterilized 5–20ml syringe (with eccentric nozzle if preferred).
Needle (serum or No. 1).
Spirit lotion in container⎫
Sterile cotton wool balls ⎭ *or* Mediswabs.
Receptacle for soiled swabs.

Additional requirements:
Appropriate specimen bottle.
Laboratory form.

VENEPUNCTURE
A vein in the antecubital fossa, either the cephalic or median basilic, is usually selected and the elbow hyperextended. The vein may be made more prominent by warming the limb and asking the child to clench his fist or grasp an object, and by constricting the dependent arm above the site with the hand of the assisting nurse. A pocket tourniquet or length of rubber tubing may be applied over an older child's sleeve to achieve the same result. At no time should the constriction be tight enough to occlude the radial pulse. If a vein on the dorsum of the hand is used, digital constriction is applied around the wrist until the vein has been entered.

The skin is cleansed and allowed to dry. Once the vein has been entered, the pressure is released and the blood specimen withdrawn. On withdrawal of the needle, firm pressure is applied over the injection site with a dry sterile swab and the limb raised for about one minute.

When the superficial veins of an infant are inaccessible, a specimen of blood may be withdrawn from the jugular or femoral vein.

JUGULAR VEIN PUNCTURE
The restrained infant is placed in a supine position with the shoulders to the edge of a mattress or table. The head is extended and rotated 90° to one side of the mid-line and supported in position by the assisting nurse (FIG. 78). Crying distends the vein which can then be located.

On withdrawal of the needle, the infant is sat up and comforted for three minutes while a dry sterile swab is maintained firmly over the site.

FEMORAL VEIN PUNCTURE
Only as a last resort is this site used. Adequate restraint and asepsis are impera-tive. The buttocks and groins are thoroughly cleansed and dried before the infant is placed supine across a firm mattress or table. The assisting nurse positions herself at the infant's head, splints the infant's trunk with her forearms,

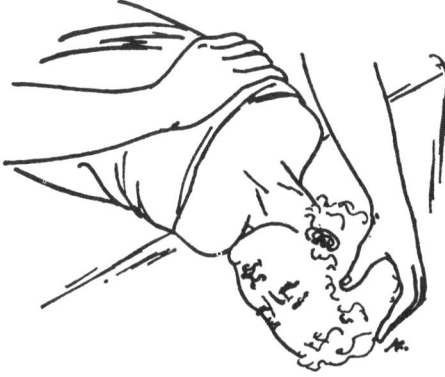

Fig. 78. Position of a child for jugular vein puncture.

and places a hand on each flexed knee. The hips are externally rotated and abducted to an angle of 45° and the knees flexed to 90° and maintained in contact with the firm surface (Fig. 79).

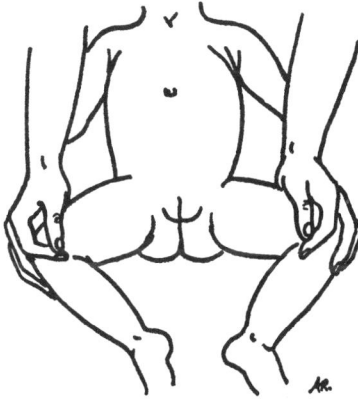

Fig. 79. Position of an infant for femoral vein puncture.

On withdrawal of the needle, firm digital pressure is applied over a dry sterile swab for three minutes.

CHAPTER TWENTY

Assisting with Diagnostic and Therapeutic Procedures

Biopsies

A biopsy is the removal of living tissue for diagnostic purposes.

Bone Marrow Biopsy

Red cell production (haemopoiesis) takes place in the red bone marrow located in the medullary cavity of long bones during infancy and in the ends of long bones, vertebrae, ribs, cranium, sternum and pelvic bones throughout life. Red bone marrow is required for cytology in the diagnosis and assessment of progress in blood disorders such as leukaemia and aplastic anaemia.

REQUIREMENTS

The basic trolley is prepared, as described on page 258 with the addition of the following equipment:
A Bard Parker handle and blade (sterile).

Bottom shelf:
Mask ⎫
Sterile gloves ⎬ for the doctor.
2-2ml syringes ⎫
Nos. 17 and 12 ⎪
  hypodermic needles ⎬ for local anaesthetic.
Lignocaine 1% ⎪
Hyaluronidase ⎭
Sterilized Salah needle.
2ml syringe.
Nobecutane.
Narrow adhesive tape.
Specimen containers, slides, fixatives, supplied by the laboratory.

PREPARATION OF THE CHILD

The procedure is frightening and painful to the small child who requires adequate sedation. The sleeping child is placed on a firm surface, the position depending on the doctor's choice of site for puncture:

1 Tibia (used in first two years of life)—supine with a sandbag placed underneath the site.

2 Iliac crest (used at any age)—lateral position.

3 Sternum (used in older children)—recumbent position.

METHOD

While the doctor puts on his mask, washes and dries his hands and puts on sterile gloves, the nurse ensures that everything required for the procedure is on the top of the trolley.

Working together, the doctor and nurse check, prepare and prime the syringe with a mixture of lignocaine and hyaluronidase (used to promote rapid far-penetrating local anaesthesia).

With the child held firmly in position, the doctor cleanses the area, administers the local anaesthetic and drapes the site. After assembling the equipment, a small incision is made in the skin (if necessary) and the needle inserted. A specimen of red bone marrow is withdrawn into the syringe and the needle is removed.

Pressure is applied over the site for one or two minutes before the area is sprayed with Nobecutane and/or a firm dry dressing applied.

Care of the specimen is the responsibility of the laboratory staff.

AFTER CARE

The puncture wound is dressed and the child made comfortable in bed. The dressing is removed and the puncture site is inspected forty-eight hours later.

Jejunal Biopsy

This test is carried out to diagnose coeliac disease. Children with this disease are unable to metabolize gluten—the protein portion of wheat and rye flour. As the result of this intolerance, the normal long villi forming the jejunal mucosa are flattened, with consequent decrease of the absorptive surface. A special intestinal tube containing a small capsule enclosing a blade, e.g. a Crosby capsule, is used to obtain the specimen.

REQUIREMENTS

Tray.

For passage of the tube:
A fully assembled Crosby capsule.
Water soluble lubricating jelly.

Short length of anti-static pressure tubing (10cm).
Gauze swabs.
10ml syringe.
10ml normal saline or water.
pH indicator paper.
Waterproof protection for the bed or table.
Vomit bowl.

For collection of specimens:
Sterile kit containing forceps and scissors.
2 specimen bottles containing normal saline.
Silver foil and dry ice.

PREPARATION OF THE CHILD

As most of the patients undergoing investigation for coeliac disease are of the younger age group, a good sedative is usually prescribed, to be given half to one hour before intubation is attempted, or rectal thiopentone may be administered immediately prior to passing the tube. Preparation is, therefore, as for patients prior to general anaesthesia.

For children of ten-years-of-age or more, fluids and diet are withheld overnight and the throat may be sprayed with a local anaesthetic immediately prior to passage of the tube. A simple explanation is necessary and the child's full co-operation obtained.

METHOD

The assembled intestinal tube is threaded through the pressure tubing on which the child can safely bite. The lubricated capsule is passed over the back of the tongue into the oro-pharynx and quickly advanced into the oesophagus and stomach. A further 5–10cm or 2–4 inches of tubing is passed and the child is turned on to his right side to encourage the capsule towards the pyloric sphincter. Alternatively, the radiologist may assess the position of the capsule and attempt to direct it through the pylorus, under X-ray control.

Once the capsule has passed through the pyloric sphincter, it is advanced to the site of choice for biopsy, confirmed by X-ray examination. The capsule is 'fired' and the biopsy collected. The negative pressure created by a 10ml syringe attached to the free end of the tube draws a small portion of jejunal mucosa into the capsule and releases the blade. With the biopsy specimen safely encapsulated, the intestinal tube and capsule are slowly withdrawn.

The capsule is opened and the specimen carefully removed with the sterile instruments. Specimens are cut for:
1 Histology—for microscopic examination of the mucosal structure.
2 Bacteriology—for the presence of Giardia lamblia (a protozoal infestation of the small intestine causing steatorrhoea).

3 Biochemistry—for estimation of tryptic activity. (Specimen placed on dry ice.)

A differential diagnosis of giardiasis or cystic fibrosis is excluded by examinations (2) and (3) respectively.

AFTER CARE

The child is nursed in bed for the rest of the day.

Jejunal perforation and haemorrhage are rare, but possible complications, therefore:

  i   the pulse rate is recorded at half-hourly intervals for twelve hours;

  ii any complaint of abdominal discomfort must be reported;

  iii any vomit is inspected for the presence of blood;

  iv stools are tested for occult blood;

  v   only clear fluid is given for the first feed/drink, followed by fluids only for twenty-four hours.

Renal Biopsy

Microscopic examination of a specimen of renal tissue will confirm a diagnosis and help a doctor to decide on the appropriate treatment and prognosis for a child with a kidney disorder. An intravenous pyelogram is performed prior to a percutaneous renal biopsy to determine the position and efficiency of the kidneys. These films must accompany the child to the operating theatre or X-ray department.

The child is prepared as for any child going to the operating theatre and the procedure is performed under a general or local anaesthetic.

After care

For the rest of the day, the child is nursed in the left lateral position if biopsy is taken from the left kidney, and right lateral position if the right kidney has been punctured, and is under constant observation until consciousness is regained. The main complication of percutaneous renal biopsy is concealed haemorrhage, therefore:

  i   loin pain, local swelling or discolouration must be reported;

  ii haematuria is common, therefore to be expected in the first urine voided, and all urine passed in the following twenty-four hours must be inspected. The amount of blood passed should diminish steadily;

  iii a record of the pulse rate is maintained at half-hourly intervals for twelve to twenty-four hours;

  iv hourly–four hourly recording of blood pressure is maintained. A fall in the blood pressure, particularly if associated with a rising pulse rate, is indicative of haemorrhage. The blood pressure may rise in response to the production of renin by a failing kidney.

Collection of Cerebrospinal Fluid

Cerebrospinal fluid, the crystal clear secretion produced by the choroid plexus in the four cerebral ventricles, is contained within the ventricular system, central canal of the spinal cord and subarachnoid compartment of the brain and spinal cord. Reabsorption into the blood stream is through the arachnoid granulations protruding into the superior sagittal sinus. Production and reabsorption is continuous. The volume of cerebrospinal fluid in circulation varies with body size—an adult has 100–150ml and children proportionately less.

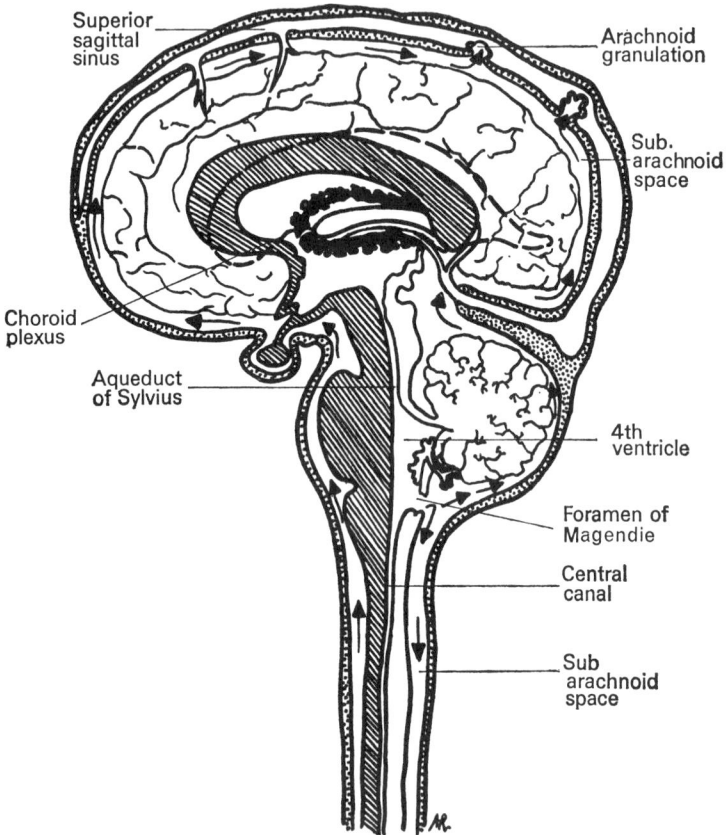

FIG. 80. Circulation of cerebrospinal fluid.

Normal constituents of cerebrospinal fluid:
Protein 20–40mg/100ml
Sugar   45–85mg/100ml
0–5 lymphocytes per cu. mm. (up to 30 in newborn infants)
Pressure 70–200mm water

Cerebrospinal fluid may be collected by:
1 Lumbar puncture.
2 Cisternal puncture.
3 Ventricular puncture.

Lumbar puncture

Lumbar puncture is the procedure most commonly used to collect a specimen of cerebrospinal fluid. The spinal cord terminates at the level of the third lumbar vertebra in infancy and the lower border of the first lumbar vertebra in older children. Cerebrospinal fluid contained in the subarachnoid compartment below this point can be safely tapped by inserting a needle between the third and fourth, or second and third lumbar vertebrae of a firmly controlled child.

A lumbar puncture may be performed for the following reasons:

1 DIAGNOSTIC
    i To collect a specimen of cerebrospinal fluid to isolate the causative agent and to assess progress in meningitis. Specimens are collected for microbiology and/or virology and for biochemical analysis.
    ii to inject contrast medium prior to radiological studies:
    a. Filtered air or oxygen for pneumoencephalography.
    b. Iodized oil for myelography.
    iii To estimate the pressure of cerebrospinal fluid. A lumbar puncture is contra-indicated in the presence of papilloedema associated with a raised intracranial pressure. Consequent herniation of the brain stem into the foramen magnum (coning) results in respiratory failure and death.

2 THERAPEUTIC
    i To inject intrathecal antibiotics in tuberculous and pyogenic meningitis.
    ii To inject chemotherapeutic agents, e.g. methotrexate in leukaemic infiltration of the meninges.

3 TO INDUCE SPINAL ANAESTHESIA (rare in childhood)

REQUIREMENTS
The basic trolley is prepared, as described on page 258 with the addition of the following equipment:

Selection of lumbar
  puncture needles
Spinal manometer   } These may be included in a composite pack.
2–3 sterile screw-cap
  laboratory containers

Bottom shelf:

Mask
Sterile gloves } for the doctor.

Tincture of iodine.

2ml syringe
Nos. 12 and 17 hypodermic needles } for local anaesthetic.
Lignocaine 1%

Nobecutane.

Narrow adhesive tape.

Appropriate laboratory forms and labels.

Additional requirements:
A stool for the doctor.

PREPARATION OF THE CHILD

Sedation may be given to an infant. The co-operation of an older child is sought. He should be given opportunity to empty his bladder before being dressed in an open-back gown. The child is placed in the lateral position with his arched back to the edge of a firm narrow mattress or table. Complete control of the child is imperative for the safety and success of this procedure. Control is maintained by the assisting nurse who directs one arm around his flexed knees, grasping her hands in front of the child. Care must be taken to ensure that the vertebral column remains parallel with the firm surface and that respiratory and circulatory embarrassment is not caused by over-flexion of the neck (FIG. 81).

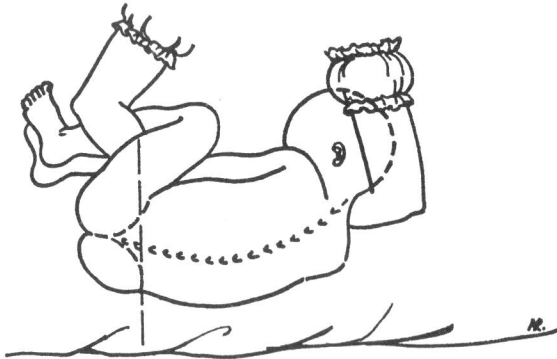

FIG. 81. Position of a child for lumbar puncture.

METHOD

To allow the nurse to give her undivided attention to her patient, a second person is required to assist the doctor with this procedure. If this is not practical, then doctor and nurse working together ensure that all is prepared before the nurse positions her patient.

While the doctor puts on his mask, washes and dries his hands and puts on sterile gloves, the nurse ensures that everything required for the procedure is on the top of the trolley. The local anaesthetic, if used, is checked by both doctor and nurse before a small quantity is drawn into a 2ml syringe. If the specimen containers have been pre-sterilized so that the outside is sterile as well as the inside, these are put on to the trolley top, otherwise it is essential for a third person to be available to collect the specimens of cerebrospinal fluid. Whichever alternative is used, it is advisable to ensure that the caps are loosened before the procedure is commenced.

A stool is provided for the doctor and the trolley is conveniently placed.

Once the child is securely restrained, the doctor cleanses the area, administers the local anaesthetic (if required) and drapes the site. The lumbar puncture needle is inserted, the stilette removed and specimens of cerebrospinal fluid are collected into two specimen containers.

Before collection of the specimens, the doctor may wish to estimate the pressure of cerebrospinal fluid in circulation. This he does by attaching the Luer attachment of the manometer to the lumbar puncture needle. With the manometer in an upright position, the level to which the cerebrospinal fluid rises is noted. Queckenstedt's test may then be performed.

PRINCIPLE OF QUECKENSTEDT'S TEST

The nurse is asked to compress a jugular vein by placing the side of her hand between the sternomastoid muscle and the trachea. Jugular vein compression increases venous congestion within the skull and the fluid level in the manometer will rise markedly. Following quick release of jugular compression, the fluid level quickly falls. If there is interruption to the flow of cerebrospinal fluid, there will be diminished or no increase in pressure during jugular compression. Crying induces the same response.

Following removal of the needle, iodine, if used, is removed with a spirit lotion and a small, firm dressing is applied. Leakage from the puncture site can be controlled by application of Nobecutane.

The specimen containers are clearly labelled and immediately dispatched with their appropriate forms to the laboratories. The first specimen collected is usually sent to the biochemistry department and the second for bacteriological investigation.

AFTER CARE

The child is warmly dressed and returned to his bed to rest in a recumbent position. Complications are rare in childhood. Elevation of the foot of the bed will control headache or vomiting. Complaints of tingling in the legs must be reported. The dressing covering the site is removed the following day.

Cisternal Puncture

When there is obstruction to the flow of cerebrospinal fluid between the basal cistern of the brain and the spinal theca, cerebrospinal fluid may be collected by cisternal puncture. Because of the close proximity of the medulla, this procedure is only attempted when complete immobilization of the patient can be guaranteed.

REQUIREMENTS
As for lumbar puncture. A long spinal needle is necessary.

Additional requirements:
Electric hair cutters and razor   *or*   Gauze swabs.
                                         Razor and blade.
                                         Soap solution.

PREPARATION OF THE CHILD
The occipital region of the scalp is shaved to the occipital protuberance. The child is placed in the lateral position with the neck moderately flexed. Alternatively, an older child may be sat astride a chair, his head resting on his arms placed on the back of the chair. Both positions widen the space between the occipital bone and the first cervical vertebra.

METHOD
The procedure is essentially as for lumbar puncture. A local anaesthetic is given unless general anaesthesia has been induced.

Ventricular Puncture

This procedure can only be carried out in infants where an anterior fontanelle or coronal suture has not closed, or following bi-parietal trephining (burr-holes) in an older child. It is the method of choice for obtaining a specimen of cerebrospinal fluid from a child when the intracranial pressure is raised and the method by which cerebrospinal fluid is replaced by filtered air or oxygen prior to ventriculography.

REQUIREMENTS
As for lumbar puncture. A calibrated brain needle may be preferred.

Additional requirements:
As for cisternal puncture.

PREPARATION OF THE INFANT
The infant's head is prepared by shaving a 5cm or 2 inches area round the anterior fontanelle or coronal suture. The restrained infant is placed supine across a firm mattress or table with his head to the edge. The assisting nurse

positions herself at the infant's feet, splints his body with her forearms, and supports his head so that his nose remains perpendicular to the mattress (FIG. 82).

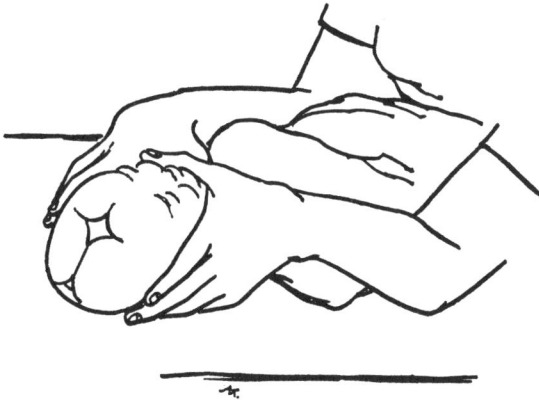

FIG. 82. Position of an infant for ventricular puncture.

METHOD

The procedure is essentially as for lumbar puncture. Neither sedation nor local anaesthetic is usually necessary. Following withdrawal of the needle, firm pressure is applied to the puncture site while the child is supported in an upright position.

When it is necessary to remove cerebrospinal fluid from the ventricular system at frequent intervals, or when there is a need for chemotherapeutic agents to be instilled to control infection, a ventriculostomy reservoir may be inserted or incorporated into a Holter drainage system. A short, fine perforated catheter connects one lateral ventricle to the small reservoir lying just below the skin surface. The skin overlying the 'button' is cleansed and a No. 1 hypodermic needle inserted into the reservoir to withdraw cerebrospinal fluid or to instil drugs.

Subdural Tap

Normally only a small amount of clear fluid is contained in the closed subdural compartment. Post meningitic effusions and haemorrhages associated with injury are diagnosed and drained by subdural tap. A short needle is necessary.

Requirements, preparation of the child, and procedure are as for ventricular tap.

Removal of Excess Extracellular Fluid

Oedema is swelling due to excess fluid in the tissue spaces. Oedema may affect the whole body, or may be localized to one area.

With reference to FIG. 83, it will be seen that tissue fluid will accumulate:

i   if there is a general increase in the systemic venous pressure due to con-
    gestive heart failure. Occlusion of a localized vein, e.g. the portal vein by
    cirrhosis of the liver, or the femoral vein by a thrombus, will cause ascites
    and distal dropsical swelling (oedema) respectively;

ii in hypoproteinaemia due to:
    a. nutritional lack of protein as in kwashiorkor;
    b. loss of protein from the kidneys as in nephrotic syndrome;

iii in salt, therefore water retention associated with inadequate renal function
    (page 402);

iv with occlusion of localized lymphatic vessels as in cystic hygroma.

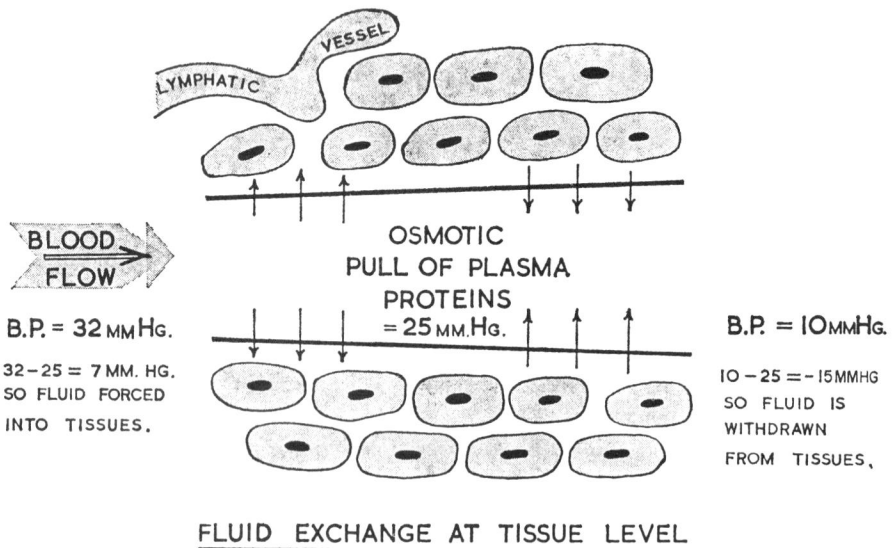

FLUID   EXCHANGE   AT   TISSUE   LEVEL

FIG. 83.

The measures adopted to relieve the condition depend on the cause of the
oedema. One or more of the following may be employed:

i   Treatment of the cause.
ii Restricting dietary salt.
iii Reducing the fluid intake.
iv Increasing the urine output by the administration of diuretics.
v   Removing the fluid by mechanical means:
    a. Abdominal paracentesis to relieve ascites.
    b. Use of Southey's tubes to relieve generalized oedema (anasarca).

Abdominal Paracentesis

The two layers of peritoneum, the parietal and the visceral, enclose a thin layer of serous fluid, thus allowing free movement of the abdominal contents. An excess of serous fluid within the peritoneal cavity is called ascites and may be associated with portal hypertension, or with generalized oedema as in congestive heart failure and nephrotic syndrome. With the effective use of diuretics, mechanical measures for the relief of generalized oedema are now used infrequently. An abdominal paracentesis may, however, be necessary to relieve respiratory embarrassment caused by gross ascites.

A Southey's tube is usually preferred for this procedure. This is a fine perforated silver cannula with a shield and sharp stilette. A length of narrow tubing connects the cannula to a collecting bag, thus creating a closed drainage system avoiding the risk of ascending infection.

REQUIREMENTS

The basic trolley is prepared as described on page 258 with the addition of the following equipment:

Southey's tube with shield
Stilette and length of narrow tubing, *or* } All sterile.
Trocar and cannula } (These will be included in a composite
Bard Parker handle and blade } pack.)

Bottom shelf:
Masks for all participants.
Sterile gloves for the doctor.
Lignocaine 1%
2ml syringe } for local anaesthetic.
Nos. 12 and 17 hypodermic needles
Sterile screw-cap laboratory container.
Completed laboratory form and label.
Collecting bag (urine collection) and bracket.
Flow regulator.
Many-tailed bandage (abdominal binder).
Narrow adhesive tape.
Safety-pin.
Waterproof protection.

PREPARATION OF THE CHILD

The child is usually very ill. A sedative is necessary to overcome agitation and anxiety. A simple explanation of what is about to happen will help to give an older child confidence. Dressed only in a pyjama jacket, the child is made comfortable in an upright position as required by his dyspnoea and to allow the ascitic fluid to gravitate.

The bladder should be emptied before the cannula is inserted to one side of the mid-line, mid-way between the umbilicus and the symphysis pubis. The child is, therefore, encouraged to pass urine. Failing this, the doctor may request that the bladder is catheterized.

The many-tailed bandage is placed behind the child so that the tails can be subsequently brought around the abdomen to support his decreasing girth. The chest is protected with a treatment blanket and the bedclothes turned down to the upper thighs. If a second nurse is available, the child's attention is distracted from the doctor's activities.

METHOD

While the doctor puts on a mask, washes and dries his hands and puts on sterile gloves, the nurse ensures that everything required for the procedure is on the top of the trolley. The local anaesthetic is checked and drawn into the syringe.

Using a strict aseptic technique, the doctor cleanses the area, administers the local anaesthetic and drapes the site. The equipment is assembled, a small incision is made in the skin and the Southey's tube inserted. The stilette is removed to allow ascitic fluid to flow down the length of tubing to the collecting bag suspended at the side or end of the bed. The tubing, secured to the drawsheet with a safety-pin, is partially occluded with a flow regulator to prevent sudden collapse of the child, due to rapid reduction of intra-abdominal pressure. The cannula is maintained in position with lengths of adhesive tape and the many-tailed bandage is fastened firmly across the abdomen. This serves two useful purposes. First and foremost, it gives firm support to the abdomen and requires re-adjustment as the intra-abdominal pressure falls. It also provides a useful barrier between the intraperitoneal cannula and exploring fingers.

AFTER CARE

As the fluid may continue to flow for up to twenty-four hours, all basic nursing care must continue. A bed-cradle is used to raise the bedclothes off the abdomen. Restraint should not be necessary—diversional therapy being preferable. If the child is particularly restless, it may be necessary to secure his hands to the sides of the cot during the night. The child should be carefully observed for signs of distress, and the abdominal binder tightened at intervals. The rate of ascitic drainage should be regulated as necessary and the collecting bag exchanged as it becomes full. The child is usually considerably relieved by this procedure and becomes noticeably happier as drainage progresses.

REMOVAL OF THE CANNULA

When drainage has ceased and on instruction from the doctor, the cannula is gently withdrawn and the wound covered with a dry dressing. Leakage may persist for a day or two, but closure of the perforation is usually rapid.

Subcutaneous Drainage of Oedema (Southey's Tubes)

As mentioned above, generalized oedema can now be effectively controlled by increasing the urine output with the use of diuretics. Very occasionally, drainage may be needed in addition to diuretics.

REQUIREMENTS

The basic trolley is prepared as described on page 258 with the addition of the following equipment:

Southey's tubes with stilette   } All sterile.
    and lengths of narrow tubing } (These will be included in a composite pack.)

Bottom shelf:
Masks for all participants.
Sterile gloves for the doctor.
2ml syringe   }
Nos. 12 and 17 hypodermic needles } For local anaesthetic (if necessary).
Lignocaine 1%   }
Crêpe bandages.
Narrow adhesive tape.
Collecting bags and brackets.
Safety-pins.
Waterproof protection.

PREPARATION OF THE CHILD

Excess tissue fluid is encouraged to gravitate to the dependent legs. The child is, therefore, nursed in a cardiac bed or an armchair.

METHOD

The procedure and after care is essentially as described in the preceding section. A fine Southey's tube is inserted into the outer aspect of each leg just above the ankle. The narrow tubing secured to the draw sheet with safety-pins connects each tube to a collecting bag suspended at the end of the bed. The tubes are secured in position with lengths of adhesive tape and crêpe bandages. The bed-clothes are arranged to avoid pressure over the oedematous legs. Prophylactic antibiotics diminish the risk of bacterial invasion of the devitalized tissues.

Aspiration of the Pleural Cavity

The two layers of pleura, the parietal and the visceral, enclose a thin layer of serous fluid allowing for free, painless movement of the thoracic contents. Because pressure in the pleural cavity is sub-atmospheric or negative, care has to be taken to ensure that air does not enter the pleural space during aspiration.

A special chest aspiration cannula or needle is attached to a two-way tap and syringe, each with a self-locking device. A length of tubing is attached to the second arm of the two-way tap.

A chest aspiration is usually both diagnostic and therapeutic. In most instances a specimen of pleural fluid is retained for bacteriological examination. Aspiration may be performed:

i   to relieve dropsical hydrothorax (transudate);

ii to aspirate inflammatory exudate (pleural effusion) complicating pneumonia or pulmonary tuberculosis;

iii to aspirate a pyothorax (empyema);

iv to relieve a haemothorax ⎫
          a pneumothorax ⎭ following injury or surgery.

REQUIREMENTS

The basic trolley is prepared as described on page 258 with the addition of the following equipment:

20 or 50ml syringe ⎫
2-way tap ⎪
Length of narrow tubing ⎬ All sterile.
Selection of aspiration needles ⎪ (These will be included in a composite pack.)
Jug or receiver ⎭

Bottom shelf:

Masks for all participants.
Sterile gloves for the doctor.
Collodion.
2ml syringe ⎫
Nos. 12 and 17 hypodermic needles ⎬ For local anaesthetic.
Lignocaine 1% ⎭
Narrow adhesive tape.
Sterile screw-cap laboratory container.
Completed laboratory form and label.
Waterproof protection.

PREPARATION OF THE CHILD

Although the child will be greatly relieved by the removal of a large collection of pleural fluid, the procedure is unpleasant. A sedative is necessary to overcome agitation, and a linctus may be prescribed to depress the cough reflex. The child is placed in a suitable position in which the intercostal spaces are enlarged and in which he can comfortably remain or be restrained. This is best achieved by sitting a big child on the side of his bed or the examination couch with his feet resting on a stool and his arms and head resting on a pillow placed on a bed-table in front of him (FIG. 84). Alternatively, he may sit up in bed and similarly lean forward over a bed-table, but his position is difficult to maintain in comfort for more than a few minutes.

A small child is either similarly positioned on the nurse's knees or on his non-affected side over a pillow with the upper arm elevated over the head. The nurse should see that the X-ray films are available for study.

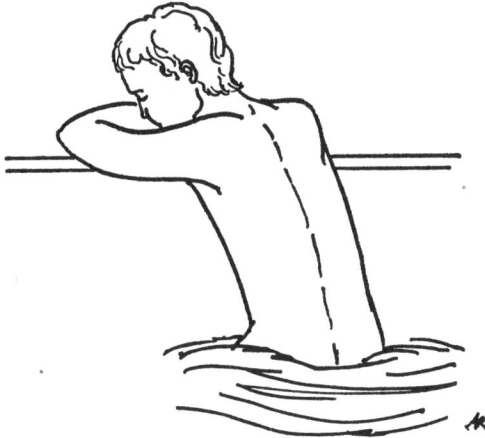

FIG. 84. Position of a child for aspiration of the pleural cavity.

METHOD

While the doctor puts on a mask, washes and dries his hands and puts on sterile gloves, the nurse ensures that everything required for the procedure is on the top shelf of the trolley. The local anaesthetic is checked and drawn into the syringe.

Using a strict aseptic technique, the doctor cleanses the area, administers the local anaesthetic and drapes the site. The equipment is assembled and the needle inserted. Pleural fluid is withdrawn by negative pressure in the syringe. The tap is then turned through 90° and the contents of the syringe expelled by the second arm and tubing into a jug. The tap is turned to its former position and the procedure is repeated for as long as necessary.

Throughout the procedure the nurse must observe, comfort and reassure the child. The doctor must be told of any deterioration in the child's condition and forewarned of anticipated movement and coughing so that he can take the appropriate precautions to prevent visceral injury.

On completion of the procedure, the needle is withdrawn and the puncture wound sealed with collodion or covered with a dry dressing, secured with lengths of adhesive tape. The child is made comfortable in an upright position and allowed to rest, while remaining under close observation. A warm, soothing drink is often appreciated.

Venesection

Polycythaemia in childhood is limited for practical purposes to the secondary changes occurring in severe (cyanotic) congenital heart disease. Polycythaemia increases the viscosity of the blood and the tendency to intravascular clotting, and is aggravated by dehydration. Venesection is sometimes used in such cases. Negative pressure is necessary as the blood is usually too viscid to flow freely from a cannulated vein.

REQUIREMENTS

The basic trolley is prepared as described on page 258 with the addition of the following equipment:

Bottom shelf:
Several 20ml syringes with eccentric nozzles.
Needle or cannula (as large calibre as possible).
Bottle of heparinized saline.
Padded splint and bandage.
Waterproof protection for the bed.
It may be necessary for a vein to be dissected if the child is small, when the necessary instruments should be supplied.

METHOD

A sedative is usually prescribed and given an hour before withdrawing blood. While the doctor washes and dries his hands, the nurse ensures that everything required for the procedure is on the top of the trolley.

A vein in the antecubital fossa is usually selected and the elbow splinted and rested on the waterproof protection. The vein is made more prominent by constriction of the arm above the site, using a pocket tourniquet, sphygmomanometer cuff or with the hand of the assisting nurse, and an older child is asked to clench his fist or grasp an object.

The skin is cleansed and allowed to dry. The needle is inserted and the pressure released. Withdrawal of blood may prove slow and difficult. Heparinized saline is necessary to prevent clotting. Once each syringe is full or blocked, another is substituted until the required amount of blood has been withdrawn, or the attempt abandoned. On withdrawal of the needle, firm pressure is applied over the site and the limb is raised.

Throughout the procedure, the child is closely observed for signs of blood loss, i.e. a rapid weak pulse, pallor and a feeling of faintness.

Blood Transfusion

All human beings inherit one of the following blood groups AB, A, B or O according to the antigen present in the red blood cells. The serum contains natural antibody which is the opposite to the antigen in the cells.

TABLE 17. A B O Blood-group System

Group	Antigen in red blood cells	Antibody in serum
AB	A and B	Neither
A	A	anti-B
B	B	anti-A
O	Neither	anti-A and anti-B

Approximately 85% of all Europeans, in common with the Rhesus monkey, carry an additional antigen in the red blood cells and are referred to as Rhesus positive. Naturally occurring antibody is not present in the serum of Rhesus negative subjects, but a Rhesus negative person may be sensitized to produce Rhesus antibodies by transfusion of Rhesus positive blood or bearing a Rhesus positive child.

In the presence of an antigen in the red blood cells of the donor and the appropriate antibodies in the serum of the recipient, the red blood cells clump together (agglutinate) and subsequently release haemoglobin (haemolyse). The patient should be transfused with donor blood of his own group, though in an emergency, group O Rhesus negative blood may be transfused to any patient of any blood group as long as the anti-A and anti-B titre of the donor blood is not of a high level.

Blood and Blood Fractions

Whole blood or the constituent parts of blood are available for a variety of uses. Blood is donated freely by a small percentage of healthy adults. Venesection of the donor allows 420ml of blood to be freely mixed with 120ml of anticoagulant, usually sodium citrate, in a sterile pyrogen-free glass bottle or polythene bag, referred to in the text as a unit of blood. Following tests made on the blood sample trapped in the pilot tubing, it can be stored for up to three weeks at a temperature of 4°C.

Whole blood. This is a valuable source of red blood cells and is used extensively to replace blood loss due to haemorrhage. During infancy when the blood volume forms approximately 8% of the body weight (80ml/kg) a transfusion of 20ml/kg will raise the haemoglobin level approximately 25%.

Packed cells. To avoid overloading the circulation of small children, packed cells are used to replace blood loss due to haemolysis and to counteract inefficient erythrocyte haemopoiesis (red cell production). Under sterile laboratory conditions, the supernatant plasma from a unit of whole blood is removed within twelve hours prior to use.

Settled cells. Used for the same purpose as above, but the whole unit of blood is erected. To avoid unsettling the cells, the air-inlet of the recipient set must extend above the level of the blood. Only the precipitated cells are administered.

Fresh donor blood. During storage, the potassium contained in the red blood cells gradually leaks, increasing the potassium content of the plasma. Where increase in the serum potassium level could prove dangerous, recently donated blood is used, e.g. to small infants with inefficient renal function, for exchange transfusions and for heart surgery involving cardio-pulmonary by-pass.

Platelet rich plasma and platelet concentrate. Used when the platelet level is dangerously low.

Leucocyte rich plasma. Used to replace the essential white cells destroyed by the administration of cytotoxic chemotherapy. The leucopenia experienced by a child with leukaemia undergoing intensive drug therapy may be treated with this blood fraction.

Plasma and plasma fractions. These can be administered to children of all blood groups. The pooled dried plasma stored in a cool place is reconstituted with 400 ml of sterile distilled water immediately prior to use. It is useful in the replacement of the protein fraction of blood in children suffering from extensive burns. It has little value as a means of nourishment. A record of the batch number is kept for subsequent reference if necessary.

Fresh frozen plasma. The over-cooled supernatant plasma taken from a unit of freshly donated blood is a rich source of the globulins essential for clotting of blood. Bleeding in both haemophilia and Christmas disease can be controlled by prompt transfusion of fresh frozen plasma containing all the clotting factors. The sealed unit is warmed in a bowl of water, temperature 36·8°C or 98·4°F. Rapid thawing and administration are necessary to achieve full benefit from the transfusion.

Cryoprecipitate. A concentrated source of anti-haemophilic globulin (AHG), cryoprecipitate is produced by reducing the temperature of fresh plasma to $-70°C$ to allow the AHG to be precipitated—hence its name. The AHG contained in one unit of blood is then contained in about 10ml of plasma, thus reducing the necessity to transfuse large quantities of whole plasma to boys with haemophilia during a bleeding crisis. With the introduction of cryoprecipitate, the necessity to use AHG of bovine or porcine origin has been obviated. When surgery is undertaken, the AHG level of the blood is maintained with sufficient doses of cryoprecipitate administered by intravenous injection every twelve to twenty-four hours.

Albumin. This may be transfused to reduce the oedema caused by hypoprotein-aemia.

Pooled gamma globulins. Given by intramuscular injection in selective instances to give temporary passive immunity (page 23).

Precautions Taken Prior to Blood Transfusion

Following a request for blood, the child's blood group is determined and a few cells of the donor blood are mixed with the serum of the recipient and examined for agglutination twenty minutes later. This is called cross-matching of blood, and if no agglutination occurs, the unit of blood is carefully labelled and reserved in the blood bank refrigerator until required for the child.

Blood should be collected from the blood bank within half-an-hour of being required on the ward or in theatre and should never be warmed prior to transfusion. Blood not used within half-an-hour must be discarded, as the risk of contamination and multiplication of micro-organisms in this ideal medium is too great to allow the blood to be returned to cold storage for use at a later date.

Collection of blood from the blood bank is a responsible task. The child's name, hospital registration number, A B O and Rhesus group and serial number of the blood unit should be carefully checked against the patient's records, according to hospital policy. The blood unit is then carefully carried upright to the ward to avoid damage to the red blood cells, and checked again at the child's bedside with a second senior nurse. Administration of the wrong blood to the patient could result in death.

Vitamins, drugs and electrolytes should never be introduced into blood for transfusion. A chelating agent—desferrioxamine—is sometimes given, either before or following a transfusion of whole blood, to prevent accumulation of iron in the tissues (haemosiderosis) in children with blood disorders, such as aplastic anaemia and thalassaemia major, demanding repeated transfusions.

Care of the Child During Blood Transfusion

With careful selection of donors and collection of donor blood, meticulous cross-matching and double checking of blood prior to transfusion, reactions during administration are minimal. A child receiving a blood transfusion requires careful observation, particularly in the first hour or so of the transfusion. Signs of incompatibility, allergy, infection or overloading of the circulation should be reported immediately.

Incompatibility results in agglutination of red blood cells and blockage of the small capillaries of the brain, lungs, kidneys and extremities. Any complaint of *pain in these areas or 'pins and needles' in the extremities* demands immediate discontinuation of the transfusion. *Jaundice, haemoglobinuria and anuria* are later signs, due to haemolysis of the agglutinated cells.

Use of disposable polythene recipient sets has reduced the incidence of allergy to bacterial products (pyrogens) manifesting as *urticaria*, a *rise in temperature* or a *rigor*.

Infection is rare and usually presents as serum hepatitis some months later.

Overloading the circulation is prevented by administering the blood at the rate requested by the doctor, recording the *pulse rate* and carefully observing the child for *signs of dyspnoea*. It is advisable, therefore, to maintain a quarter to half-hourly recording of the pulse and respiration rates, to record the temperature hourly and to maintain an accurate fluid balance chart for all children receiving a transfusion.

On completion of the transfusion, the unwashed blood bottle or bag is retained for laboratory tests should an untoward reaction occur.

Several methods are available to the doctor who wishes to increase the rate of transfusion:

1 A second vein may be cannulated.

2 The recipient set tubing may be passed around the rollers of a hand operated Martin pump.

3 A Baxter type recipient set incorporating a pressure chamber may be used. A ball valve prevents reverse flow of the blood (FIG. 85).

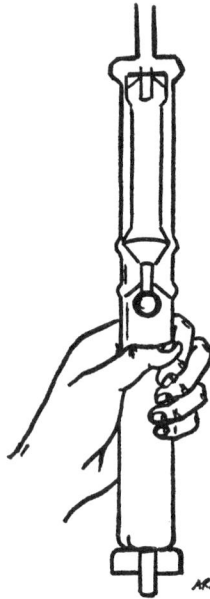

FIG. 85. Pressure chamber as incorporated in a recipient set produced by Baxter Laboratories Ltd. A ball valve prevents reverse flow of blood.

4 Increased positive pressure may be exerted on the blood contained in a polythene envelope by squeezing the bag until empty.

Exchange Transfusion

Exchange transfusion is a relatively safe method of exchanging a large proportion of the circulating blood of an infant with fresh blood from an appropriate donor. Its use is indicated in haemolytic disease of the newborn due to Rhesus (or O–A and O–B) incompatibility and in severe physiological jaundice of prematurity. Exchange transfusions have also been used in poisoning by iron and salicylates, but simpler alternatives are usually employed.

In Rhesus incompatibility, the infant's red blood cells carry the Rhesus D antigen, thus making him Rhesus positive. In addition, there has been transplacental passage of Rhesus antibodies from the previously sensitized Rhesus negative maternal circulation into the foetal circulation. Agglutination and haemolysis of red blood cells result in anaemia and liberation of excessive amounts of toxic insoluble unconjugated bilirubin into the foetal circulation. Much less frequently, a foetus of group A or B may be similarly affected if carried by a mother of group O with immune anti-A or anti-B antibodies.

In an older person, unexcretable unconjugated bilirubin undergoes glucuronic conjugation in the liver and the bilirubin is excreted from the body (FIG. 86). In Rhesus incompatibility, the glucuronyl transferase system is unable to fulfil the demands put on it, causing the unconjugated bilirubin level of the serum to rise to toxic levels. This enzyme system is relatively ineffective in infants of low birth weight, giving rise to severe physiological jaundice with an associated high serum unconjugated bilirubin value.

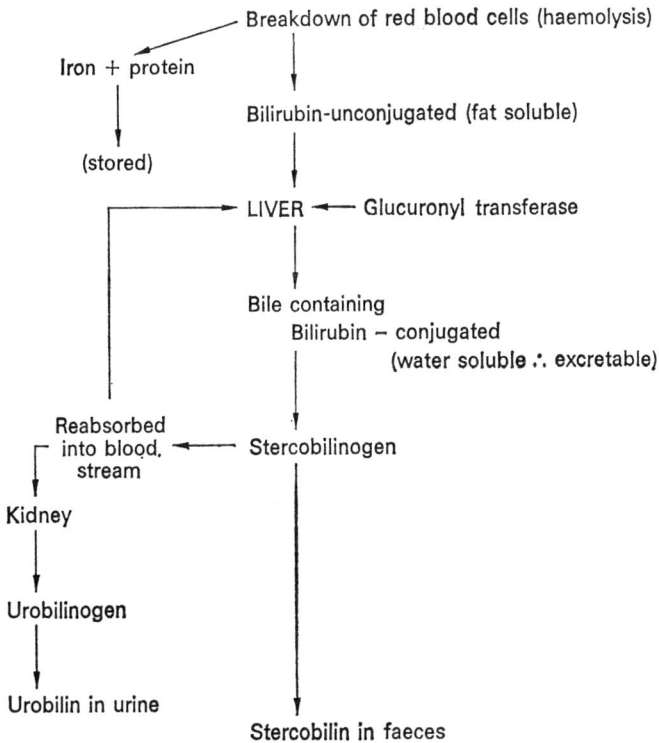

FIG. 86. The circulation and excretion of bilirubin.

With the introduction of intra-uterine transfusions of blood into the peritoneal cavity of the unborn child and the more recent opportunity to immunize a Rhesus negative mother following delivery of a Rhesus positive infant with gamma globulins from hypersensitive male volunteers, haemolytic disease of the newborn is now being prevented rather than cured.

Indications for Exchange Transfusion

1   At birth:
     i   When the haemoglobin level is 15g/100ml or less.
    ii   When the serum bilirubin level exceeds 5mg/100ml.
   iii   When the Coombs' test is positive.
2   Subsequently:
To maintain the unconjugated bilirubin level of the serum below 20mg/100ml to prevent kernicterus.

Principle of the Procedure

Freshly donated Rhesus negative blood of group O, or preferably the ABO group of the infant and compatible with the mother's serum, is used to replace the Rhesus positive red cells and remove antibodies and toxic unconjugated bilirubin from the infant's circulation. Following umbilical cannulation, successive quantities of the infant's blood are removed and replaced with the same volume of Rhesus negative blood in 20, 10 or 5ml cycles. If the infant's condition remains satisfactory, approximately 160ml/kg is exchanged at a rate not exceeding 1·6ml/kg/minute to effect an 80% exchange of blood.

REQUIREMENTS
The trolley is prepared as in the operating theatre, the top shelf being covered with sterile waterproof and draped with large towels.

Top shelf:
Waterproof protection.
4 large dressing towels.
1 dressing towel with centre window.
Gallipot.
Gauze swabs.
2 towel clips.
1 Bard Parker handle and blade.
1 pair heavy non-toothed dissecting forceps.
1 pair heavy toothed dissecting forceps.
1 pair fine toothed dissecting forceps.
1 pair stitch scissors.

1 pair iridectomy scissors.
3 pairs straight mosquito forceps.
1 pair Spencer Wells artery forceps.
1 fine silver probe.
1 needle holder.
1 metal rule.
1 aneurysm needle.
1 umbilical obturator.

Bottom shelf:
Masks for all participants.
'Scrubbing up' brush.
Sterile gown and gloves for the doctor.
Lotions for cleansing the skin.
Recipient set.
Disposable exchange transfusion set consisting of:
    20ml syringe.
    Two 2-way taps.
    Length of tubing.
Umbilical catheters of various sizes.
Bottle clip(s).
Urine collection bag (continuous bladder drainage) and bracket for discarded
    blood).
Tray containing:
    10ml syringe.
    No. 1 needle.
    Ampoules of calcium gluconate 10%.
    File.
    Mersuture.
    Mediswab.
    Narrow adhesive tape.
    Cross-match form.
    2 Sequestrene tubes for haemoglobin estimation.
    2 specimen tubes for clotted blood for bilirubin estimation.
Completed laboratory forms and labels.
Infants teat and gauze or dummy.
Requirements for restraint.

Additional requirements:
Intravenous stand.
Resuscitation equipment.
Anglepoise lamp.
Stethoscope.
Stop watch.

Blood warming apparatus set at 35°C.
Special chart.

PREPARATION OF THE INFANT

Chilling of the infant must be avoided. The room temperature is maintained at around 30°C or 80°F and its occupants suitably dressed for comfort. The infant is nursed in an incubator until preparations have been made. Parental consent is obtained. Weight and height should be known and antibiotics, sedatives and other drugs administered as prescribed by the doctor.

The procedure may take several hours to complete and stools should be provided for the participating staff. Two nurses are essential to assist the doctor with this procedure; one has the sole responsibility of the observation and care of the infant, while her colleague assists the doctor and maintains accurate records.

When all is prepared, the infant is dressed in suitable clothing to allow just the abdomen and face to be exposed, and with his arms and legs restrained. He is kept warm throughout the procedure in an open incubator or by means of protected hot-water bottles. The infant may find comfort in sucking a teat occluded with cotton wool. A urine collection bag may be placed in position to avoid contamination of the operation field. A lubricated electronic temperature probe is inserted into the rectum. The diaphragm end-piece of a stethoscope is secured over the apex of the heart, or alternatively the nurse may record the pulse rate by placing her warmed fingers over the apex or a peripheral artery.

METHOD

If instructed by the doctor, the sealed unit of blood is gently warmed in a bath of water, temperature 38°C or 100°F, while the preparations are being made. Some supernatant plasma may be removed, especially if the infant is anaemic. With reference to the cross-match form, the blood is checked by the doctor and assisting nurse, the bottle seal broken, rubber cap cleansed and the needle(s) of the recipient set introduced into the inverted bottle. The recipient set tubing is passed through a thermostatically controlled blood warmer set at 35°C.

After 'scrubbing up', the doctor puts on sterile gown and gloves and prepares his sterile requirements. The assisting nurse puts the sterile contents of packs from the lower shelf on to the top shelf of the trolley.

The saline soaks are removed from the umbilical cord and the area cleansed and draped. The umbilical vein is identified and an umbilical catheter threaded 6–9cm into its lumen. The venous pressure is recorded (normal 5–7cm of blood).

The syringe and two-way tap is connected to the umbilical catheter and the recipient set carrying donor blood. (A second recipient set primed with heparinized saline may be attached to an additional two-way tap for intermittent rinsing of the syringe.) Air is withdrawn from the recipient set and the first specimen of blood is withdrawn from the infant. This is collected into the first set of specimen tubes and the length of tubing is then attached to the collecting bag.

The exchange of infant's blood for warmed donor blood continues while the infant's condition remains satisfactory or until 160ml/kg has been exchanged. 1ml calcium gluconate 10% is injected with every 100ml of blood to counteract the sodium citrate of donor blood.

Throughout the procedure the nurse caring for the infant maintains a constant vigil, noting the colour, activity and pulse and respiration rates at quarter-hourly intervals, while her colleague maintains a careful record of these observations and the rate and volume of blood exchange (FIG. 87).

The last specimen of blood withdrawn is collected into a second set of specimen tubes. It is usual to leave the infant with a 10–20ml blood deficit to avoid overloading the cardio-vascular system. On completion, the umbilical catheter is withdrawn and the vein sutured. If further umbilical cannulation is anticipated,

EXCHANGE TRANSFUSION

Infant's name: Nicholas Paul Hobbins
Date and time of birth: 15.1.71. at 15.05 hours
Birth weight: 2.8 kg
Mother's blood group: A Rhesus negative
Age at start : 2½ hours   Bilirubin: 10 mg%   Haemoglobin: 11 g%

TIME	OUT ml	TOTAL OUT ml	IN ml	TOTAL IN ml	COMMENTS:
18.00	10	10			T35.4°C Apex 140 R54
	10	20	10	10	
	10	30	10	20	
	10	40	10	30	
18.15	10	50	10	40	T35 Apex 144 R58
	10	60	10	50	
	10	70	10	60	
	10	80	10	70	
18.30	10	90	10	80	T34.8 Apex 138 R50
	10	100	10	90	
	10	110	10	100	+1ml 10% Calcium Gluconate
	10	120	10	110	
18.45	10	130	10	120	T35 Apex 140 R54
	10	140	10	130	
	10	150	10	140	
	10	160	10	150	

FIG. 87.

an umbilical obturator may be inserted. A dry dressing is secured in position with lengths of adhesive tape. The labelled specimen tubes are dispatched to the haematology department, accompanied by the appropriate forms. The unwashed blood bottle is temporarily retained on the ward.

AFTER CARE

The infant is allowed to rest for three to four hours while being closely observed for signs of distress. Recordings of pulse and respiration rates are continued quarter to half-hourly until satisfactory. The dressing covering the abdomen is inspected for bleeding.

Dialysis

Renal dialysis is an artificial means of imitating the functions of the kidneys. With reference to Fig. 88 it will be seen that dialysis may be performed for the following reasons:

1   In acute and chronic renal failure to control:

     i   hyperkalaemia (increased serum potassium) below cardiac toxicity level, i.e. about 6·5mEq/l;

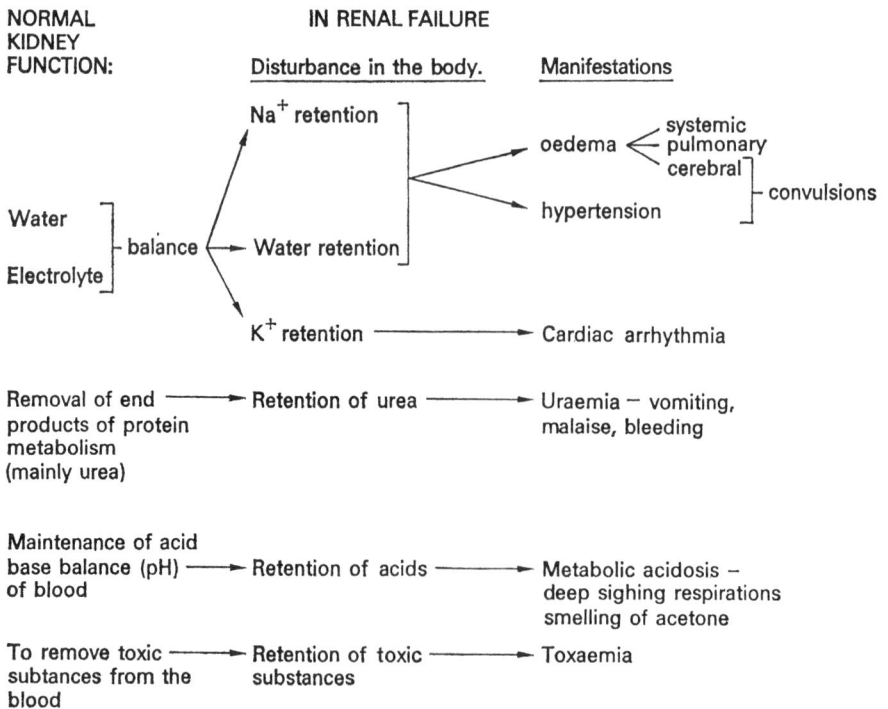

FIG. 88.

    ii   water and salt retention manifested as oedema or weight gain;

    iii acidosis (serum bicarbonate level less than 12mEq/l);

    iv azotaemia (a high level of nitrogenous waste products in the blood),
        i.e. a blood urea level about 400mg/100ml.

2   To remove toxic substances from the blood as in aspirin and barbiturate poisoning.

PRINCIPLE OF DIALYSIS

The underlying principle of dialysis is the exchange of substances in solution through a semi-permeable membrane. The two processes involved are diffusion and osmosis.

Diffusion is the passage of materials in solution from an area of high to an area of low concentration in order to equal the concentration on either side of a semi-permeable membrane.

Osmosis is the process by which water will pass through a semi-permeable membrane from an area of low concentration to an area of greater concentration of solute until equilibrium is reached (page 190).

The semi-permeable membrane may be a sheet of cellophane as in haemodialysis (artificial kidney) or the child's own peritoneum as in peritoneal dialysis. This semi-permeable membrane allows the movement of substances of small molecular size (crystalloids) such as the electrolytes, bicarbonate and urea, to move in either direction according to their percentage concentration on either side of the membrane (diffusion). For example, for the child suffering from hyperkalaemia, the use of potassium-free dialysing solution withdraws potassium from the child's circulation in order to equilibrate the concentrations on either side of the semi-permeable membrane. Substances of larger molecular size (colloids), such as protein and dextrose, are slow to pass through the membrane which is impermeable to their larger structure. These substances, therefore, exert an osmotic 'pull'. For example, if the child is overhydrated, the use of hypertonic dialysing solution exerts an osmotic 'pull' on the water in the extracellular compartment.

Haemodialysis

Haemodialysis may be used for children suffering from acute renal failure or severe aspirin or barbiturate poisoning, but is used infrequently as a long term measure in chronic renal failure. In this procedure an arterial catheter allows the patient's blood to flow on one side of a sheet of cellophane, while on the other side dialysing solution circulates. Toxic substances from the blood and fluid and electrolyte exchanges take place and the purified blood is returned to the patient via a venous catheter.

Peritoneal Dialysis

In peritoneal dialysis, the warmed dialysing solution is run via a special catheter into the peritoneal cavity where it is allowed to equilibrate for up to one hour. The solution is then syphoned into a sterile graduated bottle, and the process repeated for as long as is necessary.

Dialysing solution is essentially similar in composition to that of extracellular fluid, with the exception of omission of potassium. It is isotonic, thus avoiding overhydration. Hypertonic solutions containing 6–7% dextrose may be used when the child is overhydrated. By osmotic 'pull', the excess fluid of the body is thus drawn into the hypertonic dialysing solution. Various additives are prescribed as necessary, e.g. heparin to prevent protein exudate blocking the catheter, antibiotics to overcome bacterial intervention, and lignocaine 1% to relieve abdominal discomfort.

Sterilized pre-packed dialysis administration sets and catheters are now produced commercially (Dianeal-Baxter Laboratories Ltd.). These allow for two bottles of dialysing solution to be suspended at any one time. The solution is filtered as it passes through a drip chamber to a Y-shaped connection. The intraperitoneal catheter is attached to one arm and the drainage tube, attached to the empty graduated bottle, to the other. Flow regulators are incorporated at strategic points (FIG. 89).

REQUIREMENTS

The basic trolley is prepared as described on page 258 with the addition of the following equipment:

Bard Parker handle and blade
Spencer Wells artery forceps } all sterile.
Additional drapes

Bottom shelf:

Masks
Sterile gloves} for the doctor.
Dialysing solution.
2 bottle clips.
Mediswab.
Dialysis administration set.
Peritoneal dialysis catheter with connecting tube.
Sterile graduated bottle.
Ampoules of heparin
Ampoules of antibiotic} as required.
Selection of 2, 5, 10 and 20ml syringes.
Selection of hypodermic needles, Nos. 1, 12 and 17.
Mersuture.

Receiver for excess fluid.
Waterproof protection.
Narrow adhesive tape.
Special chart.

Additional requirements:
Intravenous stand.
Anglepoise lamp.

PREPARATION OF THE CHILD

The child is usually very ill and toxic, with a low resistance to infection. He is carefully weighed prior to commencement of the dialysis. A sedative may be necessary to overcome anxiety. The procedure may be carried out in the operating theatre, or, observing strict aseptic precautions, in the ward environment.

A check is made that the bladder is empty. As the child may well have suppression of urine, inability to micturate should not be interpreted as a need for a catheter to be passed. The doctor will decide if prior catheterization is necessary.

Following a simple explanation and reassurance, the child is made comfortable in a semi-recumbent position. The bedclothes are turned down to the upper thighs and protected with a waterproof covering. The chest is covered with a treatment blanket.

METHOD

Both doctor and nurse put on masks, and wash and dry their hands. Both check the dialysing solution to be used. The bottle seal is broken and the rubber cap cleansed prior to introduction of the needle of the dialysis administration set into the inverted bottle. The flow regulators are opened to allow the air to be displaced from the whole apparatus, then closed until ready for use. The sterile Luer fitting for insertion into the intraperitoneal catheter is re-covered by its protective sheath.

The doctor washes and dries his hands and puts on sterile gloves while the nurse ensures that everything required for the procedure is on the top of the trolley. The local anaesthetic is checked and drawn into the syringe.

Using a strict aseptic technique, the doctor cleanses the area, administers the local anaesthetic and drapes the site. The equipment is assembled and a small incision is made through the skin and linea alba between the umbilicus and the symphysis pubis—usually one-third of the way down. The trocar is then inserted, the stilette withdrawn and the catheter threaded deep into the peritoneal cavity to one or other side of the mid-line through the lumen of the trocar. The trocar is then withdrawn, leaving the peritoneal catheter for attachment to the dialysis administration set.

The catheter is maintained in position with lengths of adhesive tape. Leakage around the catheter is not uncommon and may be controlled by a purse-string suture. No tension should be applied to the indwelling catheter and a small child may need restraint to resist interference with the catheter.

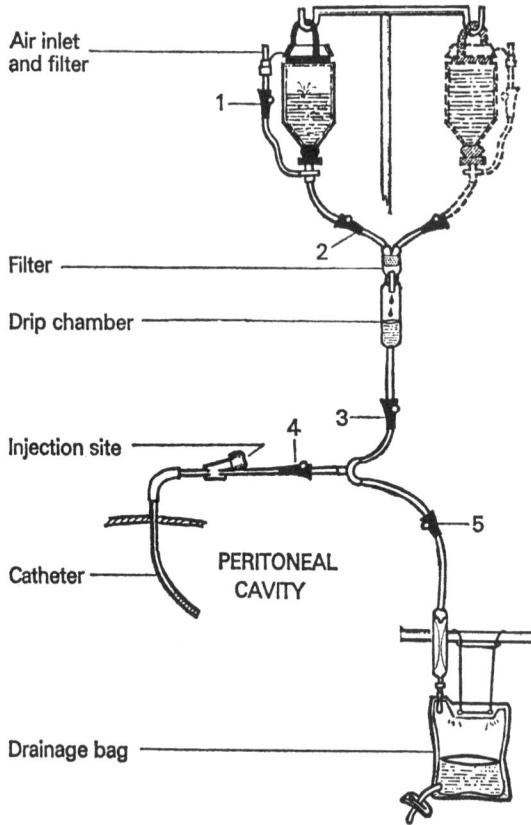

FIG. 89. Peritoneal dialysis. (Flow regulators marked 1–5.)

About 15–25ml/kg of body weight of dialysing solution is allowed to flow by gravity into the peritoneal cavity. This is achieved by opening flow regulators 1–4 and ensuring that 5 is securely closed. This phase usually takes five to ten minutes to complete. All the flow regulators are then closed for about forty minutes to allow the extracellular fluid and dialysing solution to equilibrate. With flow regulators 1–3 still closed, 4 and 5 are opened to allow the dialysing solution to syphon through the closed system into an empty sterile graduated container. Such gravity drainage should cause a steady return of the fluid over the following five to ten minutes. Flow regulator 5 is then closed and the cycle repeated continuously for twelve to thirty-six hours. Specimens of dialysate are sent for culture and biochemical analysis as requested by the doctor.

MANAGEMENT OF PERITONEAL DIALYSIS

When the doctor is satisfied that the dialysis is functioning adequately, maintenance is continued by the nursing staff. Constant observation is essential. It is imperative that the nurse delegated to this duty has been fully initiated into the regime prescribed by the doctor.

A strict aseptic technique must be adopted at all times, i.e. in preparation of the dialysate, changing the bottles and in caring for the area around the catheter. The bottle of solution may be warmed by standing in a bath of warm water (38°C or 100°F). The outside of the bottle must then be thoroughly dried to prevent unsterile water trickling down the outside of the administration set into the peritoneal cavity. Dry warming is preferable.

The cycle is continued as above.

At least the same volume of solution administered should be recovered at the end of each cycle. Should drainage stop before most of the solution has been recovered, gentle lower abdominal pressure or alteration of the child's position usually results in further drainage. The dialysate should be clear, although possibly blood-stained during the first few cycles. Opacity of the solution could be the first indication of the presence of infection, and a specimen should be retained for bacteriological as well as biochemical examination, and the doctor informed.

Careful measurement and recording are necessary.

PERITONEAL DIALYSIS

Patient's name : Timothy Wild
Age : 8 years 5 months
Weight : 25.4 kg
Date : 21.1.71

Diagnosis : Renal failure
Prescription : Isotonic Dialysing Solution 1 litre
               Heparin   500 I. U.
               Tetracycline   10 mg
Cycle : 500 ml/hour for 6 hours, then review.

NUMBER	TIME				FLUID VOLUME IN ML				REMARKS:
	ADMINISTRATION		RECOVERY		PRESENT CYCLE			CUMULATIVE BALANCE*	
	Commenced	Completed	Commenced	Completed	In	Out	Balance*		
1	10.00	10.10	10.45	11.00	500	480	+20	+20	Very restless
2	11.00	11.10	11.45	12.00	500	510	−10	+10	More settled
3	12.00	12.15	12.45	13.00	500	500	0	+10	
4	13.00	13.10	13.45	14.00	500	520	−20	−10	Sleeping
5	14.00	14.10	14.45	15.00	500	510	−10	−20	
6	15.00	15.10	15.45	16.00	500	500	0	−20	

*Patient deficit or excess

FIG. 90.

OBSERVATION

The child must be carefully observed for signs of distress and the doctor informed accordingly. Abdominal distension may cause respiratory embarrassment during the 'in' phase. Discomfort and restlessness may occur at any time, particularly during the first few cycles and if solutions of room temperature are dialysed.

A half-hourly record of the pulse and blood pressure is made at the same times during each cycle, e.g. fifteen and forty-five minutes past each hour. A cold, clammy, pale skin, associated with a rise in pulse rate and a fall in blood pressure, requires immediate medical attention and the 'out' phase of the cycle should be continued until arrival of the doctor. Shock is usually associated with the use of hypertonic dialysing solutions—the osmotic 'pull' of the dextrose having drawn fluid from the circulation at a greater rate than it can be replaced by fluid from the tissues.

A strict fluid balance chart is maintained and the urine output is measured and retained. A urine collection bag may have to be used. The child is weighed at intervals throughout the period of dialysis as requested by the doctor.

GENERAL CARE

This very sick child requires meticulous nursing care and attention during the trying hours of dialysis. The skin, pressure areas and mouth need frequent attention, and his bed should be kept fresh and clean.

Diet is usually of low fluid, potassium and protein content, but rich in carbohydrates—a modified Giovanetti diet (page 181).

He may appreciate a story during some of his better moments and would welcome the company of his mother sitting quietly at his bedside, participating in some of his nursing care.

REMOVAL OF THE CATHETER

When dialysis is completed, the catheter is gently removed, the puncture wound closed with one or two butterfly dressings and covered with dry gauze, secured with lengths of adhesive tape.

Physiotherapy

It is only following a highly specialized training that a person is qualified to competently carry out physiotherapy, but a nurse must be able to carry out simple procedures in her absence. These fall into two categories: those related to the respiratory system, and preventive measures taken to reduce the incidence of postural deformity.

Related to the Respiratory System

In carrying out basic nursing procedures, the nurse is encouraging lung expansion and loosening of pulmonary secretions. For those children who are up and about, there is no problem, and a frequent change of position is usually sufficient to prevent pulmonary complications developing in those confined to bed. Following an inflammatory condition of the respiratory passages, and lungs, the thickened mucus secretions may block the small air passages, causing consolidation or segmental collapse of a lobe, or lobes, of the lung. Similarly, the inevitable shallow respiratory effort following major thoracic or high abdominal surgery may cause pulmonary collapse, unless the necessary precautions are taken.

Intensive physiotherapy involving one or all of the following procedures may be requested for children with bronchitis, unresolved pneumonia, bronchiectasis, pulmonary collapse, asthma or cystic fibrosis, and following major thoracic or upper abdominal surgery.

DEEP BREATHING EXERCISES

Unless a child is old enough to understand and obey the command 'take a deep breath in', deep breathing is encouraged during play. The prolonged expiratory effort required to blow a piece of cotton wool or ping-pong ball along a flat surface or to blow big bubbles, demands an increased inspiratory effort, thus expanding the lungs and encouraging the child to cough. Diaphragmatic breathing can be encouraged by placing the child supine with his knees flexed and together. A favourite small toy placed just below the xiphisternum will be seen to rise and fall as the diaphragm flattens and rises.

Following a short period of deep breathing, i.e. both in and out, the child coughs and is encouraged to expectorate loosened mucus secretions, while any wound is adequately supported.

POSITIVE PRESSURE INFLATION

If life is maintained by intermittent positive pressure ventilation, the lungs are inflated with air or oxygen via a tracheostomy or endotracheal tube as described on page 306. Unless this procedure is carried out at frequent regular intervals, irreversible, secondary atelectasis may occur, especially in the very young child.

CHEST WALL PERCUSSION 'CLAPPING'

To help relieve pulmonary secretions from an affected area of lung, the overlying chest wall is 'clapped', using short, sharp claps with a cupped hand. To the uninitiated, this appears most distasteful and indeed it is, unless carried out in the correct manner. The cushion of air retained between the palm of a cupped hand and the chest wall considerably reduces discomfort. Loosened secretions are expectorated or aspirated as necessary.

POSTURAL DRAINAGE

The aim of postural drainage is to use gravity to encourage drainage of the secretions from the periphery of the lungs to the air passages, from whence they are expectorated or aspirated. The child is positioned as instructed by the physiotherapist. This depends on the area of lung necessitating drainage, and basically involves elevation of the foot of the bed for drainage of the lower lobes and sitting the child up for drainage of the apical lobes, with the affected lobe or segment always uppermost.

Following a short period of postural drainage, the child is encouraged to expectorate the loosened secretions.

Prevention of Deformity

Unconscious and paralysed children are prone to flexure deformity unless the appropriate precautions are taken. Neither group is able to carry out active exercises so that their limbs have to be put through a full range of movements by a physiotherapist or nurse. If soft tissue contractures are allowed to occur, the underlying joint becomes deformed, particularly during the years of rapid skeletal growth.

One of the cardinal aims in the nursing care of both unconscious and paralysed children is to prevent deformity. This is achieved by careful positioning of the child as a whole and particularly the limbs, a frequent change of position, use of pillows, bed-cradles, splints as necessary and passive exercises four or five times a day.

Exercises—both active and passive—not only help to maintain a normal range of movement and to prevent deformity, but encourage venous return of blood to the heart. The hip, knee, ankle, shoulder, elbow, wrist and inter-phalangeal joints require exercise. With the exception of the hip and shoulder joints, all are hinged joints, capable of flexion and extension only. Both the hip and the shoulder joints can, in addition, be abducted and adducted and the shoulder joint rotated.

Irreparable damage can be done if passive exercises are given carelessly and without instruction, and the reader is strongly advised to consult a more experienced person if confronted with any of the procedures described in this section with which she is not familiar, Physiotherapy is prescribed by the doctor and, like drugs, should only be given following a written request by the doctor.

For Further Reading

HILSON D. (1964). *Practical Paediatrics* 1st edition. Staples Press, London.
HUGHES W. T. (1964). *Paediatric procedures* W. B. Saunders Company, Philadelphia and London.

HUTCHINSON J. H. (1962). *Practical Paediatric Problems,* 2nd edition. Lloyd-Luke, London.
JOLLY H. (1968). *Diseases of Children*, 2nd edition. Blackwell Scientific Publications, Oxford.
'Physiotherapy for Nurses'. *Nursing Times Reprint* 1962.

CHAPTER TWENTY-ONE

Tests Carried Out by the Nursing Staff

Some tests performed by the nursing staff involve testing a random specimen of, for example, urine or blood. Other more intricate tests used to evaluate metabolic activities or to assess the efficiency of a single organ require a fairly rigid programme of events over a period of several hours. The satisfactory completion of these tests depends to a large extent on the nurse's ability to achieve the co-operation of the child and to carry out explicit instructions in every detail.

This chapter contains particulars related to the tests which a nurse may be asked to perform. Other tests carried out by the medical or laboratory staffs are included elsewhere in the text or will be found in the books listed at the end of this chapter.

Routine Ward Examination of Urine

A urine specimen for ward testing should be a fresh, clean specimen collected in an uncontaminated bedpan, urinal or collecting bag. It is poured into a clearly labelled specimen glass and tested as soon as possible. The results of the test should be recorded in the patient's records and any abnormalities reported.

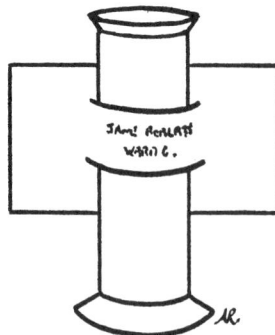

FIG. 91. A clearly labelled specimen of urine for ward testing.

With the advent of reagent sticks and tablets, urine testing is now both quick and simple. The Ames Co. tests are quoted throughout the text. Care should be taken to see that the reagents are stored in a cool, dry, locked cupboard, that the inside of the bottles do not become contaminated, and that the lid is securely fastened after use, as deterioration caused by moisture on the poisonous sticks and tablets may give inaccurate results.

General Examination

APPEARANCE

Urine is usually clear and pale amber in colour. Concentrated urine is darker in colour. Normally there is no sediment, but when urine is left to cool, a deposit of urates of phosphates may be seen. Opacity may be due to the presence of pus or blood. Urine containing larger amounts of blood is red. Ingestion of some sweets containing colouring agents, and beetroot affect the colouring of urine.

ODOUR

Fresh urine has a typical aromatic smell. If the specimen is allowed to stand, decomposition gives it an ammoniacal smell. The presence of ketones gives the odour of new-mown hay. A fishy smell may indicate the presence of infection. Other rare but typical smells can be detected in the urine excreted by children suffering from such inborn errors of metabolism as maple syrup disease.

REACTION

Urine is usually acid, thus converting blue litmus paper to red. There is no need to acidify alkaline urine prior to testing with Ames reagent sticks and tablets. pH indicator paper is used if a more definite result is required, as for example, when a child is receiving therapeutic doses of mist. potassium citrate or other alkaline solution in the treatment of urinary infection, or sodium bicarbonate for the control of thrombotic crises in sickle-cell anaemia.

SPECIFIC GRAVITY

This is the relative density of a solution compared with that of water. 1ml of water weighs 1 gramme and is expressed as 1 or more conveniently as 1·000.

Urine must be allowed to cool to room temperature before the urinometer is immersed in the specimen. The scale is then read at eye level. The normal range of specific gravity is 1·005–1·030 expressed as 1005 to 1030. If there is insufficient urine to allow the urinometer to float, the chemical tests for abnormalities are carried out. An equal quantity of water is then added to the remaining urine contained in a narrow receptacle, the specific gravity is estimated and the last two figures on the scale are doubled. For example, if 40ml of water and 40ml of urine have a specific gravity of 1010, the specific gravity of the urine is 1020.

The specific gravity is low during infancy if the fluid intake is excessive and in renal failure and diabetes insipidus. The specific gravity is raised when the fluid intake is restricted or fluid loss excessive and in diabetes mellitus when a large amount of sugar is excreted.

Chemical Tests for Abnormalities

Abnormal substances are found in urine for the following reasons:
  i   When the substance is present in excess in the blood.
 ii   When the kidneys are damaged by disease.
iii   Following injury or infection of the kidneys or urinary tract.

SUGAR

The renal tubules are able to re-absorb glucose at a constant rate equivalent to a blood sugar level of approximately 180mg/100ml—the so-called renal threshold for sugar. When this level is exceeded as in diabetes mellitus, sugar is excreted in the urine. Children who are unable to utilize a particular sugar or group of sugars due to an inborn error of metabolism, excrete the sugar in their urine, e.g. galactose in galactosaemia.

Clinitest. These reagent tablets are used to detect the presence of sugars in the urine. These tablets readily turn blue and ineffective in the presence of moisture, and contact with a wet skin will cause a burn. These points observed by the nurse must be conveyed to the diabetic child and his parents.

5 drops of urine and 10 drops of water are dropped into a test-tube. A clinitest tablet is dropped in with dry fingers. 15 seconds after boiling has ceased, the tube is gently rotated and the colour of the contents compared with the colour chart.

The detectable range of sugar is from 0% which gives a blue colouring, through green to orange which indicates 2% sugar or more.

Clinistix. A test for glucose, only. The test end of the stick is dipped in the specimen of urine. In the presence of glucose, the test end is coloured blue after one minute.

Should both the Clinitest and Clinistix give a positive result, glucose is present in the urine. Clinitest is positive, but Clinistix is negative in galactosaemia.

KETONES

These are the end-products of fat metabolism excreted in the urine when excessive amounts of fat are being used for the production of heat and energy. Ketones will be found in the urine when the carbohydrate intake is poor or when vomiting is excessive. In the absence of insulin in diabetes mellitus, glucose cannot be utilized. Heat and energy required by the body are produced by the breakdown of fat, and both sugar and ketones are excreted in the urine.

An *Acetest* tablet is placed on a clean piece of dry white paper. 1 drop of urine is placed over the surface of the tablet. 30 seconds later, the colour of the tablet is compared with the colour chart. The intensity of the mauve colouring indicates the quantity of ketone in the urine, recorded as a trace, moderately or strongly positive.

PROTEIN

Proteinuria always requires investigation, though it may not always be important. Orthostatic proteinuria is a common cause of proteinuria. It is a non-pathological state where the urine is protein-free on waking, but protein is excreted when the child is up. Large amounts of protein are excreted in the urine of children suffering from nephrotic syndrome. If blood is present in the urine, the protein test will be positive.

An *Albustix* test stick is highly sensitive to the presence of protein in a single or twenty-four hour specimen of urine. The test-end of the stick is dipped in the urine and immediately compared with the colour chart. Yellow colouring indicates a negative result. Shades of green indicate the presence of protein in increasing amounts.

Other Urine Tests

TEST FOR CHLORIDES

Where laboratory facilities are not readily available, an estimation of the urinary chlorides will give the doctor an approximation of the degree of fluid and salt loss of a dehydrated infant. The normal range of urinary chlorides after the first few weeks of life is 3–5g/litre of urine.

The Fantus test for chlorides. 1 drop of 20% potassium chromate is added to 10 drops of urine. Silver nitrate 2·9% is added drop by drop. The number of drops required to turn the colour of the solution to brick-red indicates the number of grammes of sodium chloride per litre of urine.

TEST FOR UROBILINOGEN

Urobilinogen is a constituent of normal urine (FIG. 86, page 395). The absence of urobilinogen is an indication of hepatic or biliary obstruction.

Ehrlich's test for urobilinogen. 1ml of fresh Ehrlich's reagent is added to 10ml of urine in a clean, dry test-tube. The colour is noted after allowing the tube to stand for 5 minutes. A deep pink or red colouring indicates the presence of excessive amounts of urobilinogen present as seen in haemolytic jaundice. Normal amounts produce a faint pink colouring. Urobilinogen is absent if there is no colour change to pink.

TEST FOR BILIRUBIN

Bilirubin is found in the urine when there is obstruction to the flow of bile in the liver or biliary system (FIG. 86, page 395). The kidneys are unable to excrete unconjugated (insoluble) bilirubin.

Ictotest. 5 drops of urine are dropped onto a special test mat and an Ictotest tablet is placed in the centre of the wet area. The tablet is covered with 2 drops of water. In the presence of bilirubin, a bluish-purple colouring occurs around the tablet within 30 seconds. The amount of bilirubin present is proportional to the speed and intensity of the colour change.

TEST FOR BLOOD

Haematuria is a serious sign and may occur for the following reasons:
  i In disease or injury of the kidney or urinary tract.
 ii In disorders of the bleeding and clotting mechanisms as in thrombocyto-
     penia and leukaemia.
iii Due to local lesions of the genitalia, e.g. meatal ulcer.

Hemastix. The test end of the stick is dipped into the urine and compared with the colour chart exactly 30 seconds later. In the presence of blood, the test end turns blue within 30 seconds.

TEST FOR PHENYLPYRUVIC ACID

The *Phenistix* test has been widely used for the early detection of phenylketon-uria, but has been largely replaced by the Guthrie test (page 417). A freshly wet napkin or a urine specimen is required and the test end of the stick compared with the colour chart 30 seconds after wetting with urine. A colour change ranging from grey to green indicates a positive result.

The Phenistix test may also be used to assess whether P.A.S. (para-amino-salicylic acid) or other salicylates such as aspirin have been ingested during the previous twelve to eighteen hours, when a colour change to brownish-red indicates a positive result.

QUANTITATIVE TEST FOR PROTEIN

In some centres, an Esbach's test is carried out daily on each twenty-four hour collection of urine to assess the progress of a child suffering from proteinuria, as in nephrotic syndrome.

The urine must be acidified, if necessary, with 2–3 drops of 10% acetic acid and must have a specific gravity of 1010 or less. A urine of high specific gravity is diluted with equal parts of water; the end result must then be doubled. The urine is poured into the Esbach's tube until it reaches the letter U. The Esbach's reagent is then poured to the letter R, the stopper inserted and the tube inverted to mix the contents. The stoppered tube is left covered and undisturbed for twenty-four hours to allow the protein to precipitate.

The reading at the end of the twenty-four hours is taken at eye-level and indicates the number of grammes of protein per litre of urine.

Renal Function Tests

In addition to the chemical tests carried out on urine by the nursing staff, specific tests are performed to assess the efficiency of the kidneys to concentrate and dilute urine and to clear the blood of waste products. .

CONCENTRATION TEST

The child is starved of food and fluid from 18.00 hours until the test has been completed at 08.00 hours the following day.

At 20.00 hours, the child is encouraged to pass urine and the specimen is discarded. Specimens of urine passed between 06.00 and 08.00 hours the following morning are allowed to cool to room temperature and the specific gravity is estimated.

With unimpaired renal function, at least one specimen will have a specific gravity of 1024 or more. If renal function is impaired, the highest specific gravity will lie between 1024 and 1010.

DILUTION TEST

At 08.00 hours, the child is encouraged to pass urine and the specimen is discarded. A measured amount of water, i.e. 300–900ml (the amount of water given depending on the age of the child) is given within half-an-hour. The child is then encouraged to empty his bladder at hourly intervals during the next four hours. The volume and specific gravity of each specimen are measured.

With unimpaired renal function, the 300–900ml of fluid is excreted and the largest specimen will have a specific gravity of about 1002. If renal function is impaired, there is a decrease in the total output of urine and a tendency for the specific gravity to remain constant at about 1010.

ENDOGENOUS CREATININE CLEARANCE TEST

The renal clearance of substance is the volume of blood which is completely cleared of it in one minute and can be calculated if the blood level and the amount excreted in the urine in a given time is known. In this test, the clearance of creatinine derived from the breakdown of proteins built within the body, is assessed. Clearance is dependent on the glomerular filtration rate, which is dependent on the quantity of functional glomerular tissue.

The child is weighed and measured and the results are recorded. Normal activity, diet and fluid intake are encouraged on the day before the test. A light breakfast containing no animal protein other than milk is given on the day of the test and the child remains resting on his bed, suitably occupied with a variety of quiet games.

To ensure an adequate flow of urine, 10ml of flavoured water per kilogramme of body weight is given during the hour before commencement of the test, i.e. between 08.00 and 09.00 hours and at half this volume, i.e. 5ml/kg/hour given as drinks at approximately half-hourly intervals throughout the test. A biscuit may be given with the drinks if hunger causes the child to become restless and unco-operative.

At approximately 09.00 hours, the child is encouraged to pass urine and this specimen is discarded and the exact time of voiding is recorded. Thereafter, all urine passed is saved and the time of each voiding is recorded. Complete emptying of the bladder is vital to accuracy and nervous inhibition should be avoided by allowing older children the privacy of the toilet.

Two urine collections, each of approximately three hours, are made. The last specimen is added to the first collection at approximately 12.00 hours. All the urine passed between 12.00 and 15.00 hours forms the second collection. 5ml of blood is withdrawn on completion of the first three hour collection.

The normal value is 123 ($\pm 30\%$) ml/minute/1·73m^2 body surface area.

Test for Malabsorption

D-XYLOSE EXCRETION TEST

This simple test is used in the diagnosis of malabsorption syndrome and to evaluate the results of therapy.

The child is starved of food and fluid, overnight. At 08.00 hours he is encouraged to empty his bladder and the urine is discarded. 5g of d-xylose in 100ml of water is then given followed by 150ml of water during the next hour. All urine passed within the 5 hours following administration of d-xylose is collected and sent to the laboratory.

Absorption of d-xylose is dependent on a healthy intestinal mucosa and not on any process of digestion. Normally 25% of the oral dose is excreted within five hours of administration. Levels of below 15% are indicative of malabsorption.

Test on Faeces

TEST FOR BLOOD

The presence of blood in the stools may be obvious, giving a tarry stool with or without fresh blood. It is sometimes necessary for a stool to be tested for blood when its presence is suspected, but not obvious (occult blood).

Bleeding into or on the stools occurs for three main reasons:

i Bleeding into the alimentary tract due to hiatus hernia, causing oesophageal ulceration, aspirin ingestion leading to gastric ulceration, scurvy, gastro-enteritis, intussusception, Meckel's diverticulum and following jejunal biopsy.

ii In disorders of bleeding or clotting mechanisms, such as Henoch Schönlein and thrombocytopenic purpuras and leukaemia.

iii Local lesions of the anal region, e.g. anal fissure, rectal prolapse and polypi cause the stools to be streaked with blood.

A laboratory examination will confirm the presence of hidden blood—a ward test is no longer available.

Tests on Blood

ESTIMATION OF THE BLOOD SUGAR LEVEL

Dextrostix reagent sticks give a quick easy method of estimating the approximate blood sugar level. The test is of particular value in the early detection of hypoglycaemia in susceptible newborn infants, i.e. low birth weight infants, particularly the 'small-for-dates', and infants of diabetic mothers. It may also be used to differentiate a diabetic and hypoglycaemic coma in diabetes mellitus.

A large drop of blood from a heel-prick (page 371) is allowed to flow over the test end of the Dextrostix. After exactly sixty seconds, the blood is washed off the strip with a fine jet of water. The colour of the test end is then compared with the colour chart and the result recorded.

PHENYLALANINE ASSAY

The *Guthrie test* is a screening procedure for the early detection of phenylke-tonuria. The normal phenylalanine level in the blood is 1–2mg/100ml. From the time the first milk feed is given to an infant lacking the enzyme necessary for the metabolism of phenylalanine to tyrosine, the phenylalanine level of the blood rises to 50–100mg%. When the blood level exceeds 15mg%, phenyl-pyruvic acid is excreted in the urine and may readily be detected towards the end of the sixth week of life by a positive result to the Phenistix test.

Where the procedure is in practice, the midwife collects the blood specimen when the infant is five to ten days old. Milk feeds must have been given for at least forty-eight hours prior to the collection. Specially prepared blotting paper is used, bearing the infant's name and other particulars as requested and stamped with three small circles. Blood is collected from a heel-prick (page 371) and the three circles are filled with the freely-flowing blood from the puncture wound. The blotting paper is allowed to dry prior to dispatch to the laboratory.

Tuberculin Skin Tests

These tests are used to detect evidence of tuberculosis, past or present, and usually prove negative during childhood unless:
i   the child has been given B.C.G. vaccine;
ii the child is suffering from tuberculosis.

When the child is suffering from, or has had tuberculosis, or has been immunized with B.C.G. vaccine, an allergic skin reaction results in response to the application of old tuberculin on or in the skin.

MANTOUX TEST

This test involves the intradermal injection of one of three dilutions of old tuberculin—1:10,000, 1:1,000 and 1:100. If tuberculosis is suspected, the weakest dilution is given. If the result proves negative, solutions of increasing strength are injected.

The requirements are as for any injection (page 227). A special 1ml Mantoux syringe and No. 20 hypodermic needle are used. After cleansing the flexor surface of the forearm, the needle, bevel uppermost, is inserted at an angle of 5–10° into the stretched skin. When the complete bevel-end of the needle has been inserted, 0.1ml of old tuberculin is injected to raise a definite white wheal. The area is inspected forty-eight hours later for the presence of oedema and erythema (redness). The presence of at least a 5mm diameter area of both oedema and erythema indicates a positive result. Erythema alone is negative.

HEAF TEST

A special Heaf gun is used to penetrate tuberculin purified protein derivative (P.P.D.) into the skin. Following cleansing of the skin, a small quantity of P.P.D. solution is applied to the area. The sterile end-plate of the Heaf gun is placed over the solution and the plunger is released to drive P.P.D. to a predetermined depth of 1, 2 or 3mm. The test area is inspected forty-eight to seventy-two hours later. A palpable induration at the site of at least four puncture points indicates a positive result.

For Further Reading

AMES COMPANY (Miles Laboratories Ltd. (England)) Routine Urine Tests.
EVANS D. M. D. (1969). *Special Tests and their Meanings*, 7th edition. Faber and Faber, London.
HUNTER D. (1968). *Hutchinson's Clinical Methods*, 15th edition. Baillière, Tindall, and Cassell, London.

CHAPTER TWENTY-TWO

Radiological Examinations and Investigations

X-ray examinations and investigations are a valuable means of diagnosing structural and functional disorders of the body.

There are three methods of examination with the use of X-rays:

1   Use of X-ray film direct.
2   Use of a fluoroscopic screen.
3   Use of a photographing fluoroscopic screen.

The part for examination lies between the source of the X-rays, i.e. the tube, and the film or screen.

The tissues of the body vary in their ability to absorb X-rays. Because bone and teeth contain insoluble salts of calcium, they are resistant to penetration by X-rays and can readily be detected on X-ray film. The soft tissues of the body, however, resist penetration much less and are seen as indistinct shadows on a plain X-ray. Contrast medium is, therefore, used to increase or decrease the radio-opacity of one part in comparison with the surrounding tissues, to give a clear view of the size, position and shape of body cavities and the functioning of selected organs.

Two varieties of contrast media are used:

1   Negative contrast media, that is air or oxygen. Air is less dense than soft tissues, allowing free passage of X-rays. Natural demonstration of the effectiveness of gas as a negative contrast agent is seen in:

    i   plain X-ray film of the chest (Plate 15);
    ii   plain X-ray film of the abdomen, showing fluid and gas levels in the erect child suffering from intestinal obstruction;
    iii   plain X-ray film of the abdomen, of an inverted newborn infant with rectal atresia (Plate 17).

Gas may be injected into the ventricles of the brain or spinal theca to detect disorders of the ventricular system and spinal canal.

2   Positive contrast media are more opaque to X-rays than the soft tissues of the body.

    i   Insoluble salts of heavy metals such as barium sulphate are not

419

absorbed and are used extensively to detect structural and functional defects of the alimentary tract (Plate 18).

ii Organic soluble iodides are available in various preparations to demonstrate the structure and function of selected organs and cavities of the body. They are, without exception, excreted by the kidneys. Conray 475 70%, Hypaque 25% and 45%, and Gastrografin are examples quoted in the text, but many others are available and sometimes preferred. All are reasonably safe when used with suitable precautions, but occasionally cause reactions in iodine-sensitive children.

iii Lipiodol and Myodil are examples of insoluble iodized oils used as positive contrast media in specific investigations.

When iodized preparations are to be used, parents should be carefully questioned regarding previous allergic reactions or illnesses in the child or his immediate relatives. If the information is not conclusive, a 1ml test dose of the contrast medium is given immediately prior to the X-ray examination with analeptic, antihistamine and vaso-dilator drugs available should a local reaction or circulatory collapse ensue.

The weight and height of the child should be made available to the radiologist for estimation of contrast volume. The child should be warned of a burning sensation following injection of a contrast medium into the blood circulation, as in angiography.

General Preparation for X-ray Examinations and Investigations

A visit to the X-ray department may prove an unnecessarily frightening experience to the ill-informed, unprepared child. The bewildering sight of large equipment, unfamiliar, perhaps masked faces, and the anticipation of an unpleasant experience sometimes performed in subdued lighting, all give rise to apprehension which adequate explanation and preparation may help to allay. Valuable time in the X-ray department can be lost if the child's co-operation is not forthcoming. A member of the ward staff or the child's mother should always accompany the child to the X-ray department and stay with him throughout the procedure to give constant support and reassurance.

Frequent visits of one nurse to the X-ray department should be avoided. With the use of modern X-ray equipment, the risk of radiation is minimal, but nevertheless it is the nurse who physically supports the child during his X-ray examination. The nurse should be protected with a lead-lined apron, and protective gloves may be necessary if her hands are exposed to X-rays. A small film is attached to the belt of all staff working in or visiting the X-ray department so that any exposure to scattered radiation can be measured.

Should a child be unable to visit the X-ray department for radiological examination, a portable X-ray machine is used at the bedside or in the operating theatre.

With the exception of plain X-ray examination of the skull, face, hands and feet, the child should be dressed in a gown secured by tapes at the back, warm dressing gown, socks and slippers and wrapped in a blanket. No metal buttons, hair grips, safety-pins or necklaces should be worn. An identity band is essential. A child or infant travelling to the department in his bed or incubator should be covered with an extra blanket for the journey and socks should be put on a child's feet. Opportunity should be given for the child to go to the lavatory or use a bed-pan or urinal as appropriate before leaving the ward. The child's records and previous X-ray films should accompany him to the X-ray department.

Some specific X-ray procedures are carried out with the child anaesthetized or heavily sedated. Whichever method is used, or if there is a possibility that a general anaesthetic may have to be induced, the child must be suitably prepared:

i   Parental consent obtained.
ii Starved of food for six hours, and fluid for four hours, prior to appointment time.
iii Weighed and measured for estimation of drug dosage.
iv Result of routine ward test of urine available.
v   Premedication or basal sedation given according to the written request of the doctor.
vi Mouth examined for loose teeth or orthodontic plate.
vii A check made that an infant has been baptized.
viii Contact lens, glass eyes and other artificial appliances removed.

The additional special preparations for each specific X-ray examination or investigation and after-care are discussed as appropriate.

X-ray Examination of the Skeletal System

Plain Films

Bone is comparatively opaque to X-rays compared with its surrounding soft structures, so can be examined radiologically without the use of contrast medium. A bone, or bones, may be examined for fractures, dislocation, deformities, disease, estimation of bone age, to assess the progress of callus formation in the repair of fractures, and to reveal lead lines in the diagnosis of lead poisoning.

ESTIMATION OF BONE AGE

X-ray examination is a useful aid in the diagnosis of some causes of failure to thrive. The normal rate of bone growth and development is retarded by mal-absorption and hypothyroidism (cretinism) and is affected by lack of vitamin C (scurvy) and vitamin D (rickets).

Bone age is determined by X-ray examination of specific bones for centres of ossification and union of epiphyses with the diaphysis of long bones. The effect of avitaminosis is best seen on X-ray examination of the wrist and knee. The effect of vitamin D deficiency can often be seen on a plain X-ray film of the chest, showing rickety deformity of the chondro-costal margin.

X-RAY EXAMINATION OF THE AIR SINUSES

Plain X-ray films of the frontal and maxillary bones of the face are taken to detect opacity and fluid levels of infected frontal and maxillary sinuses.

Use of Radio-Opaque Medium

ARTHROGRAPHY

Contrast medium is injected into the capsule surrounding a joint to display the positions of the articulating bones. Air or Hypaque 45% is used for the purpose. The use of arthrography in childhood is confined to X-ray examination of the hip joint to display the relationship of the head of the femur to the acetabulum of the innominate bone in congenital dislocation or subluxation of the hip joint.

A general anaesthetic is necessary as most of the children examined are between the ages of six months and two years. Plaster of Paris is removed from the area and the skin over the joint is cleansed. Radio-opaque medium is then injected by direct puncture into the hip joint, and the area is exposed to X-rays for direct films to be taken with the joint in different positions.

Care of the child following the examination is the same as for post-anaesthetic care.

X-ray Examinations of the Gastro-Intestinal Tract

PLAIN FILMS

A plain X-ray examination of the abdomen of an erect child suffering from intestinal obstruction will reveal fluid and gas levels.

When rectal atresia or imperforate anus is suspected, the infant is inverted for fifteen minutes to allow intestinal gas to enter the blind end of the rectum. With the child still inverted, a metal marker is placed over the usual site of the anus and a plain film of the inverted abdomen is taken (Plate 17).

Use of Radio-Opaque Medium

The structure and function of the alimentary tract can be examined by the introduction of barium sulphate, Gastrografin and Lipiodol. If immediate surgery is anticipated, a small amount of Gastrografin is used instead of barium sulphate for the examinations described below, as its progress through the alimentary tract and excretion from the body are rapid.

BARIUM SWALLOW

This examination may be made to detect:

i   cardio-oesophageal reflux due to achalasia of the cardia or hiatus hernia;
ii vascular ring;
iii oesophageal stricture;
iv deviation of the oesophagus due to increased heart size.

To ensure that the child is hungry and will therefore drink the barium, it is usual to starve him for four hours and to substitute the next feed with barium. The child is fed by bottle or cup and spoon, preferably at a controlled rate, while the progress of the barium is observed by direct screening.

Lipiodol is used in preference to barium to detect leakage from, and stricture of the oesophagus following repair for oesophageal atresia. Lipiodol is used because it will do no harm if it spills into the bronchial tree.

BARIUM MEAL

A barium meal may be given to demonstrate any abnormality of the oesophagus, stomach and duodenum, and to confirm the diagnosis of pyloric stenosis when only a thread of barium is seen to pass through the stenosed pyloric sphincter. Peptic ulceration is rare in childhood, but if suspected, a barium meal may outline the ulcer crater.

An empty stomach is essential for this examination, so the child is deprived of food and fluid for six hours prior to the appointment time. Barium is substituted for his next meal, and plain films are taken under screen control to record any abnormality present.

BARIUM FOLLOW-THROUGH

A barium follow-through X-ray examination may be requested to examine the structure of the small intestine and the rate of progress of barium through its lumen. X-ray films are taken at intervals requested by the radiologist and once the stomach is partially or completely emptied, food is given, usually after three hours. Films may be continued at intervals for up to twenty-four hours.

BARIUM ENEMA

Barium sulphate is injected into the rectum to detect, radiologically, abnormalities in the structure or functioning of the colon and rectum. The success of this examination invariably depends on the careful preparation of the lower alimentary tract to ensure that the child is presented for X-ray examination with the rectum and colon free from faeces, fluid and gas.

Preparation of the child includes:

i   a low residue diet for forty-eight hours prior to examination;

ii   the use of aperients, for example Senokot, seventy-two and twenty-four hours before;
iii an enema or high rectal and colonic washout, but not within four hours of examination;
iv   emptying of the bladder immediately prior to injection of barium.

Restriction of fluid and diet immediately prior to the examination is not necessary. A small child may be given a sedative to prevent voluntary expulsion of the barium during the procedure.

The child is placed in the supine position on the suitably protected X-ray examination table. A catheter is inserted into the rectum and barium sulphate is injected. Its progress into the rectum and colon is observed on a fluorescent screen, spot X-ray films being taken at selected intervals. A further X-ray of the abdomen is taken following evacuation of the bowel.

At the end of the procedure the child should be offered a bedpan, preferably before leaving the X-ray table and certainly before leaving the X-ray department.

When a diagnosis of Hirschsprung's disease or idiopathic megacolon is suspected, no preparation is given as purgation and enemas cause the distended normal bowel above the aganglionic section to deflate, giving a false impression of the diagnosis. Inspissation of barium and water intoxication are avoided by the careful use of barium. No local preparation is required if a barium enema is performed to diagnose (or in the hydrostatic treatment of) intussusception.

Care following the use of barium sulphate

Constipation following barium examinations should be avoided. Aperients and irrigation of the rectum and colon with normal saline may prove necessary. Faeces containing barium will be white.

SIALOGRAPHY
A sialogram is the special X-ray examination of a parotid salivary gland and its duct to detect blockage due to a cyst or calculus formation. Contrast medium (iodized oil) is injected through a blunt cannula inserted in the duct of the parotid gland, the entrance of which is by the second upper molar tooth. The co-operation of the child is essential as injection by the doctor is not easy. Traces of contrast medium are removed from the mouth before several plain X-ray films are taken.

CHOLANGIOGRAPHY
A cholangiogram may be carried out in the operating theatre to check the patency of the ducts forming the biliary system during an operation for relief of congenital obliteration of the bile ducts.

A cannula is inserted into a duct and a small quantity of contrast medium (Hypaque 25%) injected.

X-ray Examinations of the Respiratory System

Plain Films

Because of the distribution of air, blood vessels and other soft structures in the thorax, a plain X-ray of the chest is a common examination, revealing considerable information:

i   Lung collapse
    segmental,
    lobar.
ii Consolidation
    mottled,
    lobar,
    pneumonic.
iii Emphysema.
iv Plethoric and diminished blood supply to the lung fields.
v   Diaphragmatic hernia—when gut containing intestinal gas is seen in the thorax, often displacing the heart.
vi Swallowed or inhaled foreign bodies—radio-opaque or causing obstruction and, therefore, segmental or lobar collapse.

Use of Radio-Opaque Medium

BRONCHOGRAPHY

A bronchogram is the X-ray examination of the respiratory passages following insertion of contrast medium (iodized oil). This examination, carried out under general anaesthetic, is used to assess the degree of bronchiectatic destruction in bronchiectasis. It is essential that the respiratory passages and lungs are as free as possible from secretions so that the contrast medium completely fills the structures.

Postural drainage to drain the sputum from the affected lobe(s) of the lung(s) is combined with intensive physiotherapy to encourage coughing and expectoration of sputum. Secretions from the naso-pharynx of small children may have to be aspirated. Postural drainage should be maintained until the time of the X-ray examination. The appropriate preparations prior to induction of a general anaesthetic are made.

Iodized oil is injected into the trachea, normally through an endotracheal tube of the anaesthetized child, and the chest X-rayed with the child in various positions. The contrast medium is aspirated at the end of the examination.

On return to the ward, constant observation is required until consciousness is regained. A suction apparatus should be at the bedside and used if necessary to maintain a clear airway. Half hourly recordings of the pulse and respiration are maintained until satisfactory, and the temperature recorded four-hourly. Following recovery of consciousness, postural drainage and physiotherapy are continued four-hourly to ensure that the iodized oil is removed from the lungs. The quantity and quality of sputum is recorded.

X-ray Examination of the Cardio-Vascular System

Plain Films

Plain X-ray films of the chest show the position, size and shape of the heart and the state of the lung fields, i.e. increased pulmonary vascularity, due to a left to right shunt through a persistent ductus arteriosus or ventricular septal defect, or a reduced blood flow, due to pulmonary stenosis. The presence of distended intercostal arteries in coarctation of the aorta is seen as notching of the ribs.

Use of Radio-Opaque Medium

To study the structure and performance of the heart, contrast medium is injected into a suitable vessel (non-selective angiography) or through a selectively positioned catheter (selective angiography). Both procedures carry a slight operative risk which is increased in illness and the younger age group.

CARDIO-ANGIOGRAPHY

This is a non-selective examination of the heart used in the diagnosis of congenital heart disease. A cannula is inserted, usually into the median basilic vein in the antecubital fossa, and contrast medium (Conray 70%) is injected under pressure to travel rapidly in the venous return to the heart. Its progress through the heart and lungs is recorded on X-ray films taken in rapid succession, using a Schönander film-changer, or is seen on the fluorescent screen or television monitor and recorded on ciné film and video-tape. Preparation of the child for this procedure and his subsequent care is as for cardiac catheterization (see below).

CARDIAC CATHETERIZATION

In addition to selective angiography, this procedure entails estimation of the oxygen content and pressure of the blood in the various chambers of the heart and great vessels.

The child is prepared as for general anaesthetic, although the procedure is usually carried out with the child heavily sedated. Antibiotic cover is usual and is commenced before the procedure. Any pubic hair should be removed. A urine collection bag may be attached to an infant if a femoral vessel is to be cannulated.

The sedated child is placed in a comfortable supine position on the X-ray table and electrocardiograph electrodes attached to the skin for continuous monitoring. A small incision is made in the cleansed, anaesthetized skin of the groin or antecubital fossa to expose the femoral or brachial vein respectively. Using a strict aseptic technique and under X-ray control, a radio-opaque cardiac catheter is gently threaded into the vena cava, through the right atrium and ventricle of the heart and into the pulmonary artery. The pressure in each chamber and vessel is recorded and blood samples are collected for immediate estimation of the oxygen content. With the tip of the catheter suitably positioned, contrast medium is injected under pressure and its progress through the heart and great vessels is seen on a fluorescent screen or television monitor and image intensifier, and sometimes recorded on ciné film. Simultaneous recording on video-tape allows instantaneous replay of the procedure, as permanently recorded on the ciné film, and avoids the necessity of making a further injection and, therefore, additional exposure to radiation.

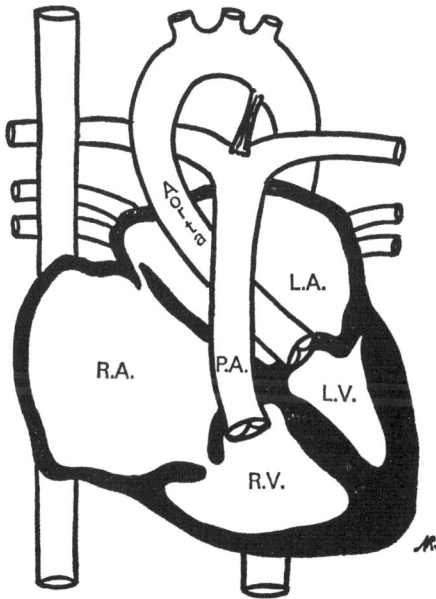

FIG. 92. Normal pressure and O_2 saturation in the different chambers of the heart.

	Pressure mmHg.	O_2Saturation ml/litre
R.A. = Right Atrium	Mean = 3	75%
R.V. = Right Ventricle	30/3	75%
P.A. Pulmonary Artery	30/10	75%
L.A. = Left Atrium	Mean = 8	95%
L.V. = Left Ventricle	100/8	95%
Aorta	100/60	95%

To catheterize the left side of the heart, a transeptal approach may be made via the foramen ovale during early infancy, or through a small opening made by the blade carried by a special cardiac catheter. The blood pressure and oxygen saturation of the blood in the left atrium and ventricle and aorta can then be assessed. Alternatively, the left side of the heart may be approached by retrograde passage of a catheter via the femoral artery and aorta.

Interference to the normal mechanism of the heart may occur resulting in bradycardia and arrhythmias. Pulmonary embolism, puncture of the heart causing blood to flow into the pericardium (tamponade), and infiltration of contrast medium into the myocardium are rare but serious complications of cardiac catheterization.

At the end of the procedure, the child is received into an oxygen tent or oxygenated incubator. A suction apparatus should be available. Electrocardiograph monitoring is continued if requested. The pulse and respiration rates and blood pressure (not in infancy) are recorded quarter to half-hourly until satisfactory. The body temperature is recorded on return to the ward and at hourly intervals until satisfactory.

The site of insertion of the catheter is inspected frequently for bleeding and the pressure bandage removed four hours or so later if no bleeding occurs. The appropriate brachial or femoral artery is checked for pulsation at the radial or dorso-pedal pulse. The limb may be cold and discoloured. To discourage venous congestion, the limb may be raised.

Fluids are encouraged as soon as consciousness has been regained, particularly if the child is cyanosed, as the risk of thrombosis is increased by polycythaemia and haemoconcentration. An infant is fed by a naso-gastric tube to ensure adequate hydration without over-exertion.

Rest is encouraged for the following forty-eight hours and then an older child is allowed up and is able to go home. A full course of antibiotics is given and the sutures are removed on the seventh day.

BALLOON SEPTOSTOMY (Rashkind Procedure)
When transposition of the great vessels has been diagnosed or suspected, a special balloon cardiac catheter, for example a Rashkind catheter, is used to traverse the foramen ovale and to break down the atrial septum, thus allowing free mixing of blood between the two atria. The care of the infant and the procedure is essentially as for cardiac catheterization. The leg is raised as it is likely to swell, especially if the femoral vein is used. The child is always an infant and invariably in poor condition, so the appropriate care and risks apply. Grouping and cross-match for one unit of blood is a necessary pre-operative procedure.

AORTOGRAPHY
An aortogram entails cannulation of a suitable large artery and the retrograde

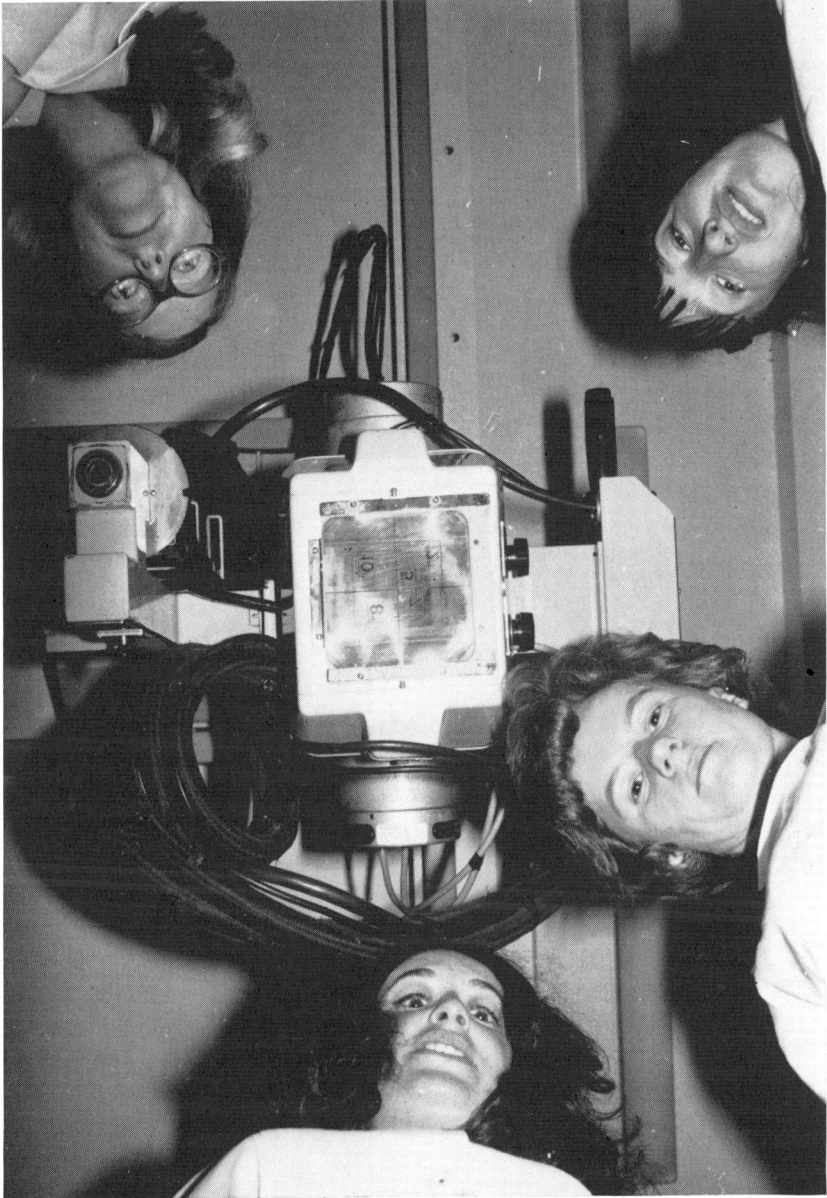

PLATE 13. A 'child's-eye' view. The bewildering sight of large equipment, unfamiliar faces, and anticipation of an unpleasant experience, all give rise to apprehension which adequate explanation and preparation may help to allay.

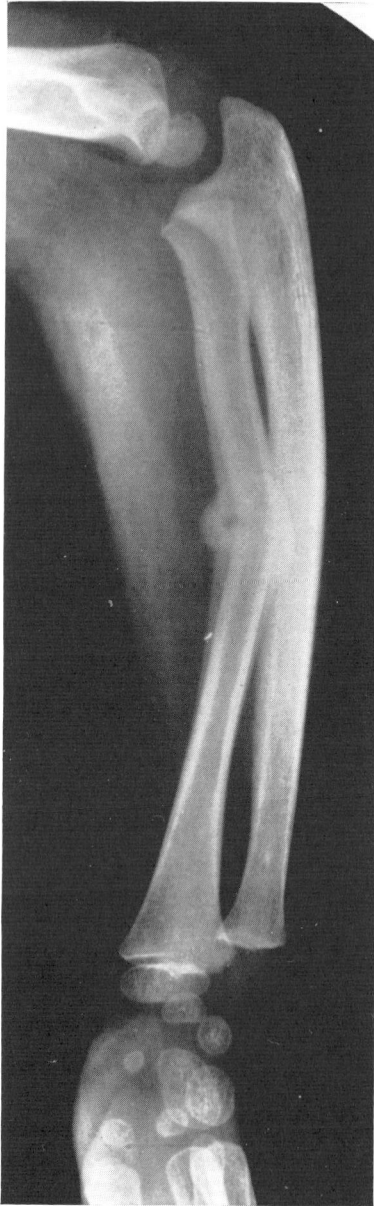

PLATE 14. Plain X-ray film showing a typical greenstick fracture of a long bone in a small child. Note the formation of callus around the healing fracture.

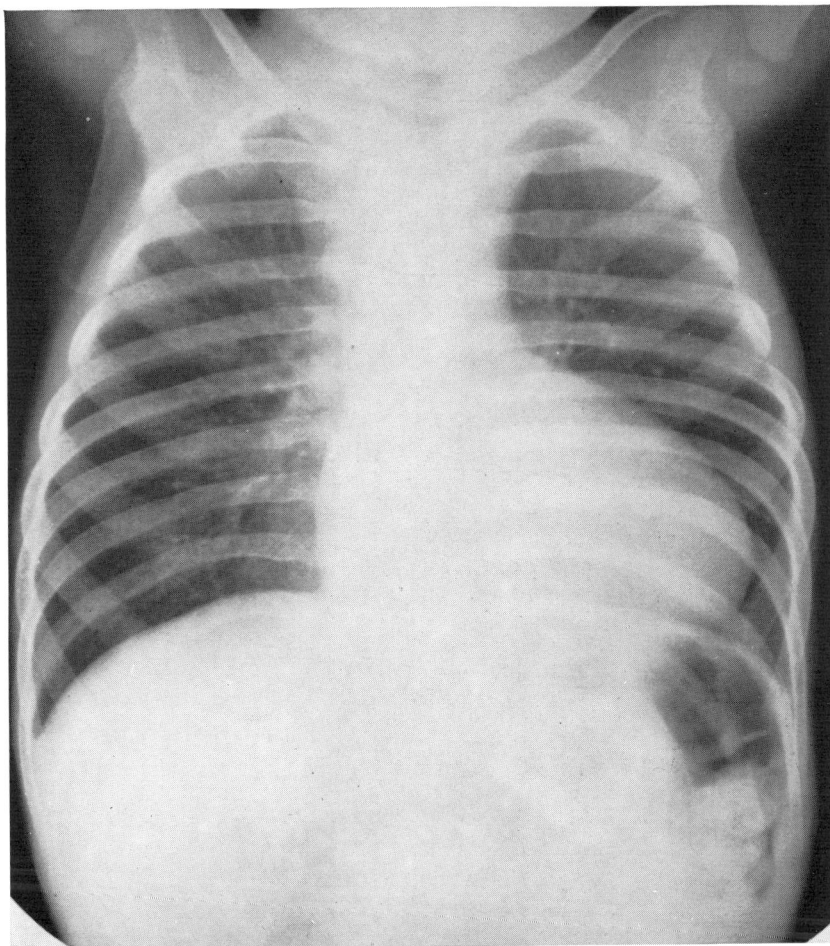

PLATE 15. Plain X-ray film of the chest of a small child with an enlarged heart—in this case due to Fallot's tetralogy. Note the typical boot-shaped heart and the plethoric lung-fields.

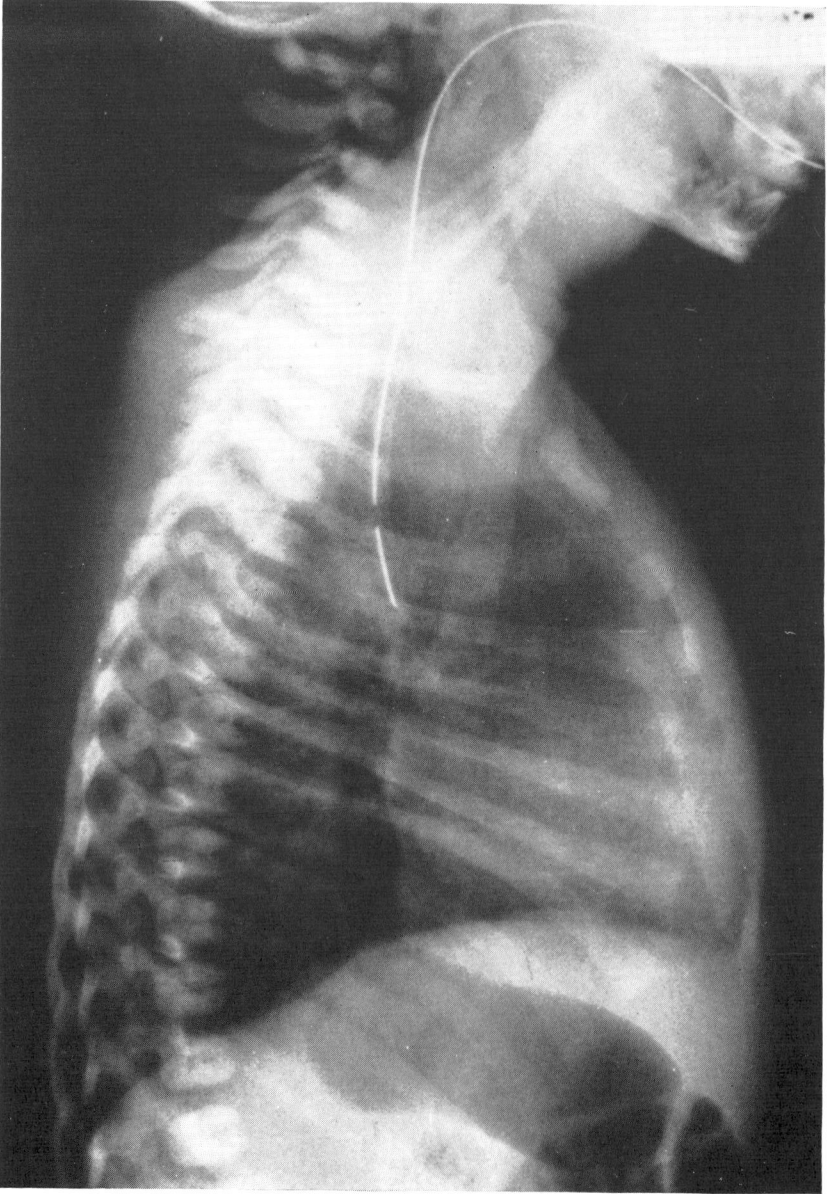

PLATE 16. Plain X-ray film showing the passage of a fairly rigid sterile radio-opaque catheter into the oesophageal pouch of a newborn infant with oesophageal atresia. Note the presence of gas in the lower oesophagus, stomach and intestine indicating the presence of a tracheo-oesphageal fistula.

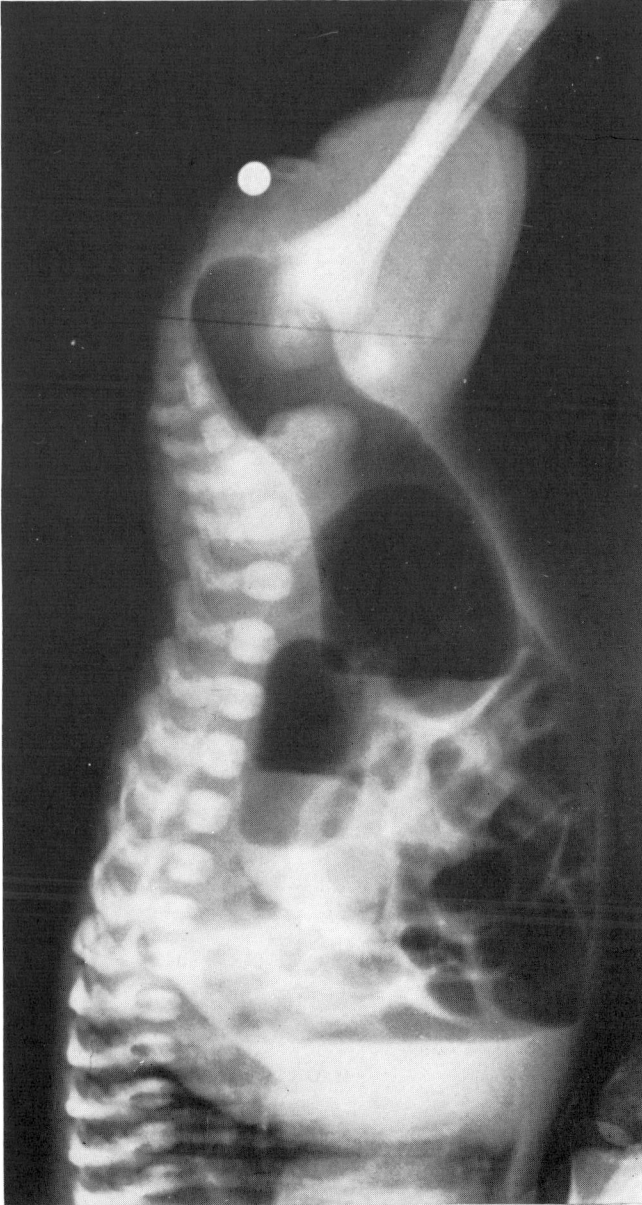

PLATE 17. Demonstration of the effectiveness of gas as a negative contrast agent. Plain X-ray film of the abdomen of an inverted newborn infant with rectal atresia. Intestinal gas fills the blind end of the rectum. A metal marker is placed over the usual site of the anus.

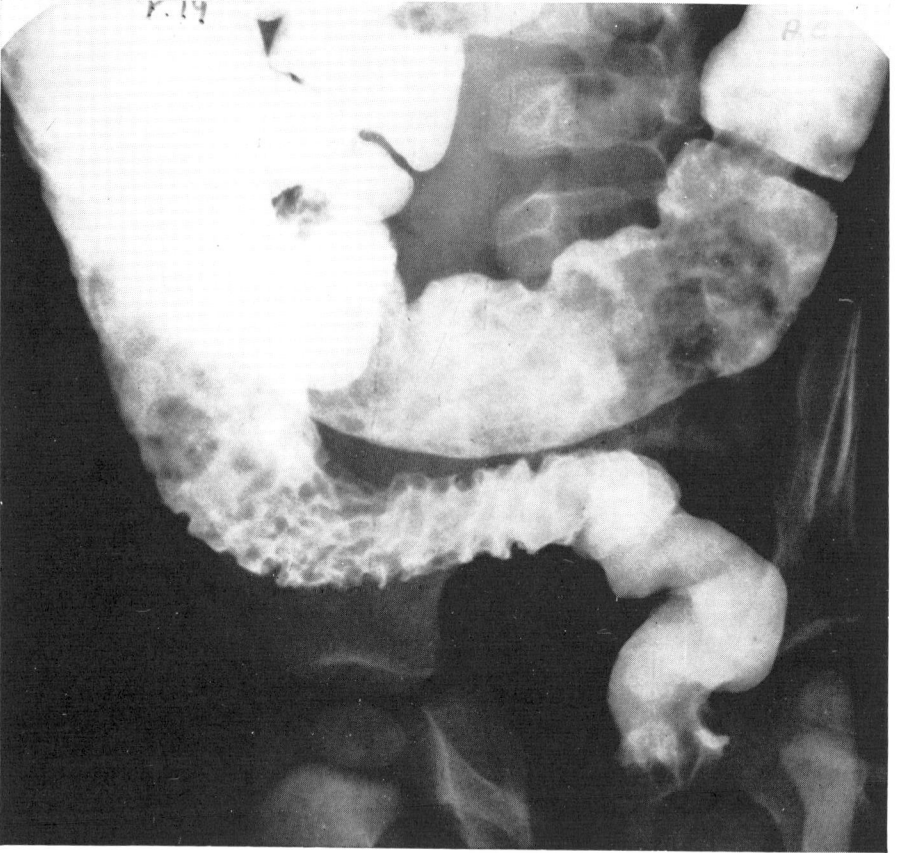

PLATE 18. Use of contrast medium. Barium enema in a two-year-old child with Hirschsprung's disease, demonstrating a dilated sigmoid colon above a narrowed rectal segment.

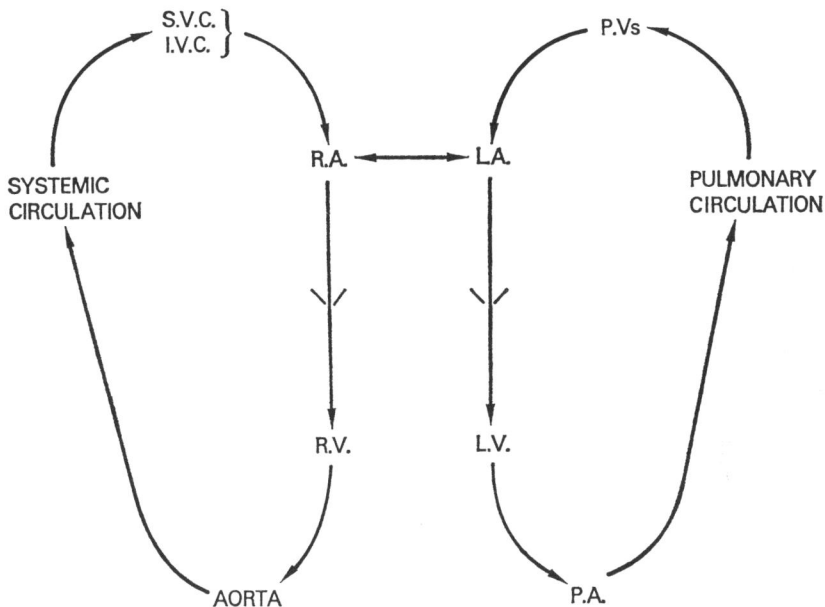

FIG. 93. Diagrammatic representation of the flow of blood in transposition of the great vessels.

←——————→ = Flow of blood allowed by balloon septostomy

R.A. = Right atrium	L.A. = Left atrium
R.V. = Right ventricle	L.V. = Left ventricle
S.V.C. = Superior vena cava	P.A. = Pulmonary artery
I.V.C. = Inferior vena cava	P.V. = Pulmonary vein

passage of a radio-opaque catheter to the appropriate level in the aorta. Contrast medium (Conray 70%) is then injected under pressure, and X-ray films are taken at a rapid exposure rate.

Preparation for the procedure and subsequent care is as for cardiac catheterization. The peripheral pulses are checked at frequent intervals.

X-ray Examination of the Urinary System

Plain Films

A plain X-ray film of the abdomen may detect the presence of a renal calculus or a renal mass, as for example, a nephroblastoma (Wilm's tumour) causing pressure on the normal abdominal contents.

Without the use of contrast medium, the renal system cannot be detected on X-ray examination.

Use of Radio-Opaque Medium

EXCRETION PYELOGRAPHY (I.V.P.)

An intravenous pyelogram is a comparatively simple X-ray examination frequently used to detect structural and functional defects of the kidneys. Contrast medium (Conray 70%) injected into a convenient vein—usually the median basilic—is subsequently concentrated and excreted by the kidneys. The examination is not carried out when renal function is impaired, manifested by a rise in the blood urea level.

Careful preparation is essential. The presence of faeces and intestinal gas obscure the view of contrast medium in the pelvis of the kidney and their presence must be eliminated by:

i   giving a low residue diet for forty-eight hours prior to X-ray;
ii   aperients, for example Senokot granules, given seventy-two and twenty-four hours prior to examination;
iii   an enema which may be given twenty-four hours before appointment time if the child has a history of constipation;
iv   allowing the child up as much as possible to disperse intestinal gas.

Fluids may be restricted, but with adequate preparation and the use of more effective contrast media, restriction of fluid is no longer necessary.

The child empties his bladder. A plain X-ray film of the abdomen is taken prior to the injection being made. In spite of careful preparation, the intestinal contents may still obscure the renal field. After the injection has been given aerated water may be given which fills the stomach, causing downward displacement of the intestine. The concentrating contrast medium can then be detected through the even distribution of the gas content of the stomach. Plain X-ray films of the abdomen are taken five, ten, fifteen and twenty minutes after the injection has been made.

If venepuncture proves difficult during infancy, radio-opaque medium (Hypaque 25%) is injected with hyaluronidase into the subcutaneous tissues of the subscapular region. The plain X-ray films of the abdomen are taken ten, fifteen, twenty and twenty-five minutes later.

RETROGRADE PYELOGRAPHY

A retrograde pyelogram is performed to outline the structure of the renal pelvis when kidney function is impaired and excretion pyelography unsatisfactory.

A general anaesthetic is required. If the bladder is not emptied prior to passage of a cystoscope, the urine is collected in a sterile container for bacteriological examination. Following cystoscopy, fine radio-opaque ureteric catheters are passed through the cystoscope into the bladder and threaded into the ureters to the left and right kidneys. Radio-opaque medium (Hypaque 25%) is injected into the pelvis of each kidney and plain films are taken. The ureteric catheters are removed at the conclusion of the X-ray examination unless further urine specimens are required. Subsequent discomfort accompanying micturition frequently results, due to the passage of the cystoscope. Fluids should be encouraged as soon as recovery from anaesthetic has been made, and a careful record of the urine output is maintained. Slight haematuria may be present at first.

CYSTO-URETHROGRAPHY

This X-ray examination, sometimes called a micturating cystogram, is used to detect structural and functional defects of the lower urinary tract. Distortion in the contour of the bladder wall, vesico-ureteric reflux and post-urethral valves can be diagnosed by this examination.

The co-operation of an older child is essential. A small child may have the examination carried out under a general anaesthetic.

Catheterization of the bladder may be carried out on the ward and the child transferred to the X-ray department for introduction of contrast medium. A strict aseptic technique is required and a specimen of urine collected for culture and sensitivity. The bladder is completely emptied.

Contrast medium (Hypaque 25%) is injected through the catheter and a plain X-ray of the bladder taken (cystogram). The catheter is then removed and the child encouraged to void urine. As the bladder contracts, X-ray films are taken to detect vesico-ureteric reflux and post-urethral valves. If a general anaesthetic has been induced, supra-pubic pressure is required to empty the bladder.

X-ray Examination of the Nervous System

Plain Films

A plain X-ray of the skull and spinal column will detect:
  i fractures;
 ii dislocation;
iii a raised intracranial pressure;
 iv premature closure of the sutures;
  v presence of a tumour, seen as enlargement of the sella turcica in a child with a pituitary tumour, or as calcification of a tumour or destruction of bone.
Detailed radiological examinations of the central nervous system can be made with the use of both negative and positive contrast media.

'Air Studies'

'Air studies' of the central nervous system involve the replacement of cerebrospinal fluid with the equivalent amount of air. This may be injected into the lumbar spinal theca or the basal cisterns when the examination is usually called pneumoencephalography, or directly into the lateral ventricles of the brain when the examination is referred to as ventriculography (page 378).

Both are used to examine the size, shape, position and patency of the ventricular system and its connecting channels. To prevent herniation of the medulla, a ventriculogram is always used in preference to a pneumoencephalogram if the intracranial pressure is raised and papilloedema is present.

VENTRICULOGRAPHY

A ventriculogram may be carried out with the child under general anaesthetic or following a strong sedative. The ventricles of the brain are approached by passing brain needles through the wide sutures or fontanelle of an infant and through bilateral posterior burr holes in an older child. This part of the procedure is carried out in the operating theatre. As a ventriculogram is frequently followed by brain surgery, the whole head is shaved.

The skin is carefully cleansed and the brain needle inserted. 20–50ml of cerebrospinal fluid is exchanged with a similar quantity of filtered air in 5 or 10ml cycles. Specimens of cerebrospinal fluid may be retained for culture and biochemical analysis for sugar and protein content. The child is maintained in a supine position for transfer to the X-ray department and a sandbag is placed on either side of the head to keep the air equally distributed between left and right sides. X-ray films are taken with the child in various positions to allow the air bubble to outline the ventricular system.

PNEUMOENCEPHALOGRAPHY

The injection of air may be made on the ward prior to transfer, or a general anaesthetic may be induced and the whole procedure carried out in the X-ray department. Air replacement of cerebrospinal fluid is usually made through a lumbar puncture needle until about 20ml of air has been exchanged for a similar quantity of cerebrospinal fluid in 5ml cycles. The cerebrospinal fluid thus collected is retained for culture and biochemical analysis.

If the cerebrospinal fluid/air exchange is to be made in the basal cisterns, the head must be shaved to 2·5cm (1 inch) above the occipital protuberance.

The child is maintained in an upright position to allow the air to travel to the ventricular system. X-ray films of the skull are taken with the child supine, prone, erect and inverted to bring the air bubble into different positions to outline the ventricular system.

CARE OF THE CHILD FOLLOWING 'AIR STUDIES' OF THE CENTRAL NERVOUS SYSTEM

Following examination of the central nervous system with the use of air, the child may feel wretched. He should be returned to a quiet corner in the ward, and the foot of the bed elevated if he complains of headache. Often the child is ill and the X-ray examination further aggravates his symptoms. Vomiting may be persistent and distressing. Pulse and respiration rates and blood pressure should be recorded at quarter to half-hourly intervals until satisfactory, when the interval between recordings may be suitably increased. The temperature-regulating mechanism may have been disturbed, so a four-hourly recording of body temperature is required. Fluid intake should be encouraged unless cerebral oedema is suspected.

Any signs of deterioration manifested by a slowing of the pulse, an increase in blood pressure, or a fall in the level of consciousness, should be reported immediately.

The scalp incisions or puncture holes should be inspected for leakage of cerebrospinal fluid, especially if the intracranial pressure is high.

Use of Radio-Opaque Medium

MYELOGRAPHY

Iodized oil may be injected into the spinal theca to localize a mechanical blockage to the flow of cerebrospinal fluid. Spinal cord tumours, prolapsed intervertebral disc (rare), spina bifida deformity, and fibrous exudate blockage of the canal in tuberculous meningitis are some of the reasons for carrying out a myelogram during childhood.

A general anaesthetic is usually preferred for this procedure during childhood. A lumbar puncture is performed and a small quantity of Myodil injected. The posture of the child is adjusted so that the iodized oil moves along the spinal canal until the obstruction is encountered. A metal marker may be placed on the skin surface at the site of the blockage. On no account should this be removed. As Myodil has an irritating effect on the brain, the child is maintained in an upright position to allow the heavier oil to settle around the cauda equina. Absorption is extremely slow, taking several years or even a lifetime. Some radiologists may attempt to remove the oil by further lumbar puncture at the end of the procedure.

CEREBRAL ANGIOGRAPHY

As its name suggests, this X-ray examination involves the injection of contrast medium (Conray 70%) into an artery supplying the brain—usually the carotid artery—and recording its progress through the cerebral vessels. Localization of a space-occupying lesion can be confirmed by an increased, decreased, or displaced blood supply to an area of the brain.

A general anaesthetic is essential to ensure that an unpredictable child remains still. Contrast medium is injected by direct puncture of the carotid artery or by a catheter in the aortic arch (see aortography) and X-ray films of its progress are taken in rapid succession.

Care of the child is as for any post-anaesthetic patient, and the puncture sites are inspected frequently for bleeding or bruising.

For Further Reading

CHESNEY D. N. and M. O. (1970). *Care of the Patient in Diagnostic Radiography*, 3rd edition. Blackwell Scientific Publications, Oxford.

CHAPTER TWENTY-THREE

Discharge from Hospital

Fortunately, most children leave hospital to go home to lead a normal life. A few have their medical and nursing care continued at home, some are transferred to special units, others spend a period of convalescence in a country or seaside environment, while a few, sadly but often mercifully, die.

Going Home

To most children, the thought of getting well enough to go home is uppermost throughout their stay in hospital, and all procedures are endured with this happy thought in mind. For the few deprived of a secure, loving home, discharge day is not so happily anticipated. Their need is particularly pathetic, and a compassionate nurse cannot help but feel utter despair over the apparent lack of parental interest.

Before a child goes home, the medical and nursing staff must be sure that the mother is capable of looking after her child. A mother may feel unable to accept an abnormal infant into her care. When this is apparent, the infant must be retained until a better relationship is established, or the health and welfare of both mother and infant are in jeopardy. Competence in handling is achieved by adequate motivation, careful instruction and practice. Most mothers are only too willing to be shown how to care for their child, and one of the essential duties of a paediatric nurse is to educate the mother in this special care. Once instructed, opportunity for practice will encourage confidence and proficiency. Instruction includes the education of a new mother in the basic care of her infant, caring for a colostomy, feeding by gastrostomy, giving or supervising the administration of hypodermic injections, preparation of special feeds and diets, as appropriate. Carefully written instructions, giving simple explanations in non-medical terms, prove their lasting worth and give an insecure or less intelligent mother something to which to refer. If the child is to continue his care under the supervision of the district nurse, she should be given the opportunity to visit the child while still in hospital and to discuss his future care with the ward staff. Changing of a gastrostomy tube or tracheostomy tube are unfamiliar procedures to the average district nurse, and opportunity to familiarize herself with the technique is usually much appreciated.

It is important that a mother is warned that her young child may not be quite himself for the first few days, or possibly weeks, following discharge from hospital. As is seen in Chapter 6, psychological trauma caused by emotional deprivation is considerably reduced by frequent contact with someone from home. The adverse effect that admission to hospital has on a child depends on his age, emotional maturity, length of stay in hospital, contact with home, his acceptance of treatment and the opportunity afforded for relief of inner aggression. Regression to an earlier stage of development is common, and manifested by thumb-sucking, soiling (encopresis) and bedwetting (enuresis). Sleep may be disturbed by night terrors, when traumatic experiences previously repressed are brought to consciousness. Distrust and fear of a repetition of maternal abandonment will make a child attention-seeking and clinging, not allowing mother out of his sight. Alternatively, a child may distrust his mother and reject her attention in sheer resentment of her previous betrayal. With patience and extra loving attention and understanding during the first few days following discharge from hospital, the child will once more be assured of his mother's love and feel secure in the home environment.

Before the day for discharge, parents should be given some idea when they can expect their child to go home so that the necessary arrangements regarding home commitments and transport can be made. Hospital transport or an ambulance may prove necessary if a private car is not available, and the child is not well enough to travel on public transport. Demands on the ambulance service are great and requests for non-urgent journeys should be made twenty-four hours beforehand, and the parents asked to travel with their child at the appointed time.

Most parents are happy to collect their child as soon as possible on the day of discharge. With a rapid turnover of bed occupancy, there is a tendency to stipulate a discharge time to suit the needs of the ward, which may prove inconvenient to the busy mother. If given the option, most mothers will make an early visit convenient.

A limited supply of drugs prescribed for the child are dispensed by the hospital pharmacy, and the mother must be carefully instructed regarding their storage and administration. Further supplies are prescribed by the family doctor.

The hospital doctor informs the appropriate family doctor of the child's treatment and progress whilst in hospital and gives details of any further treatment and follow-up. All parents should be assured of further help and advice whenever necessary and encouraged to obtain this from their family doctor and his team. Close co-operation and communication between hospital and community services help to discourage conflicting views and lack of parental faith in one or the other. The services of a district nurse, health visitor or home help may be organized by the family doctor or through the medical social worker, and continuation of the child's education is assured by transfer from the hospital school back to the local or special school or to a home teacher. The necessary out-patients follow-up appointment is made.

Parents of physically or mentally handicapped or debilitated children have a special need for moral support in their caring. This may be given by a member of a professional organization or from parents with similar needs who have formed groups for exchange of information and mutual help and support. A list of the nature and addresses of such organizations is to be found in Appendix B.

Final information is exchanged between the ward sister and the mother. The nurse attending to the child's discharge should ensure that his locker is emptied of all his belongings before he leaves the ward with his mother. The bedclothes are sent to the laundry and the waterproof mattress cover, bedstead and locker washed thoroughly with hot soapy water, rinsed and dried before the bed is made up for the next patient. Only if the child has suffered an infection is it necessary to disinfect the bedding and furniture (page 142).

Records and X-ray films are collected together for completion by the doctor prior to storage for subsequent reference.

Discharge Against Medical Advice

If parents insist on discharging their child before completion of treatment, they must be seen by a senior member of the medical staff and warned of the consequences of such behaviour, for which the hospital and its staff can take no responsibility. Parents who wish to continue their intent after discussion with the doctor and sister are asked to sign the relevant form to the effect that the above warning has been given. In so doing, the child cannot be deprived of subsequent care or admission by the hospital.

Transfer

The need for special care in one of the sparsely distributed paediatric units makes transfer from one hospital to another a very common procedure. The need for transfer should be fully discussed with the parents who should be given the opportunity to travel with their child. If they are unable to do so, information must be exchanged through the escorting nurse. Relevant notes, X-rays and letters—from doctor to doctor, and sister to sister—together with parental consent for further treatment, must travel with the child, and the nurse returns with the appropriate information for the parents regarding the local hospital arrangements.

Convalescence

Unless home conditions are very poor or if the child has suffered a debilitating illness, convalescence is not usually recommended, particularly during the vulnerable first five years of life. After a stay in hospital, most children prefer to go home, but some parents may not want their child to go home until he is really well. Both may go out to work and his unwanted presence at home may disrupt this pattern and reduce the family income. Special requests for convalescence have to be carefully considered by the doctor and medical social worker, and the parents are encouraged to accept their responsibility should this prove necessary. Two to three weeks away from the polluted city air, however, benefit all who are not of an age to suffer from prolonged separation from home, but does more harm than good to a homesick young child.

Death

Care of the Dying Child

The care of children suffering from a fatal illness calls for some of a nurse's best qualities, both in the care of the sick child and offering support to distressed relatives. Some degree of emotional involvement is necessary if both the sick child and his parents are to be helped, but one's emotions must be kept under control if the parents are to be supported. It is only natural for a young student nurse facing death of a patient for the first time to feel sad, but it is imperative that she remains composed in the ward situation. Probably at no other time will she feel so utterly helpless than at the bedside of a dying child, and there is a desire to act when inactivity is what is necessary.

The doctor usually informs the parents of their child's incurable disease. If possible, both parents are seen together and the serious nature of the information to be given inferred by the general manner in which the appointment is made. If the parents are prepared, it will lessen the shock and help them to listen to what the doctor has to say. When confronted with bad news, most parents are unable to concentrate. It is important, therefore, that the ward sister knows exactly what the parents have been told, as it is she who will have to reinforce and often repeat the doctor's explanation, and to sustain the morale of the parents during the difficult weeks ahead.

A talk together over a cup of tea will allow the parents to comfort each other and to control their grief so enabling them to return, when composed, to their sick child's bedside. Inevitable queries should be answered by the ward sister or, in her absence, by an informed senior member of the staff.

If possible, the child is allowed to go home as soon as his condition allows, and to return to hospital for further treatment and possibly for terminal care. Parents must be assured of the hospital's co-operation in this matter, and every effort should be made to ensure that the child is readmitted to the same familiar ward.

Terminal Care

Fear of death sometimes causes apprehension in adults, especially to those who do not believe in life after death. Mercifully, children lack this apprehension, making death a great deal easier. A child's natural urge to live is strong, but as disease progresses, so it wanes.

Unless the sick child is too ill to be bothered with the noisy activities of the ward, or his appearance too distressing for his fellow patients, he is happier nursed where he can watch the ward activities. When confined to a single cubicle, loneliness must be overcome. Most parents want to spend as much time as possible with their dying child and they need sympathetic support and understanding through this sometimes prolonged period. To remain hopeful and cheerful with the knowledge of the inevitable outcome, yet helpless at seeing their child's continual deterioration, puts a great strain on the family. Breaks from the bedside vigil for rest and food are essential and must be encouraged if the parents' strength is to be maintained. This is more likely to be accepted if they can be assured that a nurse will stay at their child's bedside. Separation, particularly from mother, becomes intolerable towards the end.

Most parents find it helpful to talk to their appropriate minister of religion whether normally religious or not. A visit by the hospital chaplain or the child's own minister of religion will also ensure that the child is baptized, confirmed or given the last rites as appropriate. In the absence of the chaplain, infant baptism is performed by a member of the nursing staff (page 47).

The care of a dying child aims at keeping him fresh and comfortable in every respect, his skin, mouth, bladder and bowel requiring meticulous care. Pain and restlessness need adequate analgesic and sedative relief, preferably by the oral route. Requests made by the child should be fulfilled. Maternal devotion to simple nursing needs helps the mother to feel that she is doing everything possible to help her dying child.

Anticipation of impending death is one of the nurse's primary duties. It is always important to know if the parents wish to be at their child's bedside during his last minutes of life, or if they wish to be informed of any deterioration during the night. By merely asking these questions, the severity of their child's illness will be realized and they will be prepared for the possibility of death.

A child should never be left to die alone. In the absence of his parents, a familiar nurse should remain quietly by his bedside, gently holding his hand. Attending parents welcome the presence of a nurse to give them moral support.

When all is over, the parents should be left at the bedside for a few moments and then led quietly away. The inevitable, sudden emptiness comes as a great shock however much the parents have been prepared. Words seem most inadequate when trying to comfort distressed parents. A reminder that death has relieved their little one of discomfort or disability may help. A period of time together will allow them to share their grief and to become more composed before returning home. An appointment is made for them to return to the hospital the following day to attend to the necessary formalities which a death entails. A senior nurse should escort the child's parents to the hospital entrance where a firm, friendly handshake will impart her understanding, but unspoken thoughts.

If the parents do not wish to be at their dying child's bedside, then they must be informed of his death by telephone or police message. If his death is expected, this is distressing, but not usually difficult. A sudden, unexpected death of a child is always most distressing, requiring very careful handling. The parents must be informed and this is best done by contacting them and telling them that their child has collapsed and although everything possible is being done, the outlook is grave. This prepares them for more serious news (and slightly lessens the shock) which they receive on arrival at the hospital or over the telephone a short time later, and gives them time to contact a friend or relative.

Care of the Body after Death

REQUIREMENTS
Receptacle for soiled linen.
Cotton wool.
Cotton bandages.
Small container of water.
Receiver for urine.
Tape measure.

Once the parents have left the bedside and death has been certified by the doctor, bed and personal clothing is removed and the body laid straight and flat.

Small moist pledgets of cotton wool are placed over the closed eye-lids. If a naso-gastric tube is in position, this is aspirated before withdrawal. If the coronor requires notification of the death (see below) all possible evidence may be left in the body, i.e. naso-gastric, tracheostomy, endotracheal and drainage tubes. The drooping jaw is supported by a roll of bandage or small pillow so that the lips adopt a natural closure.

Gentle suprapubic pressure should be applied to empty the bladder into the receiver placed between the thighs. According to the religious custom or hospital policy, the arms are straightened by the side of the body or crossed over the chest, or the hands are placed together by interlacing the fingers. This latter position is maintained with cotton wool and bandage, the cotton wool being used to avoid marking the skin.

Unless the legs are straight and together, cotton wool is placed between the bony prominences of the knees and ankles and the limbs are bandaged together. The body length is measured to assess the size of shroud required before covering with a sheet and leaving for half to one hour until rigor mortis is established.

LAST OFFICES

In the intervening time, the child's personal belongings are parcelled together. Occasionally, the parents may request that a particular favourite teddy bear or doll be left with their child and, of course, their request must be fulfilled.

REQUIREMENTS

As for bed bath (page 118).

Additional requirements:
Shroud of sufficient length (i.e. to cover the feet).
Narrow cotton bandage or white hair ribbon.
A small white flower.
Identification labels.

For plugging orifices:
Cotton wool.
Sinus forceps.

For discharging wounds:
Gauze dressings.
Dressing forceps.
Waterproof adhesive tape.

METHOD

Whenever possible, two nurses should carry out this procedure quietly and efficiently, the senior giving emotional support to her junior colleague.

The restraining bandages are removed and the body sponged and dried. Occlusive dressings are applied to wounds and drainage sites. The finger and toe nails are cut and cleaned as necessary. The rectum and other orifices are plugged with cotton wool, if requested or necessary. The shroud is put on and fastened at the neck. The child's hands are placed together with the fingers interlaced, clutching the small white flower. The hair is combed and styled as the parents liked to see it.

The body is identified according to the policy of the hospital, the child's full name, age, and date and time of death being the usual minimal requirements.

If an immediate visit of the parents is expected, they should see their child in the familiar ward surroundings before the concealed body is transferred to the mortuary to await burial or cremation.

Answering the Children's Questions

Answering the questions of the other children in the ward about the sudden disappearance of a child who has previously demanded a lot of attention, may not prove easy. In the majority of instances, children are satisfied with a simple, honest answer as, for instance 'Peter was too poorly to live here with us so he has gone to live with Jesus in heaven'. This must be followed by positive reassurance such as 'but this will not happen to you—your tummy is getting better, isn't it?', or words to that effect. The loss is rarely mentioned again, except perhaps in the delightful matter-of-fact casual conversation of small children.

Formalities Related to a Death

1 POST MORTEM EXAMINATION (Autopsy)
It is usual for the doctor to discuss the child's last illness with both parents and to obtain permission for a post mortem examination to be made if this is thought desirable. Parents have the right to refuse permission unless the registrar is not satisfied with the cause of death stated on the death certificate and informs the coroner, or, in Scotland, the procurator fiscal, who orders an examination.

2 REGISTRATION OF DEATH
The death certificate, signed by a registered medical practitioner, must be sent or taken to the registrar for the sub-district within five days of death. A disposal certificate is issued on satisfactory registration of the death.

3 CASES FOR THE CORONER
   The coroner's court is a court of law concerned with investigation into:
 i deaths from unknown or uncertain causes;
 ii violent or unnatural deaths or related to accident or injury, want, exposure, neglect, poisoning or drug mishap;
 iii all deaths suspected or alleged to be connected with hospital treatment or before full recovery from an anaesthetic or operative treatment.
   If the cause of the child's death falls into one of these categories or any other category specified locally, such as a child dying within twenty-four hours of admission to hospital, it is usual for the doctor to inform the coroner, but this may be done by the registrar. A death certificate is not issued by the coroner's office until the necessary enquiries and examination have been made. Sometimes, an inquest may prove necessary.

Conversion Tables

The Metric System

The units of measurement in the metric system are:
  metre (m) for length
  gramme (g) for weight
  litre (l) for capacity
With these units the following prefixes are used:
  Milli . . . meaning 0·001 (1/1000) of unit
  Centi . . . meaning 0·01 (1/100) of unit
  Deci . . . meaning 0·1 (1/10) of unit
  Unit
  Deka . . . meaning 10 times unit
  Hekto . . . meaning 100 times unit
  Kilo . . . meaning 1,000 times unit
Therefore:

Kilo	Hekto	Deka	Unit	Deci	Centi	Milli
1 =	10 or	100 or	1,000 or	10,000 or	100,000 or	1 million
	1 =	10	100	1,000	10,000	100,000
		1 =	10	100	1,000	10,000
			1 =	10	100	1,000
				1 =	10	100
					1 =	10

Micro i.e. gramme or metre means 1 millionth part of a unit
Therefore 1,000 microgrammes (mcg) = 1 milligramme (mg)

Weight

UNITS OF THE METRIC SYSTEM
1 Kilogramme (kg) = 1,000 grammes (g)
1 Gramme   = 1,000 milligrammes (mg)
1 Milligramme   = 1,000 microgrammes (mcg)

UNITS OF THE AVOIRDUPOIS WEIGHT

1 stone (st) = 14 pounds (lb)
1lb   = 16 ounces (oz)
1oz   = 437·5 grains (gr)

USEFUL APPROXIMATE METRIC AND AVOIRDUPOIS EQUIVALENTS

1g = 15·4 grains   1oz = 28·3 (30) g
1kg = 2·2lb   1lb = 0·45kg

TO CONVERT KILOGRAMMES TO POUNDS

Multiply the weight in kilogrammes by 2·2
Example: The average newborn male infant weighs 3·4kg
$$= 3·4 \times 2·2 = 7·48\text{lb} = 7\text{lb } 8\text{oz}$$

TO CONVERT POUNDS TO KILOGRAMMES

Divide the weight in pounds by 2·2
Example: The average newborn male infant weighs 7lb 8oz
$$= \frac{7·5}{2·2} = 3·4\text{kg}$$

To Convert Stones, Pounds and Ounces to Kilogrammes

st	kg	lb	kg	oz	kg
1	6·350	1	0·454	1	0·028
2	12·701	2	0·907	2	0·057
3	19·051	3	1·361	3	0·085
4	25·401	4	1·814	4	0·113
5	31·752	5	2·268	5	0·142
6	38·102	6	2·722	6	0·170
7	44·452	7	3·175	7	0·198
8	50·802	8	3·629	8	0·227
9	57·153	9	4·082	9	0·255
10	63·503	10	4·536	10	0·283
11	69·853	11	4·990	11	0·312
12	76·204	12	5·443	12	0·340
13	82·554	13	5·897	13	0·369
14	88·904			14	0·397
15	95·254			15	0·425

Correct to the nearest gramme. (Figures based on the British Standards Institution's conversion chart for weight.)

The weight on the Avoirdupois system is split into its appropriate units and the figures looked up for each. The sum is the equivalent weight in kilogrammes.

Example: A child weighs 3st 4lb 6oz. Using the table:

$$3st = 19·051$$
$$4lb = 1·814$$
$$6oz = 0·170$$
$$\overline{21·035kg}$$

Approximate Metric and Imperial Equivalents

WEIGHT

30g = 1oz	30mg = $\frac{1}{2}$gr
15g = $\frac{1}{2}$oz	20mg = $\frac{1}{3}$gr
8g = 120gr	15mg = $\frac{1}{4}$gr
4g = 60gr	10mg = 1/6gr
2g = 30gr	7·5mg = 1/8gr
1g = 15gr	6mg = 1/10
600mg = 10gr	3mg = 1/20gr
450mg = 7$\frac{1}{2}$gr	1mg = 1/60gr
300mg = 5gr	(1,000 microgrammes)
250mg = 4gr	0·6mg = 1/100gr
200mg = 3gr	0·5mg = 1/120gr
150mg = 2$\frac{1}{2}$gr	0·3mg = 1/200gr
100mg = 1$\frac{1}{2}$gr	0·2mg = 1/300gr
60mg = 1gr	0·1mg = 1/600gr
50mg = $\frac{3}{4}$gr	

Height

UNITS OF THE METRIC SYSTEM
1 kilometre (km) = 1,000 metres (m)
1 metre (m) = 100 centimetres (cm)
1 centimetre (cm) = 10 millimetres (mm)

UNITS OF THE IMPERIAL SYSTEM
1 yard (yd) = 3 feet (ft)
1 foot (ft) = 12 inches (in)

USEFUL APPROXIMATE METRIC AND IMPERIAL EQUIVALENTS
1cm = 0·39 inches (in)   1in = 2·54cm
1m = 1·1 yards (yd)   1ft = 30·48cm

TO CONVERT CENTIMETRES TO INCHES
Divide the length in centimetres by 2·54
Example: The average newborn infant measures 50·8cm.

$$= \frac{50·8}{2·54} = 20 \text{ inches}$$

TO CONVERT INCHES TO CENTIMETRES

Multiply the length in inches by 2·54.

Example: The average newborn infant measures 20 inches.

$$= 20 \times 2·54 = 50·8cm$$

To Convert Feet and Inches to Metres

ft	m	in	m
1	0·305	0·5	0·013
2	0·610	1	0·025
3	0·914	2	0·051
4	1·219	3	0·076
5	1·524	4	0·102
6	1·829	5	0·127
7	2·134	6	0·152
		7	0·178
		8	0·203
		9	0·229
		10	0·254
		11	0·279

Correct to the nearest millimetre. (Figures based on the British Standards Institution's conversion chart for height.)

The length on the Imperial system is split into its appropriate units, i.e. feet and inches, and the figures looked up for each. The sum is the equivalent length in metres.

Example: The head circumference of a newborn infant is approximately 13½in. Using the table:

$$
\begin{array}{rl}
1 \ \text{ft} &= 0·305 \\
1 \ \text{in} &= 0·025 \\
0·5\text{in} &= 0·013 \\
\hline
0·343 & \text{metres or } 34·3\text{cm}
\end{array}
$$

Surface Area

The surface area of the body cannot easily be measured directly, therefore it is generally estimated from charts of weight and height or weight alone. Body surface area is measured in square metres (m^2) and the average adult has a surface area of $1·72m^2$.

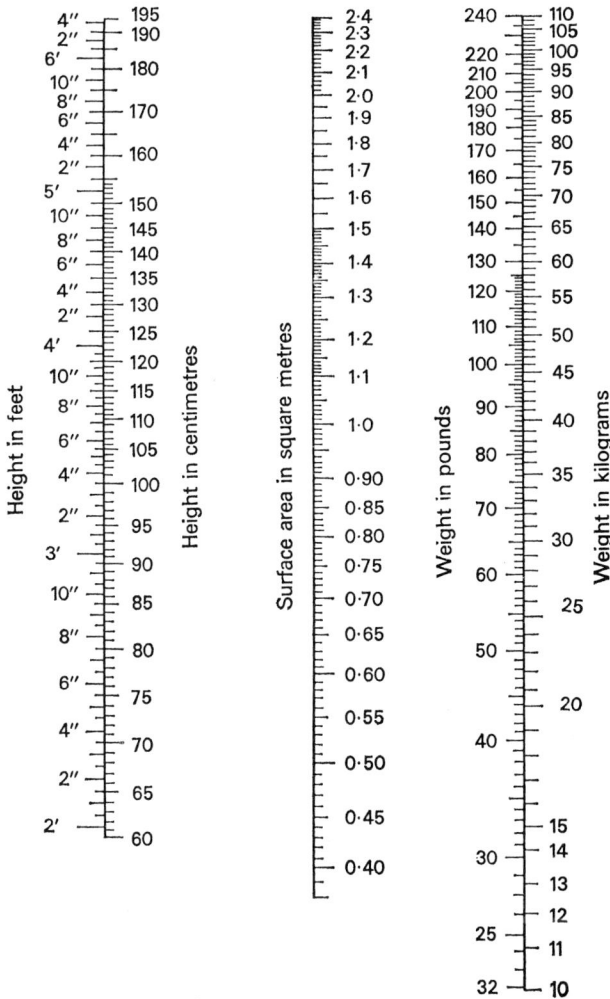

Surface area nomogram. (Adapted from J. R. Geigy, S.A., data.)

(As printed in *A Paediatric Vade-Mecum*, 7th edition (1970) by kind permission of B. S. B. Wood and Lloyd-Luke (Medical Books) Ltd.)

Capacity (Volume)

UNITS OF THE METRIC SYSTEM

1 litre (l) = 1,000 millilitres (ml)
or cubic centimetres (cm3)

UNITS OF THE IMPERIAL SYSTEM

1 gallon = 4 quarts = 8 pints

1 quart = 2 pints
1 pint = 20 fluid ounces
1 fluid ounce = 8 drachms
1 drachm = 60 minims

USEFUL APPROXIMATE METRIC AND IMPERIAL EQUIVALENTS
1 litre   = 1·75 pints
1oz   = 30ml
1 pint   = 0·568 litres or 568ml
1 gallon = 4·55 litres

CONVERSION TABLE

Litres		Pints
0·28	0·5	0·88
0·57	1	1·75
1·14	2	3·50
1·70	3	5·28
2·28	4	7·04
2·85	5	8·80
3·42	6	10·50
3·99	7	12·30
4·55	8	14·08

To read the table: 3 litres = 5·28 pints
                    3 pints = 1·70 litres

Comparative Temperature Scales

Equivalent Points on the Two Scales

	Centigrade	Fahrenheit
Boiling Point	100°	212°
Freezing Point	0°	32°

Between the two fixed points, i.e. the boiling point and the freezing point, there are:

100 divisions on the Centigrade scale
180 divisions on the Fahrenheit scale

The ratio of the number of Centigrade divisions to the number of Fahrenheit divisions is:

$$100:180$$
$$= \quad 5:9$$

Therefore   1 degree Centigrade $= \dfrac{9}{5}$ degrees Fahrenheit, and

                 1 degree Fahrenheit $= \dfrac{5}{9}$ degrees Centigrade

To Convert a Temperature on the Fahrenheit Scale to its Equivalent on the Centigrade Scale

As the comparison must be taken from the freezing point on both scales, 32 (i.e. the difference between the freezing points on the two scales) must be deducted from the temperature on the Fahrenheit scale prior to multiplying by 5 and dividing by 9.

Therefore $(°F-32) \times \frac{5}{9} = °C$

Example: 98·4°F is the average human body temperature. To convert this to the Centigrade scale:

$$(°F-32) \times \frac{5}{9}°C$$

$$(98·4-32) \times \frac{5}{9}°C$$

$$= 66·4 \times \frac{5}{9}°C$$

$$= 36·9°C$$

Or using the table below, the temperature on the Fahrenheit scale is split into tens, units and decimals and the figures looked up for each. When added, the sum is the equivalent temperature on the Centigrade scale:

Tens		Units		Decimals	
°F	°C	°F	°C	°F	°C
30	−1·1	1	0·56	0·1	0·06
40	4·4	2	1·11	0·2	0·11
50	10·0	3	1·67	0·3	0·17
60	15·6	4	2·22	0·4	0·22
70	21·1	5	2·78	0·5	0·28
80	26·7	6	3·33	0·6	0·33
90	32·2	7	3·89	0·7	0·39
100	37·8	8	4·44	0·8	0·44
110	43·3	9	5·00	0·9	0·5
120	48·9				
130	54·4				
140	60·0				
150	65·6				
160	71·1				
170	76·7				
180	82·2				
190	87·8				
200	93·3				
210	98·9				

Example: The average body temperature on the Fahrenheit scale is 98·4°F

$$90 \ \ = 32\cdot2$$
$$8 \ \ \ = \ \ 4\cdot44$$
$$0\cdot4 = \ \ 0\cdot22$$
$$\overline{36\cdot86°C}$$

To Convert a Temperature on the Centigrade Scale to its Equivalent on the Fahrenheit Scale

Similarly, to convert a temperature on the Centigrade scale to one on the Fahrenheit scale, 32 is added to the answer after the temperature on the Centigrade scale has been multiplied by 9 and divided by 5.

Therefore
$$\left(°C \times \frac{9}{5}\right) + 32 = °F$$

Example: 20°C is a suitable temperature for working conditions. To convert this to the Fahrenheit scale:

$$\left(°C \times \frac{9}{5}\right) + 32°F$$

$$\left(20 \times \frac{9}{5}\right) \div 32°F$$

$$= 36 + 32°F$$

$$= 68°F$$

Or using the table below, the temperature on the Centigrade scale is split into tens, units and decimals and the figures looked up for each. When added, the sum is the equivalent temperature on the Fahrenheit scale:

Tens		Units		Decimals	
°C	°F	°C	°F	°C	°F
0	32	1	1·8	0·1	0·18
10	50	2	3·6	0·2	0·36
20	68	3	5·4	0·3	0·54
30	86	4	7·2	0·4	0·72
40	104	5	9·0	0·5	0·9
50	122	6	10·8	0·6	1·08
60	140	7	12·6	0·7	1·26
70	158	8	14·4	0·8	1·44
80	176	9	16·2	0·9	1·62
90	194				
100	212				

Example: The average body temperature on the Centigrade scale is 36·8°C.
Taking figures from the table:

$$
\begin{aligned}
30 \ &= 86 \\
6 \ &= 10\text{·}8 \\
0\text{·}8 \ &= \underline{\ \ 1\text{·}44\ } \\
&\ \ \ \underline{98\text{·}24°\text{F}}
\end{aligned}
$$

Names and Addresses of Charitable Organizations

A list of names and addresses of organizations formed to help, advise and promote the welfare of children with specific disorders.

Association of Spina Bifida and Hydrocephalus
112 City Road, London E.C.1.

Children's Chest Circle—The Chest and Heart Association
Tavistock House North, Tavistock Square, London W.C.1.

Coeliac Society
PO Box No 181, London NW2 2QY

Cystic Fibrosis Research Foundation Trust
59 Holborn Viaduct, London E.C.1.

Diabetic Association
3–6 Alfred Place, London WC1E 7EE

Haemophilia Society
94 Southwark Bridge Road, London S.E.1.

Ileostomy Association of Great Britain
15 Witherford Croft, Solihull, Warwicks.

National Society for Autistic Children
1a Golders Green Road, London N.W.11.

National Society for Mentally Handicapped Children
85/86 Newman Street, London W.1.

Spastics Society
28 Fitzroy Square, London W.1.

Index

Main references are in **bold** type